T0228915

Advances in Cardiac Mapping and Catheter Ablation: Part I

Editors

MOHAMMAD SHENASA
AMIN AL-AHMAD

CARDIAC ELECTROPHYSIOLOGY CLINICS

www.cardiacEP.theclinics.com

Consulting Editors
RANJAN K. THAKUR
ANDREA NATALE

September 2019 • Volume 11 • Number 3

ELSEVIER

1600 John F. Kennedy Boulevard • Suite 1800 • Philadelphia, Pennsylvania, 19103-2899

http://www.theclinics.com

CARDIAC ELECTROPHYSIOLOGY CLINICS Volume 11, Number 3
September 2019 ISSN 1877-9182, ISBN-13: 978-0-323-68347-0

Editor: Stacy Eastman
Developmental Editor: Donald Mumford

© **2019 Elsevier Inc. All rights reserved.**

This periodical and the individual contributions contained in it are protected under copyright by Elsevier, and the following terms and conditions apply to their use:

Photocopying
Single photocopies of single articles may be made for personal use as allowed by national copyright laws. Permission of the Publisher and payment of a fee is required for all other photocopying, including multiple or systematic copying, copying for advertising or promotional purposes, resale, and all forms of document delivery. Special rates are available for educational institutions that wish to make photocopies for non-profit educational classroom use. For information on how to seek permission visit www.elsevier.com/permissions or call: (+44) 1865 843830 (UK)/(+1) 215 239 3804 (USA).

Derivative Works
Subscribers may reproduce tables of contents or prepare lists of articles including abstracts for internal circulation within their institutions. Permission of the Publisher is required for resale or distribution outside the institution. Permission of the Publisher is required for all other derivative works, including compilations and translations (please consult www.elsevier.com/permissions).

Electronic Storage or Usage
Permission of the Publisher is required to store or use electronically any material contained in this periodical, including any article or part of an article (please consult www.elsevier.com/permissions). Except as outlined above, no part of this publication may be reproduced, stored in a retrieval system or transmitted in any form or by any means, electronic, mechanical, photocopying, recording or otherwise, without prior written permission of the Publisher.

Notice
No responsibility is assumed by the Publisher for any injury and/or damage to persons or property as a matter of products liability, negligence or otherwise, or from any use or operation of any methods, products, instructions or ideas contained in the material herein. Because of rapid advances in the medical sciences, in particular, independent verification of diagnoses and drug dosages should be made.

Although all advertising material is expected to conform to ethical (medical) standards, inclusion in this publication does not constitute a guarantee or endorsement of the quality or value of such product or of the claims made of it by its manufacturer.

Cardiac Electrophysiology Clinics (ISSN 1877-9182) is published quarterly by Elsevier Inc., 360 Park Avenue South, New York, NY 10010-1710. Months of issue are March, June, September, and December. Subscription prices are $224.00 per year for US individuals, $366.00 per year for US institutions, $249.00 per year for Canadian individuals, $413.00 per year for Canadian institutions, $303.00 per year for international individuals, $442.00 per year for international institutions and $100.00 per year for US, Canadian and international students/residents. To receive student/resident rate, orders must be accompanied by name of affiliated institution, date of term, and the signature of program/residency coordinator on institution letterhead. Orders will be billed at individual rate until proof of status is received. Foreign air speed delivery is included in all Clinics subscription prices. All prices are subject to change without notice. **POSTMASTER:** Send address changes to Cardiac Electrophysiology Clinics, Elsevier Health Sciences Division, Subscription Customer Service, 3251 Riverport Lane, Maryland Heights, MO 63043. **Customer Service: 1-800-654-2452 (US and Canada). From outside of the US and Canada, call 314-477-8871. Fax: 314-447-8029. E-mail: JournalsCustomerService-usa@elsevier.com (for print support); JournalsOnlineSupport-usa@elsevier.com (for online support).**

Reprints. For copies of 100 or more of articles in this publication, please contact the Commercial Reprints Department, Elsevier Inc., 360 Park Avenue South, New York, NY 10010-1710. Tel.: 212-633-3874; Fax: 212-633-3820; E-mail: reprints@elsevier.com.

Cardiac Electrophysiology Clinics is covered in *MEDLINE/PubMed (Index Medicus)*.

Contributors

CONSULTING EDITORS

RANJAN K. THAKUR, MD, MPH, MBA, FHRS
Professor of Medicine and Director, Arrhythmia
Service, Thoracic and Cardiovascular Institute,
Sparrow Health System, Michigan State
University, Lansing, Michigan, USA

ANDREA NATALE, MD, FACC, FHRS
Executive Medical Director, Texas Cardiac
Arrhythmia Institute, St. David's Medical
Center, Austin, Texas; Consulting Professor,
Division of Cardiology, Stanford University,
Palo Alto, California; Adjunct Professor of
Medicine, Heart and Vascular Center, Case
Western Reserve University, Cleveland, Ohio;
Director, Interventional Electrophysiology,
Scripps Clinic, San Diego, California; Senior
Clinical Director, EP Services, California Pacific
Medical Center, San Francisco, California, USA

EDITORS

MOHAMMAD SHENASA, MD, FHRS
Heart and Rhythm Medical Group,
Department of Cardiovascular Services,
O'Connor Hospital, San Jose, California,
USA

AMIN AL-AHMAD, MD, FHRS
Texas Cardiac Arrhythmia Institute,
St David's Medical Center, Austin, Texas,
USA

AUTHORS

AMIN AL-AHMAD, MD, FHRS
Texas Cardiac Arrhythmia Institute,
St David's Medical Center, Austin, Texas,
USA

**JONATHAN P. ARIYARATNAM, MB BChir,
MA, MRCP**
Cardiovascular Sciences, University
of Manchester, Core Technology
Facility, Manchester, United
Kingdom

SAMUEL J. ASIRVATHAM, MD
Professor of Medicine and
Pediatrics, College of Medicine,
Department of Cardiovascular Medicine,
Division of Heart Rhythm Services,
Department of Pediatric and Adolescent
Medicine, Division of Pediatric
Cardiology, Physiology and

Biomedical Engineering, Mayo Clinic,
Rochester, Minnesota,
USA

HÜSEYIN AYHAN, MD
Texas Cardiac Arrhythmia Institute, St. David's
Medical Center, Austin, Texas, USA;
Department of Cardiology, Faculty of
Medicine, Yıldırım Beyazıt University, Ankara,
Turkey

RICHARD G. BENNETT, MBBS
Bristol Heart Institute, Bristol Royal Infirmary,
Bristol, United Kingdom

OMER BERENFELD, PhD
Professor of Internal Medicine and Biomedical
Engineering, Center for Arrhythmia Research,
Department of Internal Medicine (Cardiology),
University of Michigan, Ann Arbor, Michigan,
USA

MARTIN BORLICH, MD
Heart Center, Segeberger Kliniken
(Academic Teaching Hospital of the
Universities of Kiel, Lübeck and Hamburg),
Bad Segeberg, Schleswig-Holstein,
Germany

FELIX BOURIER, MD
Cardiac Electrophysiology Department,
Hôpital Haut-Lévêque, Bordeaux, Pessac,
France; Electrophysiology and Heart Modeling
Institute (LIRYC), Bordeaux University,
Talence, Pessac, France

TIMOTHY CAMPBELL, BSc
Department of Cardiology, Westmead
Hospital, Westmead Applied Research
Centre, University of Sydney, Sydney,
Australia

UĞUR CANPOLAT, MD
Texas Cardiac Arrhythmia Institute,
St. David's Medical Center, Austin,
Texas, USA; Arrhythmia and Electrophysiology
Unit, Department of Cardiology,
Hacettepe University, Ankara,
Turkey

MIHAIL G. CHELU, MD, PhD, FHRS
Comprehensive Arrhythmia Research &
Management (CARMA) Center, Assistant
Professor, Division of Cardiovascular
Medicine, Section of Electrophysiology,
University of Utah, Salt Lake City, Utah,
USA

QIONG CHEN, MD
Texas Cardiac Arrhythmia Institute, St. David's
Medical Center, Austin, Texas, USA;
Department of Cardiopulmonary Function
Test, Henan Provincial People's Hospital,
People's Hospital of Zhengzhou University,
China

GHASSEN CHENITI, MD
Cardiac Electrophysiology Department,
Hôpital Haut-Lévêque, Bordeaux, Pessac,
France; Electrophysiology and Heart Modeling
Institute (LIRYC), Bordeaux University,
Talence, Pessac, France

HUBERT COCHET, MD
Electrophysiology and Heart Modeling Institute
(LIRYC), Bordeaux University, Talence,
Pessac, France; Department of Cardiovascular
Imaging, Hôpital Haut-Lévêque, Bordeaux,
Pessac, France

DOMENICO DELLA ROCCA, MD
Texas Cardiac Arrhythmia Institute, St. David's
Medical Center, Austin, Texas, USA

ARNAUD DENIS, MD
Cardiac Electrophysiology Department,
Hôpital Haut-Lévêque, Bordeaux, Pessac,
France; Electrophysiology and Heart Modeling
Institute (LIRYC), Bordeaux University,
Talence, Pessac, France

DON CURTIS DENO, MD, PhD
Abbott Laboratories, Saint Paul, Minnesota,
USA

NICOLAS DERVAL, MD
Cardiac Electrophysiology Department,
Hôpital Haut-Lévêque, Bordeaux, Pessac,
France; Electrophysiology and Heart Modeling
Institute (LIRYC), Bordeaux University,
Talence, Pessac, France

REMI DUBOIS, PhD
Electrophysiology and Heart Modeling Institute
(LIRYC), Bordeaux University, Talence,
Pessac, France

JOSSELIN DUCHATEAU, MD
Cardiac Electrophysiology Department,
Hôpital Haut-Lévêque, Bordeaux, Pessac,
France; Electrophysiology and Heart Modeling
Institute (LIRYC), Bordeaux University,
Talence, Pessac, France

CAROLE DUMAS-POMMIER, PhD
Cardiac Electrophysiology Department,
Hôpital Haut-Lévêque, Bordeaux, Pessac,
France

IGOR EFIMOV, PhD
Alisann and Terry Collins Professor and Chair,
Department of Biomedical Engineering, The
George Washington University, Washington,
DC, USA

ANTONIO FRONTERA, MD
Cardiac Electrophysiology Department,
Hôpital Haut-Lévêque, Bordeaux, Pessac,
France; Electrophysiology and Heart Modeling
Institute (LIRYC), Bordeaux University,
Talence, Pessac, France

FADI GEARA, MD, PhD
Department of Radiation Oncology, American
University of Beirut Medical Center, Beirut,
Lebanon

CAROLA GIANNI, MD, PhD
Texas Cardiac Arrhythmia Institute,
St. David's Medical Center, Austin, Texas,
USA

MICHEL HAISSAGUERRE, MD
Cardiac Electrophysiology Department,
Hôpital Haut-Lévêque, Bordeaux,
Pessac, France; Electrophysiology and
Heart Modeling Institute (LIRYC),
Bordeaux University, Talence, Pessac,
France

SHOUVIK K. HALDAR, MD (Res), MRCP
Royal Brompton & Harefield NHS Foundation
Trust, London, England

MELEZE HOCINI, MD
Cardiac Electrophysiology Department,
Hôpital Haut-Lévêque, Bordeaux,
Pessac, France; Electrophysiology
and Heart Modeling Institute (LIRYC),
Bordeaux University, Talence, Pessac,
France

PIERRE JAIS, MD
Cardiac Electrophysiology Department,
Hôpital Haut-Lévêque, Bordeaux,
Pessac, France; Electrophysiology
and Heart Modeling Institute (LIRYC),
Bordeaux University, Talence, Pessac, France

EUGENE G. KHOLMOVSKI, PhD
Comprehensive Arrhythmia Research &
Management (CARMA) Center, Utah
Center for Advanced Imaging Research
(UCAIR), Research Associate Professor,
Department of Radiology and Imaging
Sciences, University of Utah, Salt Lake City,
Utah, USA

TAKESHI KITAMURA, MD
Cardiac Electrophysiology Department,
Hôpital Haut-Lévêque, Bordeaux,
Pessac, France; Electrophysiology
and Heart Modeling Institute (LIRYC),
Bordeaux University, Talence, Pessac,
France

NICOLAS KLOTZ, MD
Cardiac Electrophysiology Department,
Hôpital Haut-Lévêque, Bordeaux,
Pessac, France; Electrophysiology
and Heart Modeling Institute (LIRYC),
Bordeaux University, Talence, Pessac,
France

SAURABH KUMAR, MBBS, PhD
Department of Cardiology, Westmead
Hospital, Associate Professor,
Westmead Applied Research Centre,
University of Sydney, Sydney,
Australia

DECEBAL GABRIEL LAȚCU, MD
Centre Hospitalier Princesse Grace,
Monaco

THOMAS P. LADAS, MD, PhD
Department of Cardiovascular Medicine,
Division of Heart Rhythm Services,
Mayo Clinic, Rochester, Minnesota,
USA

ANNA LAM, MD
Cardiac Electrophysiology Department,
Hôpital Haut-Lévêque, Bordeaux,
Pessac, France; Electrophysiology
and Heart Modeling Institute (LIRYC),
Bordeaux University, Talence, Pessac,
France

BRYAN MACDONALD, MD
Texas Cardiac Arrhythmia Institute,
St. David's Medical Center, Austin, Texas,
USA

KARL MAGTIBAY, MASc
The Hull Family Cardiac Fibrillation
Management Laboratory,
Toronto General Hospital, University
Health Network, Toronto, Ontario,
Canada

CLAIRE A. MARTIN, MD
Cardiac Electrophysiology Department,
Hôpital Haut-Lévêque, Bordeaux,
Pessac, France; Electrophysiology
and Heart Modeling Institute (LIRYC),
Bordeaux University, Talence, Pessac,
France

STÉPHANE MASSÉ, MASc
The Hull Family Cardiac Fibrillation
Management Laboratory, Toronto General
Hospital, University Health Network, Toronto,
Ontario, Canada

NANDINI MEHRA, MD
Department of Internal Medicine, Mayo Clinic,
Rochester, Minnesota, USA

SANGHAMITRA MOHANTY, MD
Texas Cardiac Arrhythmia Institute,
St. David's Medical Center, Dell Medical
School, University of Texas, Austin, Texas,
USA

ALAN K. MORRIS, MSc
Software Developer, Comprehensive
Arrhythmia Research & Management (CARMA)
Center, University of Utah, Salt Lake City, Utah,
USA

GWILYM M. MORRIS, BM BCh, PhD, MRCP
Consultant Cardiologist and British Heart
Foundation Intermediate Clinical Research
Fellow, Cardiovascular Sciences, University of
Manchester, Core Technology Facility,
Manchester, United Kingdom

JOHN NAN, MD
Department of Cardiovascular Medicine,
Division of Heart Rhythm Services,
Mayo Clinic, Rochester, Minnesota,
USA

**KUMARASWAMY NANTHAKUMAR, MD,
FRCPC**
The Hull Family Cardiac Fibrillation
Management Laboratory, Toronto General
Hospital, University Health Network, Toronto,
Ontario, Canada

ANDREA NATALE, MD, FACC, FHRS
Texas Cardiac Arrhythmia Institute,
Center for Atrial Fibrillation at St. David's
Medical Center, Dell Medical School,
Department of Biomedical Engineering,
University of Texas, Austin, Texas, USA;
HCA National Medical Director of Cardiac
Electrophysiology, Interventional
Electrophysiology, Scripps Clinic, La Jolla,
California, USA; MetroHealth Medical Center,
Case Western Reserve University School of
Medicine, Cleveland, Ohio, USA; Division of

Cardiology, Stanford University, Stanford,
California, USA

DEEPAK PADMANABHAN, MBBS
Assistant Professor of Medicine,
College of Medicine, Department of
Cardiovascular Medicine, Division of Heart
Rhythm Services, Mayo Clinic, Rochester,
Minnesota, USA

THOMAS PAMBRUN, MD
Cardiac Electrophysiology Department,
Hôpital Haut-Lévêque, Bordeaux,
Pessac, France; Electrophysiology
and Heart Modeling Institute (LIRYC),
Bordeaux University, Talence, Pessac,
France

XAVIER PILLOIS, PhD
Cardiac Electrophysiology Department,
Hôpital Haut-Lévêque, Bordeaux, Pessac,
France

STEPHANE PUYO, PhD
Electrophysiology and Heart Modeling Institute
(LIRYC), Bordeaux University, Talence,
Pessac, France

ANDREU PORTA-SÁNCHEZ, MD, MS
Hospital Universitario Quirón Madrid y
Hospital Ruber Juan Bravo, Madrid,
Spain

**MARWAN M. REFAAT, MD, FACC, FAHA,
FHRS, FASE, FESC, FRCP**
Associate Professor of Medicine, Director,
Cardiovascular Fellowship Program,
Department of Internal Medicine, Cardiology
Division, Cardiac Electrophysiology Section,
American University of Beirut Faculty of
Medicine and Medical Center (AUBMC), Beirut,
Lebanon

FREDERIC SACHER, MD
Cardiac Electrophysiology Department,
Hôpital Haut-Lévêque, Bordeaux,
Pessac, France; Electrophysiology
and Heart Modeling Institute (LIRYC),
Bordeaux University, Talence, Pessac,
France

NADIR SAOUDI, MD, FHRS
Centre Hospitalier Princesse Grace,
Monaco

MOHAMMAD SHENASA, MD, FHRS
Heart and Rhythm Medical Group,
Department of Cardiovascular Services,
O'Connor Hospital, San Jose, California, USA

PHILIPP SOMMER, MD, FHRS, FESC, FEHRA
Clinic of Electrophysiology, Heart and Diabetes
Center NRW, University Hospital of Ruhr-
University Bochum, Bad Oeynhausen,
Germany

ALAN SUGRUE, MB, BCh, BAO
Department of Cardiovascular Medicine,
Division of Heart Rhythm Services,
Mayo Clinic, Rochester, Minnesota, USA

MASATERU TAKIGAWA, MD
Cardiac Electrophysiology Department,
Hôpital Haut-Lévêque, Bordeaux, Pessac,
France; Electrophysiology and Heart Modeling
Institute (LIRYC), Bordeaux University,
Talence, Pessac, France

CHINTAN TRIVEDI, MD
Texas Cardiac Arrhythmia Institute,
St. David's Medical Center, Austin, Texas, USA

IVANA TRIVIC, BSc
Department of Cardiology, Westmead
Hospital, Westmead Applied Research Centre,
University of Sydney, Sydney, Australia

VAIBHAV R. VAIDYA, MBBS
Department of Cardiovascular Medicine,
Division of Heart Rhythm Services, Mayo

Clinic, Rochester, Minnesota,
USA

K.L. VENKATACHALAM, MD
Associate Professor of Medicine,
College of Medicine, Department of
Cardiovascular Medicine, Division of Heart
Rhythm Services, Mayo Clinic, Rochester,
Minnesota, USA

SOHAIB A. VIRK, BMed, MD
Department of Cardiology, Westmead
Hospital, Westmead Applied Research
Centre, University of Sydney, Sydney,
Australia

KONSTANTINOS VLACHOS, MD
Cardiac Electrophysiology Department,
Hôpital Haut-Lévêque, Bordeaux, Pessac,
France; Electrophysiology and Heart Modeling
Institute (LIRYC), Bordeaux University,
Talence, Pessac, France

BASSEM YOUSSEF, MD
Department of Radiation Oncology, American
University of Beirut Medical Center, Beirut,
Lebanon

PATRICK ZAKKA, MD
Department of Internal Medicine, Emory
University Hospital, Atlanta, Georgia, USA

YOUSSEF H. ZEIDAN, MD, PhD
Department of Radiation Oncology, American
University of Beirut Medical Center, Beirut,
Lebanon

Contents

Cardiac mapping has evolved from single point-by-point registration of cardiac electrical activity to its utmost real-time multimodality of mapping and imaging for catheter ablation of arrhythmias. The technology began with electrocardiogram recordings and evolved to the simultaneous registration of depolarization and repolarization using optical mapping and real-time multimodality imaging. Zero to near-zero fluoroscopy is currently used in practice to avoid radiation exposure. Real-time noninvasive mapping, imaging, and ablation of arrhythmias are in use in practice. We present the contemporary up-to-date progress on the role of cardiac mapping and imaging in the diagnosis and management of cardiac arrhythmias.

Embryogenesis of the heart involves the complex cellular differentiation of slow-conducting primary myocardium into the rapidly conducting chamber myocardium of the adult. However, small areas of relatively undifferentiated cells remain to form components of the adult cardiac conduction system (CCS) and nodal tissues. Further investigation has revealed additional areas of nodal-like tissues outside of the established CCS. The embryologic origins of these areas are similar to those of the adult CCS. Under pathologic conditions, these areas can give rise to important clinical arrhythmias. Here, we review the embryologic basis for these proarrhythmic structures within the heart.

Knowledge of relevant cardiac anatomy is crucial in understanding the pathophysiology and treatment of arrhythmias, and helps avoid potential complications in mapping and ablation. This article explores the anatomy, relevant to electrophysiologists, relating to atrial flutter and atrial fibrillation, ventricular tachycardia relating to the outflow tracts as well as endocardial structure, and also epicardial considerations for mapping and ablation.

To characterize cardiac activity and arrhythmias, electrophysiologists can record the electrical activity of the heart in relation to its anatomy through a process called cardiac mapping (electroanatomic mapping, EAM). A solid understanding of the basic cardiac biopotentials, called electrograms, is imperative to construct and interpret the cardiac EAM correctly. There are several mapping approaches available to the electrophysiologist, each optimized for specific arrhythmia mechanisms. This article provides an overview of the fundamentals of EAM.

Novel cardiac mapping systems allow a safe and highly accurate 3-D reconstruction of cardiac structures as well as fast and accurate visualization of cardiac arrhythmias. In addition, they are increasingly reducing the need for fluoroscopy in these procedures. The current state of the art, as well as the presentation of possible uses of individual systems and their limitations, is presented in this article. Cardiac mapping systems can significantly contribute to an optimal therapeutic decision making in invasive electrophysiology. This article introduces new developments of Rhythmia, Topera, EnSite Precision, and CARTO systems and provides a look ahead to the future.

Electrocardiographic imaging is a mapping technique aiming to noninvasively characterize cardiac electrical activity using signals collected from the torso to reconstruct epicardial potentials. Its efficacy has been demonstrated clinically, from mapping premature ventricular complexes and accessory pathways to of complex arrhythmias. Electrocardiographic imaging uses a standardized workflow. Signals should be checked manually to avoid automatic processing errors. Reentry is confirmed in the presence of local activation covering the arrhythmia cycle length. Focal breakthroughs demonstrate a QS pattern associated with centrifugal activation. Electrocardiographic imaging offers a unique opportunity to better understand the mechanism of cardiac arrhythmias and guide ablation.

Radiofrequency ablation of arrhythmias depends on durable lesion formation. Catheter tip-tissue contact force (CF) is a key determinant of lesion quality; excessive CF is associated with major complications, whereas insufficient CF increases the risk of electrical reconnection and arrhythmia recurrence. In recent years, CF-sensing catheters have emerged with the ability to directly measure CF and provide operators with real-time feedback. CF-guided ablation has been associated with improved outcomes in observational studies. However, randomized controlled trials have not shown any reduction in procedural durations, fluoroscopy exposure, incidence of major complications, or long-term arrhythmia recurrence with use of CF-sensing catheters.

Noninvasive Cardioablation

Marwan M. Refaat, Patrick Zakka, Bassem Youssef, Youssef H. Zeidan, Fadi Geara, and Amin Al-Ahmad

Stereotactic body radiotherapy uses the principle of 3-dimensional localization of a target to deliver a high dose of radiation to a precise location. The aim of this technique is to ablate tissue noninvasively. Because of its high precision and target conformity, it can deliver a high dose of radiation to a specific area in a tissue without significantly affecting nearby tissues. It is being actively studied and even used in therapy for atrial fibrillation and ventricular tachycardia.

Radiofrequency Balloon Devices for Atrial Fibrillation Ablation

Carola Gianni, Qiong Chen, Domenico Della Rocca, Uğur Canpolat, Hüseyin Ayhan, Bryan MacDonald, Sanghamitra Mohanty, Chintan Trivedi, Andrea Natale, and Amin Al-Ahmad

Despite technological advancements, radiofrequency catheter ablation for pulmonary vein isolation remains a challenging procedure, as maneuvering the catheter to obtain effective lesions is technically complex and time consuming. For this reason, balloon-based ablation systems have been developed, which can quickly and easily isolate the pulmonary veins (single-shot), with outcomes comparable with point-by-point catheter ablation in the paroxysmal atrial fibrillation population. In this review, we discuss 3 balloon-based devices that use radiofrequency to obtain permanent lesions, a relatively emerging technology that may pose as an alternative option to cryoenergy or laser for single-shot pulmonary vein isolation.

Optical Mapping

Omer Berenfeld and Igor Efimov

Optical mapping of electrical activity in the heart is based on voltage-sensitive and lipophilic fluorescence dyes. Optical signals recorded from cardiac cells correlate well with their transmembrane potentials. High spatiotemporal resolution, wide field mapping, and high sensitivity to transmembrane potential enable detailed characterization of action potential initiation and propagation. Optical mapping is used to study complex patterns of excitation propagation, including propagation across the sinoatrial and atrioventricular nodes and during atrial and ventricular arrhythmias.Optical mapping is used to study the role of reentrant activity in atrial and ventricular fibrillation.

High-resolution/Density Mapping in Patients with Atrial and Ventricular Arrhythmias

Decebal Gabriel Laţcu and Nadir Saoudi

High-definition/ultra–high-definition mapping, owing to an impressive increase of the point density of electroanatomic maps, provides improved substrate characterization, better understanding of the arrhythmia mechanism, and a better selection of the ablation target in patients with atrial and ventricular arrhythmias. Despite the scarce comparative data on ablation results versus standard mapping, ultra-high-definition mapping is increasingly used by the electrophysiology community.

Reinserting Physiology into Cardiac Mapping Using Omnipolar Electrograms

Karl Magtibay, Andreu Porta-Sánchez, Shouvik K. Haldar, Don Curtis Deno, Stéphane Massé, and Kumaraswamy Nanthakumar

Omnipolar electrograms (EGMs) make use of biophysical electric fields that accompany activation along the surface of the myocardium. A grid-like electrode array provides bipolar signals in orthogonal directions to deliver catheter-orientation-independent assessments of cardiac electrophysiology. Studies with myocyte monolayers, isolated animal and human hearts, and anesthetized animals validated the tenets of omnipolar EGMs. The combination of information from omnipolar-based activation vectors and voltages may aid in localizing areas of scar, lesion gaps, wavefront disorganization, and fractionation or collision during arrhythmias. The goal of omnipolar EGMs is to better characterize myocardium through reintroducing electrogram direction related fundamentals of cardiac electrophysiology.

Cardiac MRI and Fibrosis Quantification

Eugene G. Kholmovski, Alan K. Morris, and Mihail G. Chelu

Left atrial fibrosis plays an important role in the pathophysiology of atrial fibrillation. Left atrial ablation is an effective and increasingly used strategy to restore and maintain sinus rhythm in patients with atrial fibrillation. Late gadolinium enhancement (LGE) MRI and custom image analysis software have been used to visualize and quantify preablation atrial fibrosis and postablation scar and new fibrosis formation. This article reviews technical aspects of imaging atrial fibrosis/scar by LGE-MRI; use of atrial fibrosis and scar in predicting outcomes; applications of LGE-MRI to assess ablation lesions and optimize ablation parameters while avoiding collateral damage.

Fibrosis and Ventricular Arrhythmogenesis: Role of Cardiac MRI

Mohammad Shenasa

Cardiac fibrosis is a significant increase in collagen volume fraction of myocardial tissue. It plays an important role in the pathophysiology of many cardiovascular abnormalities. Electrophysiologically, myocardial fibrosis produces anisotropic conduction, inhomogeneity, and conduction delay. Several markers are available to detect myocardial fibrosis. CMRI is the most common imaging technique; late gadolinium enhancement cardiac magnetic resonance (LGE-CMR) provides markers for tissue characterization, disease progression and arrhythmic events. LGE-CMR can be used as risk marker of occurrence of pathologic conditions. LGE-CMR demonstrates specific patterns related to different pathologic substrates. We discuss the role of CMRI in ventricular arrhythmogenesis.

CARDIAC ELECTROPHYSIOLOGY CLINICS

SERIES OF RELATED INTEREST

Cardiology Clinics
Available at: https://www.cardiology.theclinics.com/

THE CLINICS ARE AVAILABLE ONLINE!
Access your subscription at:
www.theclinics.com

Foreword
Mapping the Heart

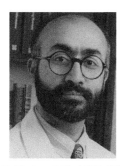   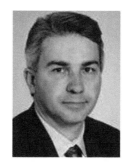

Ranjan K. Thakur, MD, MPH, MBA, FHRS   Andrea Natale, MD, FACC, FHRS

Consulting Editors

Cardiac mapping is simply the correlation of the electrical activity of the heart to the underlying anatomy. In its simplest form, placement of multipolar intracardiac catheters and induction of sustained arrhythmias are a form of mapping to determine the location of an accessory pathway or the site of origin of ventricular tachycardia, and such. Since interventional electrophysiology began in the 1980s, more and more sophisticated cardiac mapping tools as well as electrophysiologic concepts have been developed to pinpoint the mechanisms and the exact anatomic localization of susceptible arrhythmic substrates. Cardiac mapping has not been fully automated, but requires detailed electrophysiology study, the use of electrophysiologic maneuvers, and deductive reasoning.

Dr Shenasa has been active for over 2 decades in summarizing the advancements in cardiac mapping periodically. His current book, *Cardiac Mapping* is in its fifth edition. We are grateful to Drs Shenasa and Al-Ahmad for their effort of providing a summary of contemporary issues of interest in cardiac mapping for the clinical electrophysiology community. They have assembled an international panel of experts to discuss everything from anatomical considerations in mapping, the fundamentals of cardiac mapping, and unipolar mapping, all the way to the comparative advantages of the commercially available mapping systems. This issue contains useful information for electrophysiology fellows, associated professionals in electrophysiology as well as the practicing electrophysiologist.

We hope the readership will find this issue useful and informative.

Ranjan K. Thakur, MD, MPH, MBA, FHRS
Sparrow Thoracic and Cardiovascular Institute
Michigan State University
1200 East Michigan Avenue, Suite 580
Lansing, MI 48912, USA

Andrea Natale, MD, FACC, FHRS
Texas Cardiac Arrhythmia Institute
Center for Atrial Fibrillation at
St. David's Medical Center
1015 East 32nd Street, Suite 516
Austin, TX 78705, USA

E-mail addresses:
thakur@msu.edu (R.K. Thakur)
andrea.natale@stdavids.com (A. Natale)

https://doi.org/10.1016/j.ccep.2019.06.004
1877-9182/19/© 2019 Published by Elsevier Inc.

cardiacEP.theclinics.com

Preface

Advances in Cardiac Mapping: Part 1

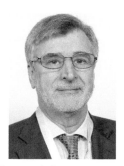   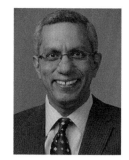

Mohammad Shenasa, MD, FHRS   Amin Al-Ahmad, MD, FHRS

Editors

Cardiac mapping has come a long way, and it has been an integral part of interventional cardiac electrophysiology. Cardiac mapping started with direct single-analogue point-by-point registration of cardiac electrical activity to its utmost complex online multimodality mapping and imaging. Technological advances in cardiac mapping and ablation allowed rhythmologists and interventional electrophysiologists to better understand the mechanisms and management of arrhythmias. Despite the unprecedented technological advances in the diagnosis and management of cardiac arrhythmias, such as atrial fibrillation, epicardial ventricular tachycardias, and arrhythmias in congenital heart disease, challenges remain ahead.

The future lies in the noninvasive mapping and imaging in the diagnosis of cardiac arrhythmias, such as electrocardiographic imaging, in even a single cardiac beat to the noninvasive ablation techniques, such as noninvasive cardiac radiation and zero to near-zero fluoroscopy, to avoid radiation exposure.

We are pleased that the consulting editors of *Cardiac Electrophysiology Clinics*. Ranjan K. Thakur, MD, and Andrea Natale, MD, invited us to serve as editors for this important topic. In addition, we are delighted that a group of pioneers in the field of cardiac mapping and ablation has unanimously accepted our invitation to contribute their state-of-the-art articles for this and the next issue of *Cardiac Electrophysiology Clinics*, both on advances in cardiac mapping.

We initially planned to have a single issue dedicated to this topic. However, due to important topics that needed to be covered, we were obliged to include a 2-issue comprehensive review. Part 1 covers the basic concepts, including cardiac embryology and anatomy relevant to cardiac mapping and ablation, followed by novel mapping and imaging techniques, such as cardiac computed tomography and MRI, and catheter and energy sources. Part 2 discusses mapping and ablation of particular arrhythmias in specific substrates, such as atrial fibrillation, ventricular tachycardia, and fibrillation.

We are confident that these 2 issues on advances in cardiac mapping will be useful to clinical cardiac electrophysiologists, fellow trainees, attending, and allied professionals who participate in the management of patients with complex arrhythmias, and we hope that it improves patients' quality of life and survival.

Mohammad Shenasa, MD, FHRS
Department of Cardiovascular Services
O'Connor Hospital
Heart and Rhythm Medical Group
105 North Bascome Avenue
San Jose, CA 95128, USA

Amin Al-Ahmad, MD, FHRS
Texas Cardiac Arrhythmia Institute
St David's Medical Center
Austin, TX 78705, USA

E-mail addresses:
mohammad.shenasa@gmail.com (M. Shenasa)
aalahmadmd@gmail.com (A. Al-Ahmad)

Card Electrophysiol Clin 11 (2019) xvii
https://doi.org/10.1016/j.ccep.2019.06.003
1877-9182/19/© 2019 Published by Elsevier Inc.

cardiacEP.theclinics.com

Historical Perspectives on Cardiac Mapping and Ablation

Mohammad Shenasa, MD, FHRS[a],*, Amin Al-Ahmad, MD, FHRS[b]

KEYWORDS

• Ablation • Cardiac mapping • Electrophysiology • History • Imaging

KEY POINTS

- Cardiac mapping has evolved from single point-by-point registration of cardiac electrical activity to a real-time multimodality of mapping and imaging for catheter ablation of arrhythmias.
- Cardiac mapping and ablation provide us tools to reach areas of the heart that once were considered inaccessible.
- Many imaging techniques such as cardiac MRI and computed cardiac tomography alone or in hybrid form are being used.
- Noninvasive mapping and ablation are being investigated and will be available the near future. Zero to near-zero fluoroscopy is also currently used in practice to avoid radiation exposure.
- Real-time noninvasive mapping and imaging as well as ablation of a variety of arrhythmias are already in practice.

INTRODUCTION

Cardiac mapping has always been an integral part of rhythmology and cardiac electrophysiology. Indeed, direct cardiac mapping has been investigated before intracardiac electrocardiography. Cardiac mapping has evolved from direct single point-by-point registration of cardiac electrical activity, to the utmost complex digital mapping, such as optical mapping with simultaneous depolarization and repolarization of electrical activation in a variety of arrhythmias. In today's world, technological advances have afforded interventional electrophysiologists to use hybrid technologies such as cardiac MRI with PET/computed tomography scans and others to better understand the mechanisms and improved management of cardiac arrhythmias. Historical perspectives on cardiac mapping have been described in detail previously and the readers are referred for further information to other sources.[1-7]

MILESTONES IN CARDIAC MAPPING

Basic electrophysiology
1. In 1883, Gaskell reported on innervation of the heart in tortoise.[7]
2. Waller in 1887 investigated the electromotive changes induced by heartbeat.[8]
3. Sir Thomas Lewis in 1915, has used direct point-by-point registration of epicardial surface in a dog heart.[9]
4. In 1913 and 1914, George R. Mines demonstrated evidence of reentrant waves in jellyfish and its relation to tachycardia.[10,11]
5. In 1914, Walter Garrey provided evidence on the nature of fibrillatory contraction of the heart and its relation to tissue mass and form.[12]

Disclosures: No relevant disclosures.
[a] Heart and Rhythm Medical Group, Department of Cardiovascular Services, O'Connor Hospital, 105 North Bascom Avenue, San Jose, CA 95128, USA; [b] Saint David's Medical Center, 919 East 32nd Street, Austin, TX 78705, USA
* Corresponding author.
E-mail address: mohammad.shenasa@gmail.com

Card Electrophysiol Clin 11 (2019) 405–408
https://doi.org/10.1016/j.ccep.2019.06.001
1877-9182/19/© 2019 Elsevier Inc. All rights reserved.

6. In 1954, Puech reported on the normal auricular activation in the dogs heart using measurements of 0.005-second intervls.[13]
7. In 1964, Moe and colleagues[14] presented the classical work of computer model of atrial fibrillation where he demonstrated the multi-wavelet theory.
8. In 1973, Allessie and colleagues[15] reported the circus movement reentry in rabbit atrial muscle as a mechanism of tachycardia. They further introduced the concept of the leading circle as a model of reentry for atrial fibrillation.[16]

Clinical investigations

9. With the advent of electrocardiogram (ECG) by Willem Einthoven in 1903 a new door to registration of electrical activity of the heart was opened.[17] Today, the ECG is one of the most commonly used tests in the world. Furthermore, the ECG is used as a mapping tool for a variety of arrhythmias.[18,19]
10. In 1970, Durrer and colleagues[20] demonstrated the total excitation of the isolated human heart.
11. Wellens and colleagues[21] in 1974 reported on epicardial mapping to interrupt accessory pathways in patients with Wolff–Parkinson–White syndrome.
12. Subsequently, Gallagher and colleagues[22] reported on epicardial mapping in the Wolff Parkinson White syndrome in 1978.
13. Josephson and colleagues[23–25] in a series of reports demonstrated reentry as the mechanism of ventricular tachycardia (VT) in patients with coronary artery disease. They also reported that reentry circuits were localized subendocardially and endocardial resection eliminated the arrhythmia.[26]
14. In 1991, Kaltenbrunner and colleagues[27] reported on the simultaneous computerized epicardial and endocardial mapping of VT in patient with myocardial infarction.
15. Shenasa and colleagues[28] reported the use of subthreshold electrical stimulation in mapping and surgical ablation of VT in humans.
16. In 1998, Haissaguerre and colleagues[29] reported their seminal work on catheter ablation of atrial fibrillation. Since this initial report, a mountain of experience and knowledge has been produced on the role of catheter ablation in atrial fibrillation.

Technological Advances

Multiple imaging techniques are now available in mapping and ablation of cardiac arrhythmias that include:

1. In 1987 Borggrefe and colleagues[30] reported on ablation of an accessory pathway in humans using high frequency alternating current.
2. Electroanatomic mapping is the cornerstone of mapping technologies in catheter ablation of arrhythmias.[31]
3. Noncontact mapping.[32–34]
4. High-resolution mapping.[35]
5. Noninvasive body surface ECG mapping.
6. Noninvasive cardiac radiation for the ablation of VT.[36]
7. Nonfluoroscopic sensor-guided navigation of intracardiac electrophysiology catheters within prerecorded cine loops.[37]
8. Robotic catheter ablation of VT.[38]
9. Zero x-ray cardiac resynchronization therapy device implantation guided by a nonfluoroscopic mapping system.[39]
10. Fluoroless catheter ablation of cardiac arrhythmias.[40]

Multimodality imaging using integration of different systems is now available. summarizes the currently available hybrid systems.

EVOLUTION OF MAPPING AND IMAGING IN CARDIAC ARRHYTHMIAS AND INTERVENTIONAL ELECTROPHYSIOLOGY

In the last 2 decades, unprecedented advances in technology provided tools for mapping and imaging of complex arrhythmias including those with congenital heart disease. summarizes the different imaging modalities useful in ablation of VT in different substrates. Noninvasive cardiac radiation for ablation of VT in patients is recently reported by Cuculich and colleagues.[36,41] One of the limitations of interventional electrophysiology is the patient and staff exposure to radiation. Razminia and colleagues[40] have reported on fluoroless catheter ablation of cardiac arrhythmias, which will be the way of the future.

SUMMARY

Cardiac mapping and imaging has evolved from a direct single point-by-point registration of cardiac electrical activity to utmost complex multimodal real-time techniques. These investigations have afforded the cardiac electrophysiologists for better understanding of the mechanisms of arrhythmias and their management. Today, cardiac mapping is the cardiac electrophysiologist's guidance system.

ACKNOWLEDGMENTS

The authors wish to thank Dr Seyed-Mostafa Razavi and Sarah J. Honoré for their assistance in preparation of this article.

REFERENCES

1. Janse MJ. Some historical notes on the mapping of arrhythmias. In: Shenasa M, Borggrefe M, Breithardt G, editors. Cardiac mapping. London: Futura Publishing; 1993. p. 3–10.
2. Janse MJ. Historical notes: George Ralph Mines. In: Shenasa M, Borggrefe M, Breithardt G, editors. Cardiac mapping. 2nd edition. London: Futura Publishing; 2003. p. 3–11.
3. Wellens H. Historical perspectives, cardiac activation mapping: the Amsterdam years. In: Shenasa M, Hindricks G, Borgrefe M, et al, editors. Cardiac mapping. Wiley Blackwell; 2009.
4. de Bakker JM, Vos MA. Evolution of cardiac mapping: from direct analog to digital multidimensional recording. In: Shenasa M, Hindricks G, Borgrefe M, et al, editors. Cardiac mapping. 4th edition. Oxford (England): Wiley-Blackwell; 2013. p. 3–11.
5. Zellerhoff S, Eckardt L, Breithardt G. History of cardiac mapping. In: Shenasa M, Hindricks G, Borgrefe M, et al, editors. Cardiac mapping. 5th edition. Oxford (England): Wiley-Blackwell; 2019.
6. Lüderitz B. Historical perspectives of cardiac electrophysiology. Hellenic J Cardiol 2009;50:3–16.
7. Gaskell WH. On the innervation of the heart with special reference to the heart of the tortoise. J Physiol 1883;4:43–230.
8. Waller AD. A demonstration on man of electromotive changes accompanying the heart's beat. J Physiol 1887;8:229–34.
9. Lewis TR, Rothschild MA, Starling EH. The excitatory process in the dog's heart. Phill Trans Roy Soc London 1915;206:181–226.
10. Mines G. On dynamic equilibrium in the heart. 1913;46:349–83.
11. Mines G. On circulating excitations in heart muscles and their possible relation to tachycardia and fibrillation. Trans R Soc Can 1914;8:43–52.
12. Garrey W. The nature of fibrillary contraction of the heart - its relation to tissue mass and form. Am J Physiol 1914;33:397–414.
13. Puech P, Esclavissat M, Sodi-Pallares D, et al. Normal auricular activation in the dog's heart. Am Heart J 1954;47:174–91.
14. Moe GK, Rheinboldt WC, Abildskov JA. A computer model of atrial fibrillation. Am Heart J 1964;67(2):200–20.
15. Allessie MA, Bonke FI, Schopman FJ. Circus movement in rabbit atrial muscle as a mechanism of tachycardia. Circ Res 1973;33:54–62.
16. Allessie MA, Bonke FI, Schopman FJ. Circus movement in rabbit atrial muscle as a mechanism of tachycardia. III. The 'leading circle' concept: a new model of circus movement in cardiac tissue without the involvement of an anatomical obstacle. Circ Res 1977;41:9–18.
17. Einthoven W. Le telecardiogtamme. Arch Int Physiol 1906;4:132–64.
18. Valles E, Bazan V, Marchlinski FE. ECG criteria to identify epicardial ventricular tachycardia in nonischemic cardiomyopathy. Circ Arrhythm Electrophysiol 2010;3(1):63–71.
19. Bazan V, Marchlinski FE. Usefulness of the 12-Lead ECG to Identify Epicardial Ventricular Substrate and Epicardial Ventricular Tachycardia Site of Origin. In: Shenasa M, Hindricks G, Borgrefe M, et al, editors. Cardiac Mapping. 5th Edition. Oxford (England): Wiley; 2019. p. 1028–49.
20. Durrer DR, Freud GE, Janse MJ, et al. Total excitation of the isolated human heart. Circ 1970;41:899–912.
21. Wellens HJJM, Van Dam RT, van Capelle FJ, et al. Epicardial mapping and surgical treatment in Wolff-Parkinson-white syndrome type A. Am Heart J 1974;88:69–78.
22. Gallagher JJKJ, Sealy WC, Pritchett EL, et al. Epicardial mapping in the Wolff-Parkinson-White syndrome. Circ 1978;57:854–66.
23. Josephson M, Horowitz LN, Farshidi A, et al. Recurrent sustained ventricular tachycardia: 1. Mechanisms. Circ 1978;57:431–40.
24. Josephson ME, Horowitz LN, Farshidi A, et al. Recurrent sustained ventricular tachycardia: 2. Endocardial mapping. Circ 1978;57:440–7.
25. Josephson MEHA, Horowitz LN. Endocardial excision: a new surgical technique for the treatment of recurrent ventricular tachycardia. Circ 1979;60:1430–9.
26. Shenasa M, Miller JM, Callans DJ, et al. Conquest of Ventricular Tachycardia: Insights Into Mechanisms, Innovations in Management: Contribution of Mark E. Josephson, MD, to Clinical Electrophysiology. Circ Arrhythm Electrophysiol 2017.
27. Kaltenbrunner W, Cardinal R, Dubuc M, et al. Epicardial and endocardial mapping of ventricular tachycardia in patients with myocardial infarction: is the origin of the tachycardia always subendocardially localized? Circ 1991;84:1058–71.
28. Shenasa M, Cardinal R, Kus T, et al. Termination of sustained ventricular tachycardia by ultrarapid subthreshold stimulation in humans. Circ 1988;78:1135–43.
29. Haissaguerre M, Jais P, Shah D, et al. Spontaneous initiation of atrial fibrillation by ectopic beats originating in the pulmonary veins. N Engl J Med 1998;339:659–66.
30. Borggrefe M, Budde T, Podczeck A, et al. High frequency alternating current ablation of an accessory pathway in humans. J Am Coll Cardiol 1987;10:576–82.

31. Al-Ahmad A, Callans D, Hsia H, et al. Electroanatomical mapping: an atlas for clinicians. Oxford (England): Wiley-Blackwel; 2009. p. 1–268.

32. Packer DL. Three-dimensional mapping in interventional electrophysiology: techniques and technology. J Cardiovasc Electrophysiol 2005;16(10):1110–6.

33. Sabouri S, Matene E, Vinet A, et al. Simultaneous epicardial and noncontact endocardial mapping of the canine right atrium: simulation and experiment. PLoS One 2014;9(3).

34. Packer DL. Evolution of mapping and Anatomic imaging of cardiac arrhythmias. J Cardiovasc Electrophysiol 2004;15(7):1045–3873.

35. Latcu DG, Saudi N. High resolution/Density mapping in patients with atrial and ventricular arrhythmias. In: Advances in Cardiac Mapping and Catheter Ablation: Part I. EP Clinic 2019. Elsevier. In press.

36. Cuculich PS, Schill MR, Kashani R, et al. Noninvasive cardiac radiation for ablation of ventricular tachycardia. N Engl J Med 2017;377(24):2325–36.

37. Piorkowski C, Hindricks G. Nonfluoroscopic sensor-guided navigation of intracardiac electrophysiology catheters within prerecorded cine loops. Circ Arrhythm Electrophysiol 2011;4(4):e36–8.

38. Valderrabano M, Dave AS, Baez-Escudero JL, et al. Robotic catheter ablation of left ventricular tachycardia: initial experience. Heart Rhythm 2011; 8(12):1837–46.

39. Colella A, Giaccardi M, Colella T, et al. Zero x-ray cardiac resynchronization therapy device implantation guided by a nonfluoroscopic mapping system: a pilot study. Heart Rhythm 2016;13(7):1481–8.

40. Razminia M, Willoughby MC, Demo H, et al. Fluoroless catheter ablation of cardiac arrhythmias: a 5-year experience. Pacing Clin Electrophysiol 2017; 40(4):425–33.

41. Refaat M, Zakka P, Youssef B, et al. Noninvasive Cardioablation. In: Advances in Cardiac Mapping and Catheter Ablation: Part I. EP Clinic 2019. Elsevier. In press.

Embryology of the Cardiac Conduction System Relevant to Arrhythmias

Gwilym M. Morris, BM BCh, PhD, MRCP*,
Jonathan P. Ariyaratnam, MB BChir, MA, MRCP

KEYWORDS

- Cardiac conduction system • Embryology • Cardiac development • Arrhythmias
- Atrial tachycardia

KEY POINTS

- The cardiac conduction system is an extensive network of specialized electrical tissue; in the adult heart this is usually defined as the sinoatrial node, atrioventricular node, and the His-Purkinje system (slow nodes and the fast ventricular conduction system).
- The electrical properties of the cardiac conduction system are distinct from working myocardium and may include slow conduction, poor electrical coupling, and automaticity. These features give a propensity to proarrhythmia in the form of enhanced automaticity, triggered activity, and local micro-reentry.
- Genetic control of embryonic differentiation of the cardiac conduction system is well defined, and persistence of this gene expression can be used in the adult heart, along with histology and ion channel expression, to locate persistence of cardiac conduction system tissue away from the traditionally defined cardiac conduction system.
- Stereotyped development and folding of the embryonic heart and development of the cardiac conduction system can help to explain the distribution of many arrhythmias in the adult, which may be related to the persistence of embryonic cardiac conduction system tissue.
- This is particularly relevant to right ventricular outflow tract ventricular tachycardia and focal atrial tachycardia.

INTRODUCTION

The cardiac conduction system (CCS) comprises the specialized electrical tissues of the heart. In the adult heart it includes the "slow nodes" (sinoatrial node [SAN], and atrioventricular node [AVN]) and the rapidly conducting His-Purkinje system (HPS). Together they are responsible for initiation of the heartbeat, as well as coordinated impulse conduction through the heart to the ventricular myocardium. CCS tissue comprises of highly specialized cardiomyocytes that differentiate from working myocardium early in cardiac development. Although CCS tissue constitutes a small proportion of the heart by volume, it is widely distributed throughout the normal adult heart, and the presence of functionally redundant CCS tissue can be demonstrated away from the traditionally recognized CCS axis. The embryology and gene program directing development of the CCS is well described; knowledge of these genes and the embryonic development of the CCS can help

Disclosure: Dr G.M. Morris is supported by a British Heart Foundation Fellowship under grant number FS/18/47/33669.
Cardiovascular Sciences, University of Manchester, Core Technology Facility, 46 Grafton Street, Manchester M13 9NT, UK
* Correspondence author.
E-mail address: gwilym.morris@manchester.ac.uk

Card Electrophysiol Clin 11 (2019) 409–420
https://doi.org/10.1016/j.ccep.2019.05.002
1877-9182/19/© 2019 Elsevier Inc. All rights reserved.

to understand the distribution of the functionally redundant CCS tissue, which may be proarrhythmic. The specialized features of the CCS and their usual distribution in the adult heart help to explain the nature and distribution of many spontaneous cardiac arrhythmias in the adult.

ELECTROPHYSIOLOGY OF THE CARDIAC CONDUCTION SYSTEM

The principal functional components of the CCS in the adult heart are the SAN, AVN, and HPS. Their roles in heartbeat initiation, atrioventricular delay, and rapid coordinated conduction to the ventricles are well known.[1] These tissues are molecularly, histologically, and functionally distinct from the working myocardium through the differential expression of ion channels, calcium-handling proteins, and gap junction proteins (**Fig. 1**A–C). These important differences confer on the CCS the ability to generate and conduct electrical signals through the myocardium. For example, study of the action potential of the SAN demonstrates rhythmic phase 4 depolarization ("pacemaker potential") that triggers an action potential in contrast to the stable, hyperpolarized, phase 4 resting potential of working myocardium (**Fig. 2**A).[2] In addition to the SAN, the primary pacemaker of the heart, other components of the CCS have been demonstrated to display pacemaker activity. Phase 4 pacemaker activity is a feature of all CCS tissue to a variable extent (**Fig. 2**B), which explains the ability of subsidiary areas such as the atrioventricular junction or HPS to act as the leading heart pacemaker during periods of sinus bradycardia, sinus arrest, or even third-degree

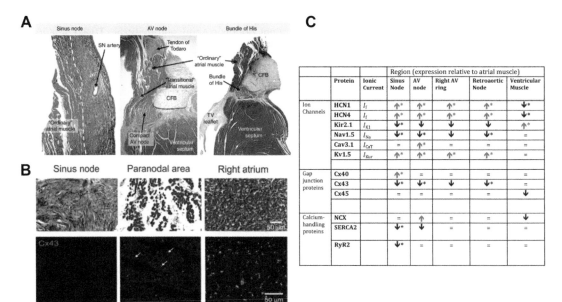

	Protein	Ionic Current	Region (expression relative to atrial muscle)				
			Sinus Node	AV node	Right AV ring	Retroaortic Node	Ventricular Muscle
Ion Channels	HCN1	I_f	↑*	↑*	↑*	↑*	↓*
	HCN4	I_f	↑*	↑*	↑*	↑*	↓*
	Kir2.1	I_{K1}	↓*	↓	↓	↓	↑*
	Nav1.5	I_{Na}	↓*	↓*	↓	↓*	=
	Cav3.1	I_{CaT}	=	↑*	=	=	=
	Kv1.5	I_{Kur}	↑*	↑*	↑*	↑*	=
Gap junction proteins	Cx40		↑*	=	=	=	=
	Cx43		↓*	↓*	↓	↓*	=
	Cx45		=	=	=	=	↓
Calcium-handling proteins	NCX		=	↑	=	=	↓
	SERCA2		↓*	↓	=	=	=
	RyR2		↓*	=	=	=	=

Fig. 1. Histologic and molecular differences between tissues of the working myocardium and the cardiac conduction system. (*A*) Low-magnification microscopy of sections of the sinus node, AVN, and Bundle of His stained with Masson's trichrome. Nodal tissues are embedded within a network of connective tissue (which stains blue) giving the nodal tissues a distinct appearance from the working myocardium. (*B*) Higher-magnification microscopy of the sinus node compared with the nearby paranodal and right atrial regions. Upper panel demonstrates Masson's trichrome staining with significantly increased collagen staining in the nodal tissue compared with working myocardium. Lower panel shows gap junction protein Cx43 immunolabeling, demonstrating significantly decreased Cx43 in the nodal tissue compared with right atrial muscle. Note that the paranodal regions exhibit an intermediate phenotype. (*C*) Significant differences in mRNA expression of ion channels, calcium-handling proteins, and gap junction proteins within tissues of the cardiac conduction system compared with atrial and ventricular working myocardium. ↑*, significant upregulation; ↓*, significant downregulation; ↑, trend to upregulation; ↓, trend to downregulation. (*From* [*A*] Sizarov A, MA, Pickoff A. Development and functional maturation of the cardiac conduction system. In: *Heart Disease in Infants, Children and Adolescents* 2013; with permission; and [*B*] Dobrzynski H, Anderson RH, Atkinson A, et al. Structure, function and clinical relevance of the cardiac conduction system, including the atrioventricular ring and outflow tract tissues. *Pharmacol Ther* 2013;139(2):260–288; with permission; and *Adapted from* [*C*] Dobrzynski H, Anderson RH, Atkinson A, et al. Structure, function and clinical relevance of the cardiac conduction system, including the atrioventricular ring and outflow tract tissues. *Pharmacol Ther* 2013;139(2):260–288; with permission.)

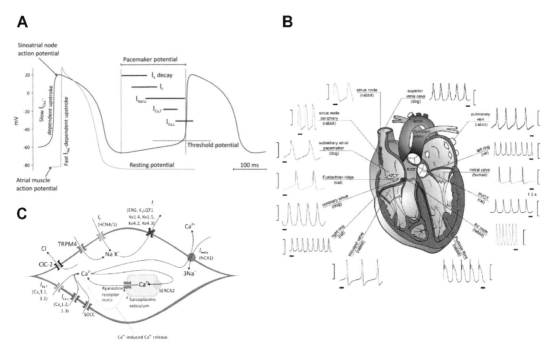

Fig. 2. Electrophysiological characteristics of the CCS. (*A*) Representative action potentials recorded from atrial tissue and the SAN. The atrial muscle action potential demonstrates a stable resting potential in phase 4. During the same period, the SAN action potential exhibits slow diastolic depolarization as a result of the presence of many ionic currents unique to the CCS. This allows for spontaneous action potential generation. (*B*) All components of the CCS (SAN, AVN, and His-Purkinje system) demonstrate diastolic depolarization when compared with atrial and ventricular working myocardium. (*C*) Representation of the interplay between the multiple ionic currents of the "membrane clock" and the intracellular "calcium clock," conferring the ability to generate the action potential within cells of the CCS. (*From* [*A*] Monfredi O, Dobrzynski H, Mondal T, Boyett MR, Morris GM. The anatomy and physiology of the sinoatrial node–a contemporary review. *Pacing and clinical electrophysiology: PACE* 2010;33(11):1392–1406; with permission; and [*B*] Dobrzynski H, Anderson RH, Atkinson A, et al. Structure, function and clinical relevance of the cardiac conduction system, including the atrioventricular ring and outflow tract tissues. *Pharmacol Ther* 2013;139(2):260–288; with permission; and [*C*] Dobrzynski H, Anderson RH, Atkinson A, et al. Structure, function and clinical relevance of the cardiac conduction system, including the atrioventricular ring and outflow tract tissues. *Pharmacol Ther* 2013;139(2):260–288; with permission.)

atrioventricular block.[1,3,4] Knowledge of the normal electrophysiology of the CCS is central to understanding the susceptibility of these regions to arrhythmia.

Of all the components, the pacemaker mechanisms of the SAN are the best studied and are an archetype of pacemaker mechanisms for all of the CCS. The molecular basis of the pacemaker potential is complex, depending on the mutual entrainment of 2 molecular clocks (**Fig. 2**C); primary membrane-generated potentials (the membrane clock), and intracellular calcium dynamics (the calcium [Ca^{2+}] clock).[2] In brief, the membrane clock depends on the interaction of the *lack* of a strong hyperpolarizing K^+ current (I_{K1}) and the *presence* of depolarizing Na^+/K^+ currents (principally the "funny current" [I_f]). SAN cells are missing the strong inward rectifier current (I_{K1}), which acts to stabilize the negative membrane resting

potential and prevents pacemaker activity in working myocytes. I_f is activated at negative membrane potentials early in phase 4 (diastole), and depolarizes the SAN cell. The molecular correlates of I_f are the HCN channels.[2]

The Ca^{2+} contributes mainly to late diastolic depolarization by processes that are linked to I_f. The Ca^{2+} clock depends on membrane channels and intracellular Ca^{2+} handling proteins. The T-type Ca^{2+} current is the first of these to be activated; the current is small but the influx of Ca^{2+} to the SAN cell recruits the Ca^{2+} clock by way of the ryanodine receptors on the sarcoplasmic reticulum and is one mechanism of initiation of the Ca^{2+} clock.[5] The Ca^{2+} clock can also initiate independently of the membrane clock through spontaneous localized Ca^{2+} sparks.[6] Elevation of intracellular Ca^{2+} generates depolarizing membrane current because of the electrogenic activity of the Na^+/Ca^{2+} exchanger, NCX1 (movement of 1 Ca^{2+} out of the cell for 3 Na^+ into the cell), generating the inward current, I_{NCX}.[6] Both the membrane and Ca^{2+} clocks are modulated by cyclic-AMP (cAMP), which mediates autonomic control at a cellular level. SAN cells depends on constitutively high levels of cAMP for normal function and so also have high expression of protein kinase A and phosphodiesterases. This allows rapid variation of heart rates over a large physiologic range.[7]

Electrical conduction through the myocardium relies on gap junctions consisting of connexin proteins. Connexin types have differing electrical resistance. The 2 cardiac high conductance connexins, Cx40 and Cx43, are not well expressed in the sinus node compared with the atrial muscle,[8] instead Cx45 is expressed in the SAN leading to poor electrical coupling and slow conduction. In some regions, including the paranodal area next to the SAN in the human, expression of ion channels and connexins is transitional, that is, part way between nodal tissue and working myocardium.[9] Understanding the effects of expression of nodal-type tissues in the working myocardium, through transitional zones or by way of embryonic remnants, helps to understand why these regions can be arrhythmogenic. For example, conduction can be slowed due to the presence of low-conductance connexins and low levels of $Na_v1.5$,

automaticity can be caused by the presence of HCN channels and afterdepolarizations can be triggered by the presence of high levels of constitutive cAMP.

DEVELOPMENT OF THE CARDIAC CONDUCTION SYSTEM

The development of the mammalian heart is well studied; most insights are derived from transgenic mice. The development of the heart begins at around the third week gestation, when the lateral plate mesoderm folds anteriorly to form the primitive gut tube. This folding process brings together the endocardial tubes, which fuse to form the pericardial cavity. Within the pericardial sac the mesenchyme differentiates into mesoderm at day 22 to allow the formation of a beating primary heart tube. Blood enters inferiorly at the inflow tract where there is also dominant automaticity.[10] This primitive heart tube forms the definitive left ventricle and atrioventricular canal (AVC), the heart tube elongates by addition of progenitor cells from the second heart field to both poles of the heart. These regions will form the definitive right ventricle and sinus venosus.[10] Cells added to the inferior pole acquire a pacemaker phenotype and the dominant pacemaker remains at the inflow

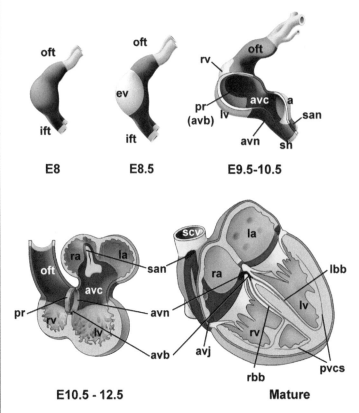

Fig. 3. Embryological development of the cardiac conduction system. Overview of the heart development in vertebrates. The early heart tube consists primarily of automatic, slowly conducting primary myocardium (purple), but as it develops, chamber myocardium (grey) expands to form the majority of the mature heart. Small areas of primary myocardium remain within the sinus venosus to form the mature sinus node and within the atrioventricular canal to form the atrioventricular node and atrioventricular ring tissues. OFT, outflow tract; IFT, inflow tract; EV, embryonic ventricle; RV, right ventricle; LV, left ventricle; A, atrium; SAN, sinoatrial node; AVN, atrioventricular node; AVB, atrioventricular bundle; RBB, right bundle branch; LBB, left bundle branch; PVCS, peripheral ventricular conduction system. (*From* Christoffels VM, Moorman AF. Development of the cardiac conduction system: why are some regions of the heart more arrhythmogenic than others? *Circulation Arrhythmia and electrophysiology* 2009;2(2):195–207; with permission.)

region.[10] Pictorial representation of the development of the heart and CCS is shown in **Fig. 3**.

Our understanding of the development of the CCS has grown with the use of both immunohistochemical and molecular markers of the CCS in embryogenesis. For example, the monoclonal antibody, HNK1, originally used as a marker of neural crest cells during embryologic development, has been found to be a particularly specific marker of the developing CCS in rat, chick, and human embryos.[11] HNK1 immunohistochemistry expanded our knowledge of the human CCS, by staining not only the established areas of the CCS (SAN, AVN, and HPS), but also additional areas such as the atrioventricular rings and the retroaortic node.

The cells of the early, primary heart tube exhibit similar features to those of the mature, adult CCS (**Table 1**). They display automaticity, slow conduction, and poor contraction. Phenotypically, the cells are small and poorly coupled (lacking gap junction proteins) with poorly developed sarcomeres and sarcoplasmic reticulum.[12] As the heart tube grows it loops, and the curvatures rapidly proliferate to form the atrial and ventricular chambers. The cellular phenotype of these chambers differentiates by expression of a "default" cardiac gene program that directs the development of chamber myocardium; a cellular phenotype that includes sarcomeric and sarcoplasmic reticulum development,[12] high conductance gap junction proteins (Cx40 and Cx43), and the cardiac sodium channel SCN5A ($Na_v1.5$), resulting in cardiac tissue with fast conduction and high contractility, but no automaticity. Most arrhythmogenic regions in the adult heart arise from areas in the embryonic heart that do not initially differentiate into chamber myocardium, namely the AVC, outflow tract, and sinus horn.

The CCS develops by suppression of this default cardiac gene program such that cellular proliferation is reduced, and automaticity and poor cell coupling is retained.[10] The SAN is best studied; the T box transcription factor Tbx18 is expressed throughout the sinus venosus, including the sinus horns and SAN, and it is necessary for the proper morphologic development of these regions.[10] Virally mediated ectopic expression of Tbx18 can induce pacemaker activity in working myocardium or subsidiary pacemaker regions.[13,14] In addition to Tbx18 expression, development of the mature SAN depends on the expression of another T box transcription factor, Tbx3, which imposes a pacemaker phenotype on myocardial cells by actively repressing working myocardium gene targets such as Cx43 and Scn5a (**Fig. 4**). The extent of expression of Tbx3 is restricted by NKX2.5 in the surrounding atrial myocardium, and left/right patterning depends on Pitx2.[10] Outside of the SAN, the remainder of the CCS also expresses Tbx3 (**Fig. 5**); Tbx3-positive cells of the AVC form the definitive AVN and atrioventricular ring bundles at the atrial side of the annulus fibrosus, and Tbx3 is important in the development ventricular conduction system. Detailed consideration of the cascades of genes involved in the development of specific components of the CCS are complex and beyond the scope of this article, but have been comprehensively reviewed by van Weerd and Christoffels.[10]

The expression of the CCS gene program is not only important in the development of the embryonic CCS but also maintains the tissue specialization in the adult heart.[15] Molecular markers specific to conduction tissues in adults, such as HCN4 and Cx45, have been used to localize CCS tissues within the adult myocardium.[16] This means that CCS tissue is distributed through a wide area of the heart, especially the atria, beyond the recognized nodes (SAN and AVN). In the late fetal heart, Tbx3 expression can be seen in extensive regions in the posterior aspects of the right

Table 1
Electrophysiological, functional and anatomic properties of myocardial cell types

	Type of Myocardium			
	Primary	Nodal	Bundle and Branches	Working
Automaticity	High	High	High	Low
Conduction velocity	Low	Low	High	High
Contractility	Low	Low	Low	High
Sarcoplasmic reticulum activity	Low	Low	Low	High

Similarities and differences in cellular properties between the primary myocardium of the developing heart and the adult CCS and working myocardium.

Data from Moorman A, Webb S, Brown NA, et al. Development of the heart: (1) formation of the cardiac chambers and arterial trunks. Heart (British Cardiac Society). 2003;89(7):806–14.

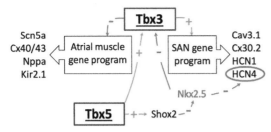

Fig. 4. Molecular determinants of atrial cardiomyocyte differentiation. The presence of Tbx3 plays a central role in maintaining a nodal phenotype in the development of the sinus node. The absence of Tbx3 results in the default differentiation to the atrial working myocyte. (*Data from* Christoffels VM, Moorman AF. Development of the cardiac conduction system: why are some regions of the heart more arrhythmogenic than others? *Circulation Arrhythmia and electrophysiology* 2009;2(2):195–207.)

atrium (RA) and around the annulus fibrosus (see **Fig. 5**). In the adult mammalian heart, cardiac tissue with attributes similar to the CCS can be demonstrated in these areas (**Fig. 6**).[4,16] Although the outflow tract is not part of the CCS, the initial common outflow tract is made up of the primary

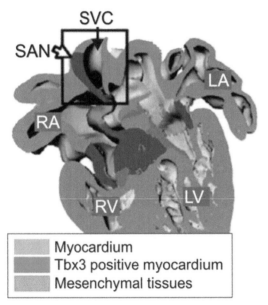

Fig. 5. Embryonic development of the cardiac conduction system. A transverse cut through a stage 23 human-embryonic heart showing Tbx3-positive myocardium in the areas of the developing sinus node and atrioventricular node. LA, left atrium; LV, left ventricle; RA, right atrium; RV, right ventricle; SAN, sinoatrial node; SVC, superior vena cava. (*From* Sizarov A MA, Pickoff A. Development and functional maturation of the cardiac conduction system. In: *Heart Disease in Infants, Children and Adolescents.*2013; with permission.)

myocardium of the heart tube. The embryonic outflow tract initially retains the embryonic phenotype and expresses markers such as minK-lacZ and Cx45, which have been associated with the CCS.[17] The distal portion of this common outflow tract is remodeled by addition of cells to form the intrapericardial arterial trunks. The proximal right ventricular outflow tract (RVOT) largely differentiates into working right ventricular myocardium with the more distal parts disappearing by apoptosis.[1] It has been proposed that some myocytes in the RVOT retain their initial nodal-like phenotype.[18]

ARRHYTHMIAS AND THE CARDIAC CONDUCTION SYSTEM

It is postulated that the CCS can promote arrhythmia by the persistence of nodal-type tissue in the working myocardium. Under normal conditions, the small numbers of slow-conducting cells are insignificant within the working myocardium. However, under certain poorly defined pathologic conditions resulting in localized cardiac remodeling, the cells become functionally significant and proarrhythmic. Regardless of the cellular mechanisms, the CCS seems to be more prone to initiating arrhythmias than the working myocardium. For example, it has been shown that Purkinje cells are more susceptible to both genetic and acquired changes in ion channel expression in comparison with cells of the working myocardium.[19] In the heritable condition catecholamine polymorphic ventricular tachycardia (CPVT), the gain-in-function mutation of the Ryanodine receptor has been shown to result in enhanced sensitivity of Purkinje cells to intracellular calcium dysregulation.[20] Triggered ventricular tachycardia (VT)/ventricular fibrillation in CPVT is therefore highly likely to be Purkinje related. In inherited long QT syndromes, Purkinje cell repolarization has been shown to be more sensitive to the genetically inherited ion channel mutations than ventricular myocytes, making them more likely to be the source of early and delayed afterdepolarization-induced ventricular arrhythmias.[21] Finally, in acquired heart failure, prolonged action potential duration within failing Purkinje cells (due to ion channel remodeling) has been well described and may result in early afterdepolarization-dependent focal VT.[22] Macroreentrant ventricular arrhythmias have also been attributed to the HPS (bundle branch reentry and fascicular reentry) in ischemic and nonischemic cardiomyopathies.[23] It may be that the CCS remnants are more prone to remodeling than the working myocardium, for example, with aging. In humans, remodeling with aging in the RA is most

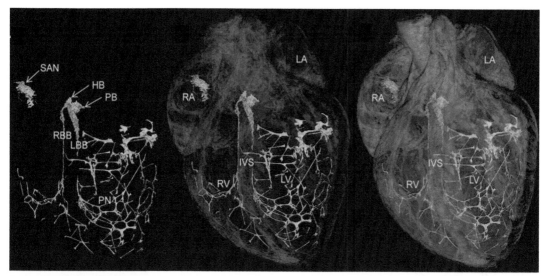

Fig. 6. Extent of the adult cardiac conduction system in the human. 3D reconstructed images of the mature rabbit cardiac conduction system (yellow) with decreasing levels of cardiac mass transparency imaged using iodine-based contrast-enhanced micro-computed tomography. Location of conduction tissues in adult heart consistent with presence of Tbx3-positive tissues in embryonic hearts. HB, his bundle; IVS, inter-ventricular septum; LA, left atrium; LBB, left bundle branch; PN, purkinje network; RA, right atrium; RBB, right bundle branch; RV, right ventricle; SAN, sinoatrial node; SVC, superior vena cava. (*From* Stephenson RS, Boyett MR, Hart G, et al. Contrast enhanced micro-computed tomography resolves the 3-dimensional morphology of the cardiac conduction system in mammalian hearts. *PloS One* 2012;7(4):e35299; with permission.)

pronounced near the crista terminalis, which is closely related to regions containing CCS-type tissue including the paranodal area and remnants of the sinoatrial ring bundle.[4,9,24] However, there is often no recognizable cause of cardiac remodeling that causes the arrhythmia.

Given this propensity toward arrhythmogenesis, it is unsurprising to note that cardiac conduction tissue is increasingly being recognized as responsible for many tachycardias arising from specific locations within the atria and ventricles.[25,26] With the advent of 3-dimensional clinical electro-anatomical mapping techniques, clinicians have been able to characterize in detail areas within the heart that are particularly susceptible arrhythmia (**Fig. 7**A, B).[27] **Table 2** summarizes arrhythmias associated with these arrhythmogenic regions of the heart, their embryonic origins, and their specific features.

The Crista Terminalis

The crista terminalis (CT) is a muscular ridge located in the RA that divides the musculi pectinati and the right atrial appendage from the smooth surface of the posterior RA. This region differs from the other regions of the RA and has molecular markers of CCS phenotype.[4] HNK1 studies and the presence of Tbx3 confirms the likely embryonic origin from the primitive sinus venosus.[25]

Histologic examination has revealed the presence of cells with an intermediate phenotype (in between nodal and working right atrial cells) with important nodal features, including small cells loosely packed in fatty tissue and reduced connexin expression.[9] Furthermore, this region has been shown to exhibit subsidiary atrial pacemaking, demonstrating spontaneous pacemaker activity.[4] These features may account for the fact that the CT is the most common site of origin for atrial tachycardia in adults; around 31% of all focal atrial tachycardias are known to arise from the CT.[28,29]

The Tricuspid and Mitral Annulus

Around 26% of focal atrial tachycardias arise from the tricuspid and mitral annuli, and the presence of CCS tissue at these locations explains this propensity to arrhythmia (see **Fig. 7**B).[28] CCS tissue extends not only to the AVN but also to the right and left atrioventricular rings surrounding the tricuspid and mitral valves, the retroaortic node, and the atrioventricular bundle (**Fig. 7**C).[1] These components of the adult CCS have been shown to arise from the primitive AVC.[12] The AVC retains a primitive nodal phenotype during embryologic development and this results in the development of the AVN. As the heart develops, however, the

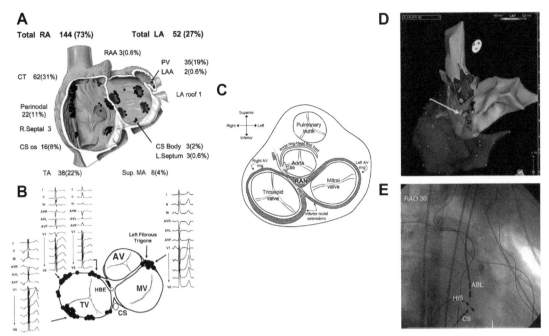

Fig. 7. Anatomic distribution of focal atrial tachycardias consistent with anatomic location of conduction tissues. (A) Schematic overview of the anatomic distribution of focal atrial tachycardias. CS, coronary sinus; CT, crista terminalis; LAA, left atrial appendage; PV, pulmonary vein; RAA, right atrial appendage. (B) Schematic overview of the distribution of focal atrial tachycardias at the atrioventricular valve annuli. AV, aortic valve; HBE, His bundle electrogram; MV, mitral valve; TV, tricuspid valve. (C) Schematic diagram demonstrating the presence of nodal-like tissue located in rings around the atrioventricular valve annuli based on the presence of HCN4 and absence of Cx43 on immunolabeling. AV, atrioventricular; LBB, left bundle branch; PB, penetrating bundle; RAN, retroaortic node. (D) Carto map from a case of focal atrial tachycardia with the point of earliest activation during tachycardia (*light blue dot*) deep within the noncoronary sinus, likely arising from the retroaortic node. (E) Fluoroscopy in RAO 30 in the same patient showing an ablation catheter at the noncoronary sinus through a retrograde aortic approach. Successful termination of the tachycardia was achieved in less than 6 seconds of ablation in this position. (*From [A, B]* Kistler PM, Roberts-Thomson KC, Haqqani HM, et al. P-wave morphology in focal atrial tachycardia: development of an algorithm to predict the anatomic site of origin. *Journal of the American College of Cardiology* 2006;48(5):1010–1017; with permission; and [C] Yanni J, Boyett MR, Anderson RH, et al. The extent of the specialized atrioventricular ring tissues. *Heart Rhythm* 2009;6:672–680; and [D, E] Beukema RJ, Smit JJ, Adiyaman A, et al. Ablation of focal atrial tachycardia from the noncoronary aortic cusp: case series and review of the literature. *Europace: European pacing, arrhythmias, and cardiac electrophysiology: journal of the working groups on cardiac pacing, arrhythmias, and cardiac cellular electrophysiology of the European Society of Cardiology.* 2015;17(6):953–961; with permission).

atrioventricular conduction axis begins to regress and becomes confined to the AVN. Markers of the embryologic conduction system (Tbx3 and minK-lacZ) begin to disappear, indicating apoptosis of the cells of the AVC.[30,31] However, there is evidence to suggest that remnants of the atrioventricular nodal phenotype continue to exist around the tricuspid and mitral valves in the mature adult heart as the atrioventricular ring bundles. This has been confirmed by molecular studies in the rat, mouse, and guinea pig, showing that rings of CCS tissue can be found around the atrioventricular valves expressing HCN4 channel and lacking Cx43.[16] Furthermore, it has been shown that these cells display nodal physiology with low resting membrane potentials, low action potential amplitudes, postrepolarization refractoriness, and Wenckebach-type responses to rapid atrial pacing. The response of these cells to adenosine is also nodal-like, exhibiting reduced action potential amplitude and dV/dt_{max} (maximum action potential upstroke velocity).[32]

An important component of the atrioventricular ring bundles is the retroaortic node, an area of CCS tissue at the junction between the right and left atrioventricular rings, superior to the compact AVN in the region of the right fibrous trigone (see **Fig. 5**). Again, it has been shown to exhibit nodal-like features with expression of HCN4 and absence of Cx43 expression.[16] It is an important area for pathogenesis of focal atrial tachycardias

Table 2
Anatomic locations of common focal arrhythmias and their relationship with the embryologic development of the CCS

Arrhythmia	Location	Embryologic Origin	Embryologic Markers of CCS	Nodal Similarities
Focal atrial tachycardia	Crista terminalis	Right horn of sinus venosus	HNK1 Tbx3 CCS-lacZ Cx43-negative	• Small cell diameter • Exhibit independent pacemaker activity • Similar ion channel and gap junction protein expression
	Interatrial groove (septum)	Left horn of sinus venosus	HNK1 Tbx3 CCS-lacZ Cx43-negative	HCN4 Cx45 Small nodal-like cells
	Coronary sinus ostium	Left horn of sinus venosus	HNK1 Tbx3 CCS-lacZ Cx43-negative	Not previously studied
	Tricuspid annulus	Atrioventricular canal	HNK1 Tbx3 CCS-lacZ Cx43-negative	• Small cell diameter • Nodal-type action potentials • Reduction of action potential amplitude with adenosine
	Superior mitral annulus	Atrioventricular canal	Tbx3 CCS-lacZ Cx43-negative	• Small cell diameter • Nodal-type action potentials • Reduction of action potential amplitude with adenosine
	Retroaortic node	Atrioventricular canal	HNK1 Tbx3	• HCN4 • Cx45
Atrial fibrillation	Pulmonary veins	Unknown	Transient HNK1 CCS-lacZ	• Clear cytoplasm, round mitochondria/few myofibrils • P cells/transitional cells/Purkinje cells
Normal heart tachycardia	Right ventricular outflow tract	Primitive outflow tract	minK-lacZ Cx45	• Cells embedded in connective tissue • Lack expression of Nav1.5, Cx43 and Kir2.1

The anatomic location of common focal arrhythmias and evidence for their association with the developing CCS and their nodal-like properties.

(**Fig. 7**D). Knowledge of the location of the retroaortic node explains the success of ablation of some focal atrial tachycardia from the noncoronary cusp by way of a retrograde aortic approach, even when the electrogram recorded at the mapping electrode is not early to the surface electrocardiogram p-wave (**Fig. 7**E).[33–35]

The Coronary Sinus Ostium

The ostium of the coronary sinus is another HNK1- and Tbx3-positive region within the RA.

HNK1 immunohistochemistry in human embryos at different ages reveals that conduction tissue exists in this region as a result of the incorporation of the primitive sinus venosus into the RA.[11] The presence of nodal tissue within this region again explains why it is one of the more common sites for focal atrial tachycardias.[28] Slow-conducting, coronary sinus musculature causes delayed activation at the coronary sinus and potentially facilitates reentrant tachyarrythmias.[36]

The Right Ventricular Outflow Tract

The RVOT represents another region of interest because of its common propensity to generate clinically significant ventricular arrhythmias.[1,17,18] The presence of nodal-like tissue within the RVOT may explain its arrhythmogenic nature. Although the developing RVOT does not express HNK1 or Tbx3, as described above, there is evidence that it arises from the primitive outflow tract (ie, primary myocardium) and therefore may retain a nodal phenotype.[17] In keeping with this, the RVOT expresses the CCS markers Cx45 and minK-lacZ.[31,37] The RVOT is also often the source of arrhythmia in the structurally abnormal heart. Conditions associated with macroscopic right ventricular disease such as arrhythmogenic right ventricular cardiomyopathy and tetralogy of Fallot often develop RVOT ventricular arrhythmias, perhaps because the embryonic origin of the RVOT is more susceptible to arrhythmogenic remodeling.

The Pulmonary Veins

There has been a great focus on the electrophysiological characteristics of the ostia of the pulmonary veins since the seminal findings of Haissaguerre and colleagues[38] that triggers for the initiation of atrial fibrillation arose from these regions. The pulmonary veins exhibit "sleeves" of myocardial tissue, and it is this tissue that is thought to be responsible for the activity initiating atrial fibrillation in 85% to 95% of paroxysmal atrial fibrillation patients. The independent pacemaker function of the pulmonary vein myocardium in rabbits and cats was first identified more than 100 years ago.[39] Subsequently, in rats, sinus node-like cells were thought to be present in these regions.[40] Despite these early discoveries, however, the precise mechanism and embryologic basis for pulmonary vein-driven atrial fibrillation has yet to be fully elucidated.

The issue of the embryologic origin of the pulmonary vein myocardium is currently unresolved. Although some evidence does exist to suggest that the pulmonary vein myocardium may originate from areas of the developing conduction system, such as the sinus venosus; this evidence is far from conclusive. For example, the expression of the marker CCS-lacZ in the pulmonary vein myocardium has led to the suggestion that these cells may originate from the developing sinus venosus and therefore exhibit nodal-like characteristics (in a similar fashion to the CT described above).[41] However, although CCS-lacZ is present within the AVN, the bundle branches, and the ventricular conduction system, it is also found in the atrial working myocardium and remains absent from the SAN.[41,42] CCS-lacZ cannot, therefore, be considered a pure marker of the embryologic CCS, and its presence within the pulmonary myocardium does not necessitate an embryologic origin from the primitive conduction system. Evidence also exists that the adult pulmonary vein sleeve myocardium does not contain nodal-like cells. For example, the cells of the pulmonary vein sleeves express Cx40 and Cx43, which are absent in CCS tissues. Furthermore, the pacemaker HCN4 channels have not been conclusively demonstrated in the pulmonary vein myocardium.[17]

SUMMARY

Many regions of the heart are particularly susceptible to arrhythmogenesis. The embryologic origins of these regions can often be traced to the CCS. Although much of the primitive CCS regresses as the embryo develops, remnants of the system remain, creating the normal adult CCS as well as additional areas of arrhythmic susceptibility. These nodal remnants have been identified through histologic, immunohistochemical, and molecular investigations of embryonic and adult hearts. Because of their embryologic origin, these regions may exhibit automaticity, afterdepolarization and slow conduction, creating the conditions for arrhythmia.

REFERENCES

1. Dobrzynski H, Anderson RH, Atkinson A, et al. Structure, function and clinical relevance of the cardiac conduction system, including the atrioventricular ring and outflow tract tissues. Pharmacol Ther 2013;139:260–88.
2. Monfredi O, Dobrzynski H, Mondal T, et al. The anatomy and physiology of the sinoatrial node–a contemporary review. Pacing Clin Electrophysiol 2010;33:1392–406.
3. Dobrzynski H, Nikolski VP, Sambelashvili AT, et al. Site of origin and molecular substrate of atrioventricular junctional rhythm in the rabbit heart. Circ Res 2003;93:1102–10.
4. Morris GM, D'Souza A, Dobrzynski H, et al. Characterization of a right atrial subsidiary pacemaker and acceleration of the pacing rate by HCN over-expression. Cardiovasc Res 2013;100:160–9.
5. Choudhury M, Boyett MR, Morris GM. Biology of the sinus node and its disease. Arrhythm Electrophysiol Rev 2015;4:28–34.
6. Bogdanov KY, Vinogradova TM, Lakatta EG. Sinoatrial nodal cell ryanodine receptor and Na^+-Ca^{2+} exchanger: molecular partners in pacemaker regulation. Circ Res 2001;88:1254–8.

7. Vinogradova TM, Bogdanov KY, Lakatta EG. beta-Adrenergic stimulation modulates ryanodine receptor Ca^{2+} release during diastolic depolarization to accelerate pacemaker activity in rabbit sinoatrial nodal cells. Circ Res 2002;90:73–9.

8. Boyett MR, Inada S, Yoo S, et al. Connexins in the sinoatrial and atrioventricular nodes. Adv Cardiol 2006;42:175–97.

9. Chandler NJ, Greener ID, Tellez JO, et al. Molecular architecture of the human sinus node: insights into the function of the cardiac pacemaker. Circulation 2009;119:1562–75.

10. van Weerd JH, Christoffels VM. The formation and function of the cardiac conduction system. Development 2016;143:197–210.

11. Blom NA, Gittenberger-de Groot AC, DeRuiter MC, et al. Development of the cardiac conduction tissue in human embryos using HNK-1 antigen expression: possible relevance for understanding of abnormal atrial automaticity. Circulation 1999;99:800–6.

12. Moorman AF, Christoffels VM. Cardiac chamber formation: development, genes, and evolution. Physiol Rev 2003;83:1223–67.

13. Kapoor N, Liang W, Marban E, et al. Direct conversion of quiescent cardiomyocytes to pacemaker cells by expression of Tbx18. Nat Biotechnol 2013; 31:54–62.

14. Choudhury M, Black N, Alghmdi A, et al. TBX18 overexpression enhances pacemaker function in a rat subsidiary atrial pacemaker model of sick sinus syndrome. J Physiol 2018;596(24):6141–55.

15. van Eif VWW, Devalla HD, Boink GJJ, et al. Transcriptional regulation of the cardiac conduction system. Nat Rev Cardiol 2018;15:617–30.

16. Yanni J, Boyett MR, Anderson RH, et al. The extent of the specialized atrioventricular ring tissues. Heart Rhythm 2009;6:672–80.

17. Christoffels VM, Moorman AF. Development of the cardiac conduction system: why are some regions of the heart more arrhythmogenic than others? Circ Arrhythm Electrophysiol 2009;2:195–207.

18. Boukens BJ, Christoffels VM, Coronel R, et al. Developmental basis for electrophysiological heterogeneity in the ventricular and outflow tract myocardium as a substrate for life-threatening ventricular arrhythmias. Circ Res 2009;104:19–31.

19. He BJ, Boyden P, Scheinman M. Ventricular arrhythmias involving the His-Purkinje system in the structurally abnormal heart. Pacing Clin Electrophysiol 2018;41:1051–9.

20. Willis BC, Pandit SV, Ponce-Balbuena D, et al. Constitutive intracellular Na+ excess in Purkinje cells promotes arrhythmogenesis at lower levels of stress than ventricular myocytes from mice with catecholaminergic polymorphic ventricular tachycardia. Circulation 2016;133:2348–59.

21. Iyer V, Roman-Campos D, Sampson KJ, et al. Purkinje cells as sources of arrhythmias in long QT syndrome type 3. Sci Rep 2015;5:13287.

22. Aiba T, Tomaselli G. Electrical remodeling in dyssynchrony and resynchronization. J Cardiovasc Transl Res 2012;5:170–9.

23. Lopera G, Stevenson WG, Soejima K, et al. Identification and ablation of three types of ventricular tachycardia involving the His-Purkinje system in patients with heart disease. J Cardiovasc Electrophysiol 2004;15:52–8.

24. Kistler PM, Sanders P, Fynn SP, et al. Electrophysiologic and electroanatomic changes in the human atrium associated with age. J Am Coll Cardiol 2004;44:109–16.

25. Jongbloed MR, Mahtab EA, Blom NA, et al. Development of the cardiac conduction system and the possible relation to predilection sites of arrhythmogenesis. ScientificWorldJournal 2008;8: 239–69.

26. Moorman A, Webb S, Brown NA, et al. Development of the heart: (1) formation of the cardiac chambers and arterial trunks. Heart 2003;89:806–14.

27. Lee G, Sanders P, Kalman JM. Catheter ablation of atrial arrhythmias: state of the art. Lancet 2012; 380:1509–19.

28. Kistler PM, Roberts-Thomson KC, Haqqani HM, et al. P-wave morphology in focal atrial tachycardia: development of an algorithm to predict the anatomic site of origin. J Am Coll Cardiol 2006;48:1010–7.

29. Morris GM, Segan L, Wong G, et al. Atrial tachycardia arising from the crista terminalis, detailed electrophysiological features and long-term ablation outcomes. JACC Clin Electrophysiol 2019;5: 448–58.

30. Hoogaars WM, Tessari A, Moorman AF, et al. The transcriptional repressor Tbx3 delineates the developing central conduction system of the heart. Cardiovasc Res 2004;62:489–99.

31. Kondo RP, Anderson RH, Kupershmidt S, et al. Development of the cardiac conduction system as delineated by minK-lacZ. J Cardiovasc Electrophysiol 2003;14:383–91.

32. McGuire MA, de Bakker JM, Vermeulen JT, et al. Atrioventricular junctional tissue. Discrepancy between histological and electrophysiological characteristics. Circulation 1996;94:571–7.

33. Das S, Neuzil P, Albert CM, et al. Catheter ablation of peri-AV nodal atrial tachycardia from the noncoronary cusp of the aortic valve. J Cardiovasc Electrophysiol 2008;19:231–7.

34. Ju W, Chen M, Yang B, et al. The role of noncoronary cusp ablation approach in the treatment of perinodal atrial tachycardias. Pacing Clin Electrophysiol 2012; 35:811–8.

35. Pap R, Makai A, Szilagyi J, et al. Should the aortic root be the preferred route for ablation of focal atrial tachycardia around the AV node?: support from intracardiac echocardiography. JACC Clin Electrophysiol 2016;2:193–9.

36. Katritsis D, Ioannidis JP, Giazitzoglou E, et al. Conduction delay within the coronary sinus in humans: implications for atrial arrhythmias. J Cardiovasc Electrophysiol 2002;13:859–62.

37. Coppen SR, Severs NJ, Gourdie RG. Connexin45 (alpha 6) expression delineates an extended conduction system in the embryonic and mature rodent heart. Dev Genet 1999;24:82–90.

38. Haissaguerre M, Jais P, Shah DC, et al. Spontaneous initiation of atrial fibrillation by ectopic beats originating in the pulmonary veins. N Engl J Med 1998;339:659–66.

39. Lauder T, Brunton JF. Note on independent pulsation of the pulmonary veins and vena cava. Proc Roy Soc Lond 1876–1877;25:174–6.

40. Masani F. Node-like cells in the myocardial layer of the pulmonary vein of rats: an ultrastructural study. J Anat 1986;145:133–42.

41. Jongbloed MR, Schalij MJ, Poelmann RE, et al. Embryonic conduction tissue: a spatial correlation with adult arrhythmogenic areas. J Cardiovasc Electrophysiol 2004;15:349–55.

42. Viswanathan S, Burch JB, Fishman GI, et al. Characterization of sinoatrial node in four conduction system marker mice. J Mol Cell Cardiol 2007;42:946–53.

Anatomic Considerations Relevant to Atrial and Ventricular Arrhythmias

John Nan, MD[a], Alan Sugrue, MB, BCh, BAO[a], Thomas P. Ladas, MD, PhD[a], Nandini Mehra, MD[b], Samuel J. Asirvatham, MD[a,c],*

KEYWORDS

- Anatomy • Cavotricuspid isthmus • Pulmonary vein ostium • Outflow tract • Endocardial structures
- Epicardial access

KEY POINTS

- Relevant anatomy for atrial flutter is based on the cavotricuspid isthmus. Variations in anatomy can include large subeustachian pouches, prominent eustachian ridges, and prominent pectinate muscles.
- Pulmonary vein isolation is a mainstay of atrial fibrillation ablation. Complications can arise from ablation of inappropriate locations. These complications include pulmonary vein fibrosis and myocardial thinning with aneurysmal dilatation.
- The anatomy of the outflow tracts and their orientation to each other and surrounding structures are important for localizing the arrhythmia, as well as avoiding inadvertent injury to nearby coronary arteries and conduction systems.
- Major endocavitary ventricular structures include papillary muscles, the moderator band, and false tendons. Ventricular arrhythmias can often originate from these structures, and mechanical complications can occur with catheter manipulation around them as well.
- The pericardial space is in close proximity to many important structures, including the diaphragm, phrenic nerves, coronary arteries, and autonomic ganglia.

INTRODUCTION

Anatomy is a central pillar in understanding and treating cardiac arrhythmias. Understanding of cardiac anatomy and function has undergone a remarkable evolution since the Egyptians first believed in the cardiocentric nature of the body circa 3500 BC. They identified the heart as the center of the vascular system, and believed that human intelligence resided in the heart.[1] Appreciation of cardiac anatomy in relation to both atrial and ventricular arrhythmias allows clinicians to gain deeper knowledge of pathophysiology and improve efficacy of treatment approaches, and enables cardiologists to anticipate and prevent potential complications. This article explores the anatomy and provides clinically important electrophysiology correlations relating to atrial flutter, atrial fibrillation, outflow tract ventricular tachycardia, and ventricular tachycardia arising from other endocardial structures, and also provides anatomic insight for epicardial access and mapping.

Disclosures: The authors have no relevant disclosures.
[a] Department of Cardiovascular Diseases, Division of Heart Rhythm Services, Mayo Clinic, 200 First Street Southwest, Rochester, MN 55905, USA; [b] Department of Internal Medicine, Mayo Clinic, 200 First Street Southwest, Rochester, MN 55905, USA; [c] Department of Pediatric and Adolescent Medicine, Division of Pediatric Cardiology, Mayo Clinic, 200 First Street Southwest, Rochester, MN 55905, USA
* Corresponding author. Department of Cardiovascular Diseases, Mayo Clinic, 200 First Street Southwest, Rochester, MN 55905.
E-mail address: Asirvatham.Samuel@mayo.edu

Card Electrophysiol Clin 11 (2019) 421–432
https://doi.org/10.1016/j.ccep.2019.04.003
1877-9182/19/© 2019 Elsevier Inc. All rights reserved.

ATRIAL FLUTTER
Introduction

Atrial flutter is the hallmark arrhythmia highlighting the important relationship and correlation between anatomy, arrhythmia, and treatment. Atrial flutter, or auricular flutter as it was initially called, was first produced by MacWilliam in 1887 by means of faradaic stimulation, and later described and named auricular flutter by Jolly and Ritchie in 1911 after they noticed rapid regular auricular contractions at 250 to 350 beats per minute associated with partial or complete heart block with a slower ventricular rate. Lewis[2] in 1913 proposed the mechanism of this arrhythmia to be intra-atrial macroreentry, but this was not universally accepted and resulted in almost 8 decades of heated assertions. It was the pivotal work by Klein and colleagues[3] that supported Lewis' original circuit movement theory, showing with atrial endocardial mapping the earliest activation of the flutter at the orifice of the coronary sinus (CS), which proceeded to the low atrial septum, high lateral right atrium, and low right atrium. Subsequently, electrical fulguration, or direct current ablation, was attempted by Chauvin and Brechenmacher[4] and Saoudi and colleagues,[6] but barotrauma concerns led to the successful application of radiofrequency energy.[4–6] Atrial flutter ablation is now considered a straightforward procedure that is generally safe.[7] However, some cases are difficult, and failure, although rare, continues to occur. Complications such as perforation, myocardial infarction, arterial damage, and inadvertent atrioventricular block are all possibilities. Understanding of key anatomic considerations can improve overall success and limit potential negative outcomes.

Anatomy

Right-sided atrial flutter

The key anatomy for atrial flutter is the cavotricuspid isthmus (CTI) (**Fig. 1**), which represents an area of viable myocardial tissue approximately 1.77 cm in length, coursing between inert anatomic obstacles, namely the orifice of the inferior vena cava posteriorly, and the attachment of the tricuspid valve anteriorly. Laterally, it is bound by the medial edge of the CS, and medially by the ostium of the CS, which is often also marked by a thebesian valve (62% of hearts in anatomic studies).[8] These myocardial fibers are oriented usually in a circumferential manner parallel to the tricuspid annulus.[9,10] The CTI is transected by the eustachian ridge, which divides the CTI into an anterior subeustachian and a posterior posteustachian isthmus. The prominence of the ridge varies and

it can be very well developed in some adult hearts. Variations of the CTI have been described, and the 2 most important to understand for electrophysiologists are the presence of a eustachian pouch, and pectinate muscles encroaching the isthmus.

A subeustachian pouch is defined as a depression in the eustachian isthmus of at least 3 mm below a plane formed by the tricuspid valve and the base of the eustachian ridge. It is present in approximately 16% of the population,[8] and generally lies in the medial two-thirds of the CTI.[9] Presence of a subeustachian pouch is strongly associated with the presence of a thebesian valve, and is less likely to occur in the presence of pectinate muscles that extend into the isthmus (25% vs 3%).[8]

Pectinate muscles fan out from the crista terminalis, or other muscle bundles on the CTI. In more than half of studied hearts, pectinate muscles cross medial to the crista terminalis and may encroach into the CTI for variable distances (0.59 ± 0.15 cm).[8] Occasionally, pectinate muscles are large and prominent on the isthmus, and may cross along the isthmus into the CS. When this occurs, the thebesian valve is either absent or vestigial.[9] In approximately one-fifth of hearts, pectinate muscles medial to the crista terminalis end in a discrete posterior atrial ridge, also referred to as a second crista terminalis.[8]

Left-sided atrial flutter

Of note, a left atrial analogous structure to the right atrial CTI is the left atrial isthmus, also known as the mitral isthmus. It is defined as the area of muscle between the orifice of the left inferior pulmonary veins (PVs) and the mitral annulus. The mean mitral isthmus length is 28.8 ± 7.0 mm, and it is smooth in 65% of hearts.[11] In addition, rather than a eustachian ridge, the left atrium (LA) contains several endocardial ridges, including interpulmonary ridges between the ipsilateral pulmonary venous orifices, as well as the posterolateral ridge between the os of the left atrial appendage and the left superior pulmonary venous orifice. Myocardial thickness of the isthmus also varies. At the level of the left inferior PV orifice, the thickness of the myocardium ranges from 1.4 to 7.7 mm. Midway along the mitral line and at the annulus the mean thickness is 2.8 mm (range, 1.2–4.4 mm) and 1.2 mm (range, 0–3.2 mm), respectively.[12,13] In cross-section analysis, this posterolateral ridge can be rounded in approximately 75% of hearts, flat in 15%, and pointed in 10% with potential implication for catheter instability when navigating in this area.[14,15]

Correlation for Electrophysiologists

Creation of a complete bidirectional conduction block across the CTI is the accepted ablation

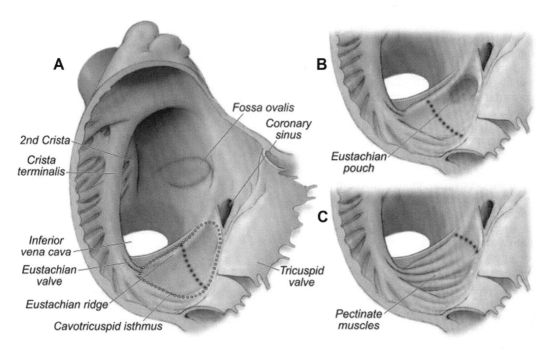

Fig. 1. Anatomy of cavotricuspid isthmus (*A, outlined in yellow*). Consider a more lateral ablation line in presence of a prominent eustachian pouch (*B, red line*), and a more medial ablation line with encroaching pectinate muscles (*C, red line*). (*Used with permission of* Mayo Foundation for Medical Education and Research, all rights reserved.)

end point for long-term success in treatment of typical atrial flutter. As mentioned, failure of flutter ablation can occur at times, because there is still continued conduction across the isthmus. Failure is often a consequence of anatomy, particularly the presence of the subeustachian pouch or pectinate muscles.

When a subeustachian pouch is present, the myocardium within it tends to be thinner, and a deep aneurysmlike recesses may form.[16] When prominent, this causes difficulty with ablation and results in lack of success. Even though the myocardium is not thick, because of poor blood flow within the pouch, power delivery is often suboptimal, with temperature and impedance variation. As a result, with poor power delivery, inadequate ablation, and gaps on the line, an incomplete bidirectional block is formed. One approach is using a larger electrode for more surface area; another is using irrigation with careful titration of energy delivery. The ablation can also be performed more laterally, because the pouch is generally found slightly to the right of the CS ostium and not in the lateral third of the CTI. Rarely, an encircling lesion around the pouch anchored to the tricuspid annulus and inferior vena cava can also be performed. In addition, catheter manipulation is more difficult within a large pouch, and, if not recognized, the electrode

will not make contact with the depth of the pouch as the catheter is drawn back in a straight line when assuming a planar CTI. The electrophysiologist can recognize the pouch preprocedurally from prior computed tomography (CT) scans, or intraprocedurally from unusual catheter tip movement, right atrial angiography, or intracardiac ultrasonography.[10,16]

Prominent pectinate muscles encroaching into the CTI may cause difficulty in creating an effective ablation lesion through the CTI. Not only is catheter stability sometimes an issue but the catheter may also become wedged between the pectinate muscles, causing inadequate power delivery with impedance increase and coagulum formation. The presence of prominent pectinate muscles may be recognized during ablation by large-amplitude atrial electrograms, characteristic catheter movement, or visualization with intracardiac ultrasonography. When this is recognized, the ablation line can be done more medially, because the pectinate muscles tend to be less prominent farther away from the crista terminalis. An irrigation catheter could also be used to enhance power delivery. However, an important consideration is that, if the ablation line is too septal, inadvertent atrioventricular node injury can occur.[10,16]

Similarly, a prominent eustachian ridge can cause difficulties in catheter manipulation and stability, because it can act as a fulcrum on which the catheter is balanced. This problem can be recognized with poor catheter contact and unexpected movement with catheter torque. In this scenario, usage of the appropriate sheath and placement of a more lateral ablation line is usually sufficient.[10,16]

It is important for electrophysiologists to recognize these anatomic variations, and modifications in ablation approach reduce instances of higher power delivery and alleviate the likelihood of direct injury to surrounding structures, including the coronary arteries (particularly the distal branches of the right coronary artery and the small cardiac veins, which lie external to the CTI), phrenic nerve, and atrioventricular node.

For left-sided mitral isthmus ablation, clinicians must be aware of surrounding epicardial structures, particularly the CS and left circumflex artery. A large CS can provide more cooling and result in inadequate ablation.[17] Furthermore, because the myocardial thickness varies, bidirectional block may be difficult to achieve, and incomplete ablation can be proarrhythmic.[14,18]

Take-home points

1. Variations in CTI anatomy can occur, including subeustachian pouches, prominent eustachian ridges, and prominent pectinate muscles. Once recognized, modifications in ablation approach should be considered:

   a. A more lateral approach for ablation in the presence of large pouches or a prominent eustachian ridge

   b. A more medial ablation for prominent pectinate muscles

   c. Irrigation with careful titration of power delivery can also be considered but can be associated with higher risk of injury to surrounding structures.

2. Left-sided isthmus ablation is affected by blood flow in the CS and can result in incomplete ablation

---

ATRIAL FIBRILLATION
Introduction

In contrast with atrial flutter, the understanding and treatment of atrial fibrillation (AF) remains largely an unconquered frontier, even since the seminal article by Haissaguerre and colleagues[19] provided the main anatomic construct on the importance of the PVs in the initiation of AF. Given

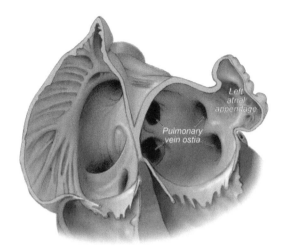

Fig. 2. The pulmonary vein ostia in the left atrium. The left atrial appendage is the only part of the left atrium with pectinate muscles. (*Used with permission of* Mayo Foundation for Medical Education and Research, all rights reserved.)

the key anatomic construct of the PVs, knowledge of these structures and their relationship to the left atrial anatomy is important for both safety and efficacy in intervention.

Anatomy

When viewed from the front aspect of the chest, the LA is the most posterior structure of the heart and has important differences from the right atrium. First, the LA is located posterior and superior to the right atrium. Second, the LA is largely a smooth surface, because embryologically the LA is derived from the primitive PV, with the primordial atrium forming the LA appendage, which is the only trabeculated part of the LA. Third, the myocardial architecture of the LA has distinct key differences compared with the right atrium.

There are usually 4 PVs, 2 on the left (superior and inferior) and 2 on the right (superior and inferior) connecting to the posterior aspect of the LA (**Fig. 2**). Anatomic variations in PVs are observed in approximately 40% of patients and include left common PV and right middle PV.[20] The left PVs are located higher than those on the right, with the inferior PV ostia more posterior and medial than the superior. Sleeves of atrial myocardium continuous with the LA wall surround the proximal portion of the PVs and this tends to be more extensive within the superior PVs compared with the inferior. The sleeves vary in thickness but are usually thickest at the proximal ends (1–1.5 mm), and gradually decrease and become irregular in the distal portions. Further, they can be replaced with fibrous tissue over time. The definition of the PV ostium is a key anatomic consideration, especially considering the catastrophic consequence of PV stenosis secondary to inadvertent ablation within the PV. There is no clear gold standard to anatomically define the PV ostium, either by imaging (CT/MRI) or histologic characteristics.[20] The transition in fiber orientation between atrial myocardium and the veins occurs gradually, without distinct anatomic landmarks or valves. Anecdotally, when different pathologists were asked to visually identify this area, wide variations were observed with up to 1.6 to 1.7 cm difference, highlighting the severe limitations of visual interpretation of this junction. As mentioned earlier, embryologically, the posterior wall of the LA is largely an extension of the PV.[20,21] As such, the best approach for defining the ostium becomes an electrical rather than visual method, which is further described later.

Myocardial thickness varies greatly within the LA, with a tendency toward paucity of myocardial fibers in the posterior and superior aspects, and thick myocardium in locations such as the mitral isthmus, the endocardial ridge separating the left atrial appendage and left pulmonary venous ostia, and the anterior atrial roof where the Bachmann bundle is located.[14,21,22] The Bachmann bundle is the primary site of interatrial conduction and is the largest of the subepicardial myocardial interatrial bundles that run circumferentially in the anterior wall. Most frequently, it is represented by parallel myocardial fibers that blend into the adjoining myocardium and play a role in propagation of sinus impulses to the LA. However, in some hearts it is very prominent. On the right side of the septum, the Bachmann bundle branches superiorly toward the sinus node and inferiorly toward the right atrial appendage. On the left side, it encircles the left atrial appendage neck. Smaller interatrial bundles are often seen alongside the Bachmann bundle, connecting the right and left atria, and occasionally there is another bundle more prominent than the Bachmann bundle.[10,23]

The CS is connected to the LA at its posteroinferior aspect. It is formed by the great cardiac vein and the vein of Marshall, and also receives left atrial as well as ventricular branches, including the posterolateral vein and the middle cardiac vein. The opening of the CS to the right atrium is demarcated by the thebesian valve. Muscle extension from pectinate muscles in the right atrium into the CS wall can be a substrate for conduction abnormalities, including focal atrial tachycardia, reentrant atrial tachycardia, and atypical atrial flutter.[22,24]

In addition, nervous tissues, which provide autonomic influences in AF, are also important anatomic elements to understand. In general, the role of autonomics in AF is not well understood but is thought to be an important entity because no AF had been observed in a denervated heart. Autonomic ganglia are located at several distinct atrial and ventricular regions. Ventricular ganglia seem to be primary located along the major coronary arteries, whereas most atrial ganglia are located near nodal tissue. The major atrial ganglia are located on the posterior surfaces of the atria and include the superior and posterior right atrial; the superior, posteromedial, and posterolateral left atrial; and the interatrial. The superior right atrial plexus is located adjacent to the junction of the superior vena cava and right atrium, and the posterior right atrial is located adjacent to the interatrial groove. The superior left plexus lies between the PVs, the posterolateral left near the atrioventricular groove, and the posteromedial left on the posterior medial surface of the LA. The interatrial plexus is a fusion of the posterior right and posteromedial left plexi, and extend anteriorly into the interatrial septum.[22,25]

Correlation for Electrophysiologists

The major element of AF ablation is isolation of the pulmonary vein ostium, because arrhythmogenic substrate seems to arise out of the depths of the PV. However, direct ablation of these areas often results in complications, including most notably pulmonary vein stenosis, and, if the ablation occurs too proximally to the ostium, thinning of myocardium and aneurysmal dilatation can result. Therefore, it is imperative that the appropriate transition area between the venous and atrial tissue be located. Preprocedural imaging from CT or MRI scans can help approximate this area, and, periprocedurally, intracardiac ultrasonography, rotational angiography, and retrograde pulmonary venography can all be helpful. Importantly, the characteristic electrogram findings include the PV potential, the presence of which suggests that the catheter is within the PV. Pacing via the ablation catheter with slow withdrawal of the catheter from the PV until the PV potentials are released can help guide the appropriate locations for ablation.[21,22]

Because of variations in myocardial wall thickness in the LA, perforation can occur, especially on the left atrial roof and posteriorly. In addition, because of the thinness of the myocardium at the posterior LA,[22] there is potential for serious esophageal trauma, including formation of esophageal fistulae. Monitoring esophageal temperature is often performed during ablation; however, because of the thickness of the anterior wall of the esophagus as well as the vascular supply, thermal injury can occur before significant increase in temperature is recorded. Monitoring of the oblique sinus, a posterior recess of the pericardial space separating the esophagus, has been used as well. Intracardiac echocardiogram is also helpful to visualize echo density or early effusions. It is critical to avoid overablation in this area. Downward deflection of the catheter and withdrawing the sheath while applying torque to go from one upper vein to the other is prudent. Ablation should only be performed at locations that show a contact near-field electrogram. In contrast, other locations, such as mitral isthmus, the Bachmann bundle region, and the endocardial ridge, may be challenging because of increased thickness of the myocardial fibers.[14,21,22]

The myocardium of the CS is sometimes targeted for ablation, and this can include ablation of the vein of Marshall and automatic foci from the CS itself, or to isolate the CS from either the LA or circumferentially to isolate it from the right atrium. Ablation within the CS carries increased risk of inadvertent injury to the coronary arteries, including the right coronary artery and the circumflex artery, and coronary angiography should be considered to assist with visualization.[21,22]

The role of targeting autonomic ganglia in the treatment of AF is not completely understood. However, studies have shown that direct stimulation of these ganglia may induce AF, and that ablation may abolish inducibility of AF during PV stimulation. This finding brings up a possible role of ganglion ablation as either a stand-alone procedure or in combination with pulmonary vein isolation in treatment of AF. Some major obstacles are still ongoing at this time. Determination of the location of specific ganglia could involve various maneuvers, including high-frequency electrical stimulation and complex fractionated electrograms. There is also complex crosstalk that may exist between ganglia, and it is unclear what extent of ablation would be required in specific patients, as well as potential increased complications with extensive ablation procedures.[22,25]

Take-home points

1. Pulmonary vein isolation is a mainstay of AF ablation. Complications can arise from ablation of inappropriate locations, including pulmonary vein fibrosis with distal ablation or myocardial thinning and aneurysmal dilatation with proximal ablation. Proper identification of the transition area between venous and atrial tissue can be determined from preprocedural and periprocedural imaging, characteristic electrograms, and specific maneuvers during ablation.

2. Due partially to variations in myocardial thickness within the LA, other serious complications involving surrounding structures, including most notably the esophagus and coronary arteries, may arise. Detailed understanding of the anatomy and intraprocedural monitoring with imaging, temperature, and electrograms can all be useful.

OUTFLOW TRACT VENTRICULAR TACHYCARDIA
Introduction

Ventricular tachycardia arising from the outflow tracts, and especially the right ventricular outflow tract, is one of the most common ventricular arrhythmias observed in a structurally normal heart. Outflow tract tachycardia is generally considered a benign arrhythmia but has been associated with malignant forms, including Brugada, or idiopathic ventricular fibrillation.

Anatomy

The outflow tracts are located at the base of the heart. The right ventricular outflow tract can be thought of as a muscular tube in a cross-section view, with the proximal right ventricular outflow tract beginning at the superior margin of the tricuspid annulus on the interventricular septum and ending at the pulmonary valve. It directs upward and leftward, with the mid and distal right ventricular outflow tract crossing the left ventricular outflow tract anteriorly. Therefore, contrary to its name, the right ventricular outflow tract is generally a left-sided structure (**Fig. 3**). For the most part, the posterior muscular wall of the right ventricular outflow tract is in continuation with the left ventricular outflow tract and aortic root. The pulmonic valve is located left and anterior (5–10 cm) to the aortic valve.[26]

The right sinus of Valsalva lies immediately posterior to the mid–right ventricular outflow tract. The anterior portion of the left sinus of Valsalva is also in close proximity to the subpulmonic right

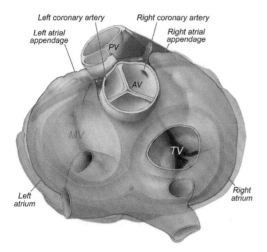

Left coronary artery Right coronary artery

Left atrial appendage

Right atrial appendage

PV

AV

MV

TV

Left atrium

Right atrium

Fig. 3. The outflow tracts. The distal right ventricular outflow tract is anterior and leftward of the left ventricular outflow tract. The ostia of the left main coronary artery and the right coronary artery are both in close proximity with the posterior wall of the right ventricular outflow tract. AV, aortic valve; MV, mitral valve; TV, tricuspid valve. (*Used with permission of Mayo Foundation for Medical Education and Research, all rights reserved.*)

ventricular outflow tract. The posterior lobe of the left atrial appendage sits on the left side of the left sinus of Valsalva.[26] It is common for myocardial tissue to extend above the semilunar valves. The myocardial extension within the aortic sinuses is usually asymmetric, and occurs most commonly at the right sinus of Valsalva and rarely at the non-CS of Valsalva. However, myocardial tissue usually is not present within the sinuses themselves. The myocardial extensions above the pulmonary valves are usually symmetric and more extensive.[27,28]

The cardiac conduction system is also in close proximity to the outflow tracts. The His bundle is identified by its encasement in the central fibrous body and location within the membranous atrioventricular septum, transitioning between the atrioventricular node and the bundle branches. The right bundle runs superficially in the right ventricular endocardium up to the level of the septal papillary muscle of the tricuspid valve, where it courses deeper in the interventricular septum before becoming superficial again to course within the ventricular trabeculations, usually traveling to the free wall in the moderator band. The left bundle emerges beneath the noncoronary cusp of the aortic valve and divides into the anterior, posterior, and often medial fascicles. The anterior fascicle crosses the left ventricular outflow tract to the region of the anterolateral papillary muscle, the posterior fascicle inserts near the base of the posterior

papillary muscle, and the median fascicle runs in the interventricular septum.[29]

Correlation for Electrophysiologists

There are 3 important correlations for electrophysiologists when it comes to outflow tract ablation: the myocardium that extends above the valves, the location of the coronary arteries, and the proximity of the conduction system. When ablating in the supravalvular portion of the left ventricular outflow tract, clinicians must be cognizant of avoiding cannulation of the ostia of the coronary arteries. However, the right coronary artery is also in close proximity to the proximal portion of the right ventricular outflow tract. In addition, the left main coronary artery is closer to the right ventricular outflow tract, and susceptible to thermal injury when ablating there. In anatomic studies, the closest myocardial sleeve to the left main coronary artery was found above the pulmonary valve rather than above the aortic valve (4.8 ± 1.7 mm vs 6.3 ± 3.3 mm).[28] Coronary angiography or the use of intracardiac ultrasonography can help decrease the likelihood of this complication. Interpretation of electrograms is also useful in this, because significant far-field atrial electrograms seen when mapping close to the pulmonary valve posteriorly may originate from the neighboring left atrial appendage, the edge of which is often near the ostium of the left anterior descending artery.[27,28]

The penetrating portion of the His bundle consistently runs in the membranous portion of the interventricular septum, which may be injured when ablating anteriorly and to the right in the noncoronary cusp region, posteriorly in the right coronary cusp region, or in the proximal portion of the right ventricular outflow tract. Appropriateness of ablation procedures should be reconsidered in these areas because complete heart block may develop with injury of the conduction system.[27,29]

Take-home points:

1. In ablating outflow tract tachycardia, it is important to recognize potential arrhythmogenic foci from above the semilunar valves

2. The anatomy of the outflow tracts and their orientation to each other and surrounding structures are important for localizing the course of the arrhythmia, as well as in avoiding inadvertent injury to nearby coronary arteries and conduction systems.

ENDOCAVITARY VENTRICULAR TACHYCARDIA

Introduction

A significant proportion of patients undergoing ventricular tachycardia ablation require specific ablation of an endocavitary structure to eliminate the tachycardia. The key endocavitary structures that need to be understood are the papillary muscles, moderator band, and false tendons (**Fig. 4**).

Anatomy

There are typically 2 papillary muscles located within the left ventricle: the anterolateral and posteromedial papillary muscles. There are 3 papillary muscles in the right ventricle: the anterior, posterior, and septal papillary muscles. The papillary muscles are connected to the atrioventricular valves via chordae tendineae. There is significant structural variation between the papillary muscles of the left ventricle and the papillary muscles of the right ventricle. In general, the right ventricular papillary muscles are less prominent and less organized. One of the septal papillary muscles often arises from the right ventricular outflow tract and is referred to as the conus papillary muscle.[30]

Another important endocavitary structure is the moderator band, which was originally described as the catena of the right ventricle by Leonardo da Vinci. It extends from the interventricular septal wall to the base of the anterior papillary muscle in the right ventricle and travels to the right ventricular free wall, containing a large portion of the distal right bundle.[31] Although most right ventricles contain a moderator band, it can vary in size, thickness, and location on the ventricular septum (mean thickness, 4.5 ± 1.8 mm; mean length, 16.2 ± 2.3 mm, ranging from 11.3 to 24.3 mm in anatomic studies).[32]

Within many left ventricles and some right ventricles, certain fibrous or fibromuscular bands can exist, extending from the septum to papillary muscles, and sometimes to the free wall, but never to the valves. These bands are called false tendons, and can contain Purkinje tissue. False tendons arise from the inner trabeculated myocardial layer, but, unlike trabeculations, these chordlike structures traverse the left ventricular cavity. They are found in approximately half of hearts examined at autopsy, and range up to 3 mm in thickness.[33,34]

Correlation for Electrophysiologists

Endocavitary ventricular tachycardia ablation is an important approach in the control of ventricular arrhythmias. Understanding of the endocavitary structural anatomy is important in avoiding the frequent difficulty seen with both interpretation of mapping data as well as catheter manipulation.

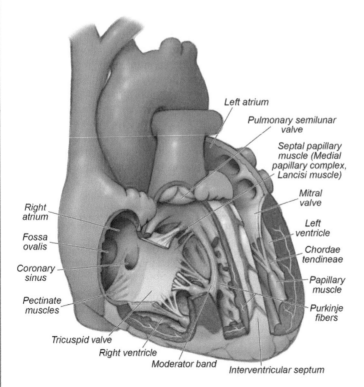

Fig. 4. Endocavitary structures, including the papillary muscles and moderator band. The conus papillary muscle (also known as septal papillary muscle, or Lancisi muscle) originates in the right ventricular outflow tract. (*Used with permission of* Mayo Foundation for Medical Education and Research, all rights reserved.)

Left atrium

Pulmonary semilunar valve

Septal papillary muscle (Medial papillary complex, Lancisi muscle)

Mitral valve

Left ventricle

Chordae tendineae

Papillary muscle

Purkinje fibers

Right atrium

Fossa ovalis

Coronary sinus

Pectinate muscles

Tricuspid valve

Right ventricle

Moderator band

Interventricular septum

Origin of arrhythmia from an endocavitary structure such as papillary muscles, moderator band, or false tendons should be suspected if no specific early site is noted. Fascicular tachycardia has also been often mapped to the vicinity of the papillary muscles. When ablating ventricular tachycardia originating from an endocavitary structure, it must be recognized that a single focus may have variable morphology because of variable exits, and the primary focus needs to be ablated or isolated rather than exit sites. In addition, catheter manipulation can be significantly hindered by the structures mechanically, and attention should be paid to the appearance and movement of the catheter on fluoroscopy, and intracardiac echocardiography can be considered.[30,31]

The conus papillary muscle, also known as Lancisi muscle or bundle, is present in 82% of human hearts, and is found adjacent to the distal bundle of His as it penetrates the membranous septum.[31] Anterolaterally, discrete trabeculations without attached chordae may be found. The conus papillary muscle may represent the origin site for ventricular arrhythmia, and can cause difficulty with ablation of right ventricular outflow tract arrhythmia as well. Simultaneous early activation sites at more than 1 location in the proximal outflow tract, varying QRS morphologies with similar coupling intervals, and Purkinje-like signals preceding ventricular activation are all clues for this cause, and use of intracardiac echocardiography can be considered to confirm location.[31]

Take-home points:

1. Major endocavitary ventricular structures include papillary muscles, the moderator band, and false tendons. Although certain patterns exist, the size, location, and presence of these structures are variable.

2. Ventricular arrhythmias can often originate from endocavitary structures, and recognition is important because exit block ablation is unlikely to be successful.

3. Mechanical hindrances and complications can occur with catheter manipulation around endocavitary structures. Awareness of this and use of imaging modalities such as fluoroscopy and intracardiac echocardiography can be useful.

EPICARDIAL ACCESS AND MAPPING
Introduction

Epicardial access, mapping, and ablation have become important components of electrophysiologists' armamentarium for ventricular arrhythmia ablation, particularly in the setting of nonischemic and ischemic cardiomyopathy, as well as arrhythmogenic cardiomyopathy.[35,36] Furthermore, some nonablation procedures, such as left atrial appendage ligation and subxiphoid pacemaker lead implantation, also require access into the epicardial space. Anatomic understanding of the regional anatomy of the epicardial space is critical to enable fluoroscopic correlation and limit potential complications.

Anatomy

Epicardial interventional procedures require access into the pericardial space (**Fig. 5**), which is defined as the potential space between the parietal and visceral layers of the serous pericardium, which is continuous with the epicardium and wraps around the roots of the great vessels to the visceral surface of the fibrous pericardium. Superiorly, the fibrous pericardium is continuous with the adventitia of the great vessels; inferiorly, it is attached to the central tendon of the diaphragm. Anteriorly, it is attached to the posterior surface of the sternum by sternopericardial ligaments, and posteriorly it approximates the bronchi, esophagus, descending thoracic aorta, and mediastinal surface of the lungs.[37]

Within the thorax, the phrenic nerves pass in front of the hilum of the lung between fibrous pericardium and the mediastinal pleura. The right phrenic nerve travels along the right anterolateral surface of the superior vena cava and descends in front of the right PVs in the lung hilum before reaching the diaphragm. The left phrenic nerve descends behind the brachiocephalic vein and may be separated from the pericardium by a layer of adipose tissue as it passes over the aortic arch, pulmonary trunk, and the pericardial wall over the left atrial appendage. It may also take a lateral or posterior course and overlie the left atrial appendage, specifically the tip (59%) or neck of the appendage (23%).[38–41]

Another important epicardial structure is the epicardial fat that is found around specific anatomic sites, which is fairly consistent among patients. These areas include the free wall of the right ventricle, left ventricular apex, atrial appendages, the grooves containing the coronary arteries, and autonomic ganglia.[38] The amount of epicardial fat is increased in patients with coronary artery disease and is positively correlated with the severity of cardiomyopathy.[42,43]

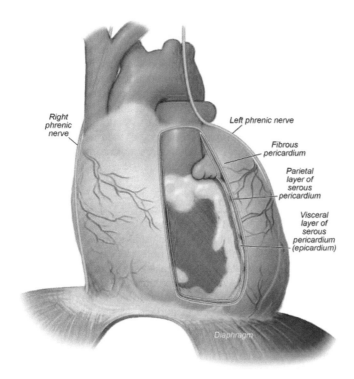

Right phrenic nerve

Left phrenic nerve

Fibrous pericardium

Parietal layer of serous pericardium

Visceral layer of serous pericardium (epicardium)

Diaphragm

Fig. 5. The pericardial space is defined as the space between the parietal and visceral layers of the serous pericardium. The phrenic nerves and diaphragm are in close proximity with this space. (*Used with permission of Mayo Foundation for Medical Education and Research, all rights reserved.*)

Correlation for Electrophysiologists

The pericardial space is accessed through a subxiphoid approach, during which the needle crosses the skin, subcutaneous tissue, and diaphragm before approaching the cardiac border, where a small amount of contrast is used as the needle enters the potential pericardial space. During this time, there is potential damage to surrounding structures, which include the myocardium, great vessels, coronary arteries, lungs, esophagus, and phrenic nerves.[37]

Although the phrenic nerves are not true intrapericardial structures, they are in close proximity to the parietal pericardium and can be damaged with epicardial ablation. There is potential for thermal injury to the right phrenic nerve when ablating at or near the right atrium, superior vena cava, or right superior PV. The left phrenic nerve may also be damaged when ablating near the ascending aorta, pulmonary trunk, or left atrial appendage. Specifically, ablating at the great cardiac vein for epicardial outflow tract tachycardia often involves energy delivery near the vicinity of the left phrenic nerve. The phrenic nerves can be identified and mapped by specific pacing maneuvers to stimulate the phrenic nerve and diaphragm. However, this requires multiple respiratory cycles because deep respiration and movement can cause absence of phrenic nerve stimulation signals. In addition, phrenic nerve stimulation cannot be recognized in patients under general anesthesia who are given skeletal muscle paralytic agents.[39,40]

Injuries to the coronary arteries during ablation are also a major concern, especially when ablating at the base of the heart. During the procedure, the mitral annulus can be outlined by a CS catheter, and the tricuspid annulus can be identified by an endoluminal right ventricular catheter. The septum is defined by the His catheter. These fluoroscopic anatomic correlations can help guide the location of the coronary arteries. Further uncertainty should prompt coronary angiography for confirmation.[38]

During epicardial mapping and ablation, the location of epicardial fat must be taken into account, because the low amplitude and fragmented electrograms that can be associated with epicardial fat may obscure interpretation of these signals that would otherwise suggest scar. Therefore, low-amplitude signals obtained near the atrioventricular grooves, as well as anterior and posterior intraventricular grooves, must be interpreted with caution, especially because coronary vessels and autonomic ganglia are frequently distributed throughout epicardial fat.[37,38]

Take-home points

1. The pericardial space is in close proximity to many important structures, including diaphragm, phrenic nerves, coronary arteries, and autonomic ganglia.

2. The right phrenic nerve travels close to the superior vena cava and right superior pulmonary vein, whereas the left phrenic nerve can overlie the LA appendage.

3. Consideration of ganglia and epicardial fat is important, especially when mapping and observing areas of low voltage.

SUMMARY

Knowledge and appreciation of intricacies in anatomy are integral in the approach and treatment of patients with atrial and ventricular arrhythmias. This article highlights and discusses key anatomic principles and take-home points, which it is hoped will provide essential understanding of regional anatomy. Application of this knowledge can enable maximal ablative efficacy and reduce complication risk.

ACKNOWLEDGMENTS

The authors thank David Factor for the medical illustrations.

REFERENCES

1. Loukas M, Youssef P, Gielecki J, et al. History of cardiac anatomy: a comprehensive review from the Egyptians to today. Clin Anat 2016;29(3):270–84.

2. Lewis T. Observations upon a curious and not uncommon form of extreme acceleration of the auricle. "Auricular flutter". Heart 1913;4(171):1912–3.

3. Klein GJ, Guiraudon GM, Sharma AD, et al. Demonstration of macroreentry and feasibility of operative therapy in the common type of atrial flutter. Am J Cardiol 1986;57(8):587–91.

4. Chauvin M, Brechenmacher C. A clinical study of the application of endocardial fulguration in the treatment of recurrent atrial flutter. Pacing Clin Electrophysiol 1989;12(1 Pt 2):219–24.

5. Cosio FG, Lopez-Gil M, Goicolea A, et al. Radiofrequency ablation of the inferior vena cava-tricuspid valve isthmus in common atrial flutter. Am J Cardiol 1993;71(8):705–9.

6. Saoudi N, Atallah G, Kirkorian G, et al. Catheter ablation of the atrial myocardium in human type I atrial flutter. Circulation 1990;81(3):762–71.

7. Patel NJ, Deshmukh A, Pau D, et al. Contemporary utilization and safety outcomes of catheter ablation of atrial flutter in the United States: analysis of 89,638 procedures. Heart Rhythm 2016;13(6): 1317–25.

8. Gami AS, Edwards WD, Lachman N, et al. Electrophysiological anatomy of typical atrial flutter: the posterior boundary and causes for difficulty with ablation. J Cardiovasc Electrophysiol 2010;21(2): 144–9.

9. Asirvatham SJ. Correlative anatomy and electrophysiology for the interventional electrophysiologist: right atrial flutter. J Cardiovasc Electrophysiol 2009; 20(1):113–22.

10. Ho SY, Anderson RH, Sanchez-Quintana D. Atrial structure and fibres: morphologic bases of atrial conduction. Cardiovasc Res 2002;54(2):325–36.

11. Holda MK, Koziej M, Holda J, et al. Anatomic characteristics of the mitral isthmus region: the left atrial appendage isthmus as a possible ablation target. Ann Anat 2017;210:103–11.

12. Pathik B, Choudry S, Whang W, et al. Mitral isthmus ablation: a hierarchical approach guided by electroanatomic correlation. Heart Rhythm 2018;16(4): 632–7.

13. Becker AE. Left atrial isthmus: anatomic aspects relevant for linear catheter ablation procedures in humans. J Cardiovasc Electrophysiol 2004;15(7): 809–12.

14. Ho SY, McCarthy KP. Anatomy of the left atrium for interventional electrophysiologists. Pacing Clin Electrophysiol 2010;33(5):620–7.

15. Ho SY, McCarthy KP, Faletra FF. Anatomy of the left atrium for interventional echocardiography. Eur J Echocardiogr 2011;12(10):i11–5.

16. Cabrera JA, Sanchez-Quintana D, Farre J, et al. The inferior right atrial isthmus: further architectural insights for current and coming ablation technologies. J Cardiovasc Electrophysiol 2005;16(4):402–8.

17. D'Avila A, Thiagalingam A, Foley L, et al. Temporary occlusion of the great cardiac vein and coronary sinus to facilitate radiofrequency catheter ablation of the mitral isthmus. J Cardiovasc Electrophysiol 2008;19(6):645–50.

18. Matsuo S, Wright M, Knecht S, et al. Peri-mitral atrial flutter in patients with atrial fibrillation ablation. Heart Rhythm 2010;7(1):2–8.

19. Haissaguerre M, Jais P, Shah DC, et al. Spontaneous initiation of atrial fibrillation by ectopic beats originating in the pulmonary veins. N Engl J Med 1998;339(10):659–66.

20. DeSimone CV, Noheria A, Lachman N, et al. Myocardium of the superior vena cava, coronary sinus, vein of Marshall, and the pulmonary vein ostia: gross anatomic studies in 620 hearts. J Cardiovasc Electrophysiol 2012;23(12):1304–9.

21. Macedo PG, Kapa S, Mears JA, et al. Correlative anatomy for the electrophysiologist: ablation for atrial fibrillation. Part I: pulmonary vein ostia,

superior vena cava, vein of Marshall. J Cardiovasc Electrophysiol 2010;21(6):721–30.

22. Macedo PG, Kapa S, Mears JA, et al. Correlative anatomy for the electrophysiologist: ablation for atrial fibrillation. Part II: regional anatomy of the atria and relevance to damage of adjacent structures during AF ablation. J Cardiovasc Electrophysiol 2010; 21(7):829–36.

23. Ho SY, Sanchez-Quintana D. The importance of atrial structure and fibers. Clin Anat 2009;22(1):52–63.

24. Noheria A, DeSimone CV, Lachman N, et al. Anatomy of the coronary sinus and epicardial coronary venous system in 620 hearts: an electrophysiology perspective. J Cardiovasc Electrophysiol 2013; 24(1):1–6.

25. Kapa S, Venkatachalam KL, Asirvatham SJ. The autonomic nervous system in cardiac electrophysiology: an elegant interaction and emerging concepts. Cardiol Rev 2010;18(6):275–84.

26. Hai JJ, Lachman N, Syed FF, et al. The anatomic basis for ventricular arrhythmia in the normal heart: what the student of anatomy needs to know. Clin Anat 2014;27(6):885–93.

27. Sehar N, Mears J, Bisco S, et al. Anatomic guidance for ablation: atrial flutter, fibrillation, and outflow tract ventricular tachycardia. Indian Pacing Electrophysiol J 2010;10(8):339–56.

28. Gami AS, Noheria A, Lachman N, et al. Anatomical correlates relevant to ablation above the semilunar valves for the cardiac electrophysiologist: a study of 603 hearts. J Interv Card Electrophysiol 2011;30(1):5–15.

29. Syed FF, Hai JJ, Lachman N, et al. The infrahisian conduction system and endocavitary cardiac structures: relevance for the invasive electrophysiologist. J Interv Card Electrophysiol 2014;39(1):45–56.

30. Abouezzeddine O, Suleiman M, Buescher T, et al. Relevance of endocavitary structures in ablation procedures for ventricular tachycardia. J Cardiovasc Electrophysiol 2010;21(3):245–54.

31. Hai JJ, Desimone CV, Vaidya VR, et al. Endocavitary structures in the outflow tract: anatomy and electrophysiology of the conus papillary muscles. J Cardiovasc Electrophysiol 2014;25(1):94–8.

32. Loukas M, Klaassen Z, Tubbs RS, et al. Anatomical observations of the moderator band. Clin Anat 2010;23(4):443–50.

33. Silbiger JJ. Left ventricular false tendons: anatomic, echocardiographic, and pathophysiologic insights. J Am Soc Echocardiogr 2013;26(6):582–8.

34. Luetmer PH, Edwards WD, Seward JB, et al. Incidence and distribution of left ventricular false tendons: an autopsy study of 483 normal human hearts. J Am Coll Cardiol 1986;8(1):179–83.

35. Maccabelli G, Mizuno H, Della Bella P. Epicardial ablation for ventricular tachycardia. Indian Pacing Electrophysiol J 2012;12(6):250–68.

36. Della Bella P, Brugada J, Zeppenfeld K, et al. Epicardial ablation for ventricular tachycardia: a European multicenter study. Circ Arrhythm Electrophysiol 2011;4(5):653–9.

37. Lachman N, Syed FF, Habib A, et al. Correlative anatomy for the electrophysiologist, part I: the pericardial space, oblique sinus, transverse sinus. J Cardiovasc Electrophysiol 2010;21(12):1421–6.

38. Lachman N, Syed FF, Habib A, et al. Correlative anatomy for the electrophysiologist, part II: cardiac ganglia, phrenic nerve, coronary venous system. J Cardiovasc Electrophysiol 2011;22(1):104–10.

39. Dib C, Kapa S, Powell BD, et al. Successful use of "cryo-mapping" to avoid phrenic nerve damage during ostial superior vena caval ablation despite nerve proximity. J Interv Card Electrophysiol 2008;22(1): 23–30.

40. Mears JA, Lachman N, Christensen K, et al. The phrenic nerve and atrial fibrillation ablation procedures. J Atr Fibrillation 2009;2(1):176.

41. Sanchez-Quintana D, Cabrera JA, Climent V, et al. How close are the phrenic nerves to cardiac structures? Implications for cardiac interventionalists. J Cardiovasc Electrophysiol 2005;16(3):309–13.

42. Silaghi A, Piercecchi-Marti MD, Grino M, et al. Epicardial adipose tissue extent: relationship with age, body fat distribution, and coronaropathy. Obesity (Silver Spring) 2008;16(11):2424–30.

43. Ahn SG, Lim HS, Joe DY, et al. Relationship of epicardial adipose tissue by echocardiography to coronary artery disease. Heart 2008;94(3):e7.

Fundamentals of Cardiac Mapping

Thomas P. Ladas, MD, PhD[a], Alan Sugrue, MB, BCh, BAO[a], John Nan, MD[a],
Vaibhav R. Vaidya, MBBS[a], Deepak Padmanabhan, MBBS[a], K.L. Venkatachalam, MD[b],
Samuel J. Asirvatham, MD[a,c,d],*

KEYWORDS

- Electroanatomic mapping • Electrogram • Signals • Filter • Arrhythmia • Activation mapping
- Substrate mapping • Mapping systems

KEY POINTS

- Characterization and subsequent ablation of arrhythmias requires an accurate cardiac electroanatomic mapping (EAM).
- The recorded cardiac biopotential (the electrogram, EGM) can be acquired as unipolar or bipolar voltages, each having different advantages and disadvantages.
- Activation mapping involves constructing a map of the activation times of a propagating wavefront at a given myocardial location about a fiducial point. For reentrant arrhythmias, first, the circuit is mapped, and second, the propagation wavefront is mapped relative to an arbitrary reference to find a sequence of activation that mirrors the tachycardia cycle length. Complex mapping maneuvers (eg, entrainment) aid in activation mapping.
- Substrate mapping is used for arrhythmias that lack stability, a clear focus, or anatomic circuit, or are hemodynamically unstable rendering mapping in arrhythmia challenging. It is based on signal amplitudes and characteristic EGM morphologies.
- Modern EAM systems allow the 3-dimensional reconstruction of cardiac anatomy and anatomic localization of catheters with minimal use of fluoroscopy.

WHAT IS CARDIAC MAPPING?

Cardiac mapping is the process of recording the electrical activity of the heart in order to create a dynamic electroanatomic picture of that activity. A map can be based on surface electrocardiogram (ECG) electrodes and epicardial or endocardial electrodes (on a catheter) to quantify the cardiac biopotential. Cardiac maps can be used to characterize the activity of normal and abnormal cardiac rhythms with sufficient spatiotemporal resolution to allow accurate diagnosis, planning, and intervention of various heart rhythm disorders.

WHAT IS NECESSARY FOR A SUCCESSFUL ELECTROANATOMIC CARDIAC MAP?

Consider the case of a simple arrhythmia, such as an automatic atrial tachycardia. The surface ECG can provide clues to the location of the tachycardia exit site, but one will not be able to determine the precise anatomic position of the origin of abnormal activity. Catheter-based intracardiac electrodes can also be used to record local myocardial activity during the arrhythmia. This signal plotted over time is the electrogram (EGM). By manipulating the catheter to different

Disclosure Statement: S.J. Asirvatham: Consultant to Aegis, ATP, Nevro, Sanovas, Sorin Medical, and FocusStart. K.L. Venkatachalam: Consultant to BioSig Technologies.
[a] Department of Cardiovascular Medicine, Division of Heart Rhythm Services, Mayo Clinic, Rochester, MN, USA;
[b] Department of Cardiovascular Medicine, Division of Heart Rhythm Services, Mayo Clinic, Jacksonville, Florida, USA; [c] Department of Pediatric and Adolescent Medicine, Division of Pediatric Cardiology, Mayo Clinic, Rochester, MN, USA; [d] Physiology and Biomedical Engineering, Mayo Clinic, Rochester, MN, USA
* Corresponding author. Mayo Clinic, 200 First Street Southwest, Rochester, MN 55905.
E-mail address: asirvatham.samuel@mayo.edu

Card Electrophysiol Clin 11 (2019) 433–448
https://doi.org/10.1016/j.ccep.2019.05.005
1877-9182/19/© 2019 Elsevier Inc. All rights reserved.

areas of the myocardium under fluoroscopic guidance, an "activation map" of the arrhythmia can be constructed and ultimately the area of abnormal cardiomyocyte activation can be honed in on, which provides a target site to deliver energy for ablation.

One can describe the location of this arrhythmia by constructing an activation map, and to do this, first needed is to establish a stable reference EGM by which local activation times (LATs) measured throughout the myocardium can be compared. This timing reference can be from a surface ECG lead or an intracardiac electrode. Next, a well-annotated EGM is needed that correctly identifies the LAT at each "point" that is taken. An EAM map is then constructed by tracking the catheter position in space over multiple such points using electrical impedance or electromagnetic fields, while storing the LAT at each catheter position. This can then be represented in a color-coded manner with the variance in color representing the variance in LAT relative to the reference point. Before this technology was available, catheter position and LAT were associated using fluoroscopy, and areas that required ablation were determined primarily by operator recall. In addition, regardless of how the map is constructed, another critical requirement for activation mapping is a stable tachycardia that has a stable cycle length. If the tachycardia cycle length or morphology changes frequently or if the arrhythmia causes hemodynamic instability, then activation mapping may not be possible. In these cases, substrate mapping may be used, whereby the endocardium can be quickly mapped in terms of the local myocardial voltage during a stable largely unidirectional wavefront. Areas of low amplitude and signal fractionation can be identified and associated with the catheter location at that site, thereby creating a voltage map. Although one may not specifically identify the abnormal electrical circuits responsible for the arrhythmia, areas of low amplitude and abnormal signals are targeted for ablation under the assumption that they may be arrhythmogenic. In such cases, it is critical to ensure that there are no inducible arrhythmias at the end of the case because this strategy by itself may also be arrhythmogenic.

If the arrhythmia is a reentrant tachycardia rather than a focal tachycardia, mapping is more difficult because there is no single site of "early" activation. One must instead use more complex maneuvers, such as entrainment mapping, whereby the response of a reentrant circuit is analyzed to overdrive pacing. However, regardless of the type of arrhythmia or the approach used to obtain the EAM, it is important to recognize that the humble intracardiac EGM forms the basis of all mapping, from the simplest to the most sophisticated technologies.

THE ELECTROGRAM

The intracardiac EGM is a critical biopotential that is fundamental to the diagnosis, mapping, and treatment of cardiac arrhythmias and represents the summed cellular biopotential from individual cardiomyocytes. This signal can be several orders of magnitude smaller than the transmembrane potential, ranging from as low as 25 μV in regions of infarcted myocardium, 1 to 6 mV for atrial EGMs, and 3 to 30 mV for ventricular EGMs.[1,2] EGMs can be recorded as either unipolar or bipolar signals, and in this section, the authors review the differences between these recording configurations and how to configure the electrophysiology (EP) laboratory setup to ensure optimal EGM signals.

Unipolar Intracardiac Recordings

In a unipolar recording, only 1 electrode, called the "exploring" electrode, actively records the EGM. However, because 2 electrodes are always required to make an EGM, a second electrode, called a "zero reference," "indifferent," or "ground" electrode, is also necessary and is assumed to be placed at a location infinitely far away from the exploring electrode. Different options exist for the choice of this indifferent reference, including using the Wilson Central Terminal[3] or an electrode on an inferior vena cava catheter. A depolarization wavefront that approaches a unipolar electrode, from any direction, will cause a positive deflection while moving toward the electrode and a negative deflection as it moves away. However, from the perspective of the unipolar electrode, the wavefront is approaching or receding with respect to infinity, and therefore, no specific anatomic localization is obtained. If the depolarization originates immediately below the exploring electrode, then the entire wavefront will move away from the electrode, and only a monophasic QS complex is seen (**Fig. 1**). The R/S ratio informs us of distance from the electrode.

Advantages of unipolar recordings

The unipolar EGM can provide precise timing of local tissue activation marked by the point of maximum negative slope,[4] and this can be determined from filtered or unfiltered signals. As noted previously, the unipolar EGM morphology informs us if the activation wavefront is moving toward or away from the recording electrode. However, this is only true for unfiltered signals or when the high pass filter cutoff frequency is 0.5 Hz or less in order

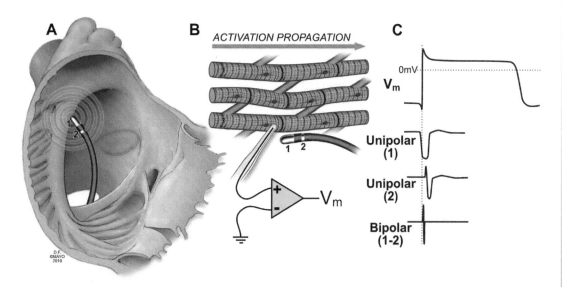

Fig. 1. (*A*) Catheter with bipolar recording electrodes measuring an intracardiac EGM that originates in the right atrium. (*B*) Highly interconnected myocardial cellular network with net activation propagation shown from left to right. Recording catheters measure from the extracellular space and therefore detect only field potentials. In contrast, intracellular recording electrodes measure individual cellular depolarization, which correlates to the EGM signal. (*C*) Temporal relationship between unipolar and bipolar EGM recordings at a particular recording location and the underlying activation of a single local cardiomyocyte. ([*A*] Courtesy of Mayo Clinic, Rochester MN.)

to prevent distortion of the EGM. A higher cutoff can cause artificial R waves to appear in the signal, even if the catheter is at the site of impulse origin.[5] The unipolar signal amplitude measured from myocardium also has value in that if the tissue is destroyed, then the amplitude will decrease, and this can be an important marker of ablation efficacy. Unipolar EGMs are also useful for mapping and ablating focal arrhythmias, allowing the operator to find a location with an appropriate QS morphology (point of origin at which the signal only travels away from the catheter). It should be noted, however, that a pure QS morphology may not be possible to find if the signal of interest originates from a midmyocardial or supravalvular location. Once at the site of origin, identifying an injury current can help ensure good electrode contact before ablating. Unipolar EGMs have also been shown to be useful for mapping accessory pathways, because both the atrial and the ventricular EGMs have an identifiable QS complex during ventriculoatrial and anterograde conduction at the ventricular insertion.[4,6]

Disadvantages of unipolar recordings

Unipolar EGMs are susceptible to noise because of differential coupling of unwanted signals, such as electromagnetic interference, myopotentials, or baseline drift at the exploring and reference electrodes[7] that may make it difficult to measure low-amplitude signals from areas of diseased tissue and scar. Furthermore, unipolar recordings are very susceptible to contamination from low-frequency far-field signals, especially when distant tissue is healthy and generates a high-amplitude signal. This can be reduced by optimizing the physical layout of the EP laboratory and decreasing noise sources, or through use of electronic filters for signal conditioning (see Supplement). Increasing the high-pass cutoff frequency to 10 Hz or even 30 Hz can be effective, with the risk of masking important low-frequency components or creating an artificial R-wave deflection due to intrinsic filter properties. When obtaining unipolar EGMs, care must also be taken to avoid poor electrode contact or even lack of contact if the catheter tip is floating in the cardiac chamber. This would manifest as a "slow" QS signal typical of a far-field potential, and ablation here would not be successful until contact is made. Another significant disadvantage to using unipolar EGM recordings is the stimulation artifact created during pacing, leading to an inability to record an accurate EGM during and immediately after pacing, and this is particularly problematic when using entrainment mapping, whereby you need to monitor the return of the tachycardia complex as well as the local EGM immediately after pacing.

Bipolar Intracardiac Recordings

Bipolar EGM recordings are obtained using 2 narrowly spaced ring electrodes (usually between 2 and 10 mm). By convention, the distal electrode in contact with the myocardium is connected to the positive input of the recording amplifier. A bipolar recording is analogous to measuring the difference potential between 2 closely spaced unipolar electrodes. In a closely spaced bipole, the far-field potentials seen by each electrode should be near similar and therefore canceled, leaving only the local myocardial signal.

Advantages of bipolar recordings

Bipolar EGMs are the most common waveform analyzed during an EP study, because cancellation of the far-field EGM results in a superior signal-to-noise ratio to accurately record near-field signals, although low-amplitude far-field signals may still be detected (**Fig. 2**). Accurate differentiation of near-field versus far-field signals is particularly important when measuring EGMs near a valve, such as when mapping ectopic beats in the right ventricular outflow tract (RVOT) that can occur above or below the pulmonary valve (**Fig. 3**). With bipolar EGMs, high-pass filters can be used with a higher cutoff frequency (30–50 Hz) to further minimize baseline shifts and low-frequency noise. This allows us to more accurately identify local activation, which is particularly helpful in areas of diseased tissue, where the amplitude may be small. The direction of wavefront propagation can be determined only by comparing times of earliest activation in successive pairs of bipolar electrodes (**Fig. 4**).

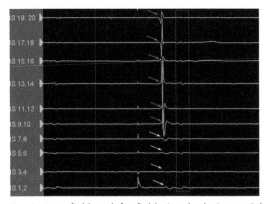

Fig. 2. Near-field and far-field signals during atrial pacing from the coronary sinus. A catheter placed across the lateral cavotricuspid isthmus shows near-field signals (*red arrows*) at electrodes (9, 10) to (19, 20). Electrodes (1, 2) to (7, 8) show far-field detection of this signal (*yellow arrows*). Of note, there are also far-field ventricular signals detected by all electrodes (*blue box*).

Disadvantages of bipolar recordings

Because the bipolar signal is calculated as the difference between the voltages seen at the 2 recording electrodes, any identical voltages will be subtracted away in the final signal. Thus, there is a dependence on the bipolar electrode orientation for signal creation. If a depolarization wavefront is propagating exactly perpendicular to the bipole axis, both electrodes will measure nearly identical voltages. The instantaneous voltage difference will remain approximately zero as the wavefront approaches and passes. Alternatively, if the direction of an advancing wavefront is exactly parallel to the bipole axis, it will be detected by 1 electrode before the other, which could potentially lead to a bipolar EGM of greater amplitude than either unipolar EGM alone.[2] Furthermore, if the distal tip is in contact with the tissue with a perpendicular orientation, then the proximal electrode will be offset from the tissue by several millimeters. In this situation, the same signal is measured from both electrodes but with the proximal electrode detecting lower overall amplitude. Although measuring the difference between the 2 electrodes removes interference, it may also remove a substantial proportion of the local signal of interest. This dependence on bipole orientation should theoretically have a large impact on creating an accurate voltage map, but this is not always seen in practice likely due to the fact that the myocardium is not a uniform, isotropic medium and the use of more closely spaced bipolar electrodes. Nonetheless, the electrophysiologist must remember that signal amplitude from bipolar EGM recordings is not necessarily a reliable indicator of myocardial function, which can be problematic when creating voltage maps using absolute amplitude cutoffs to identify areas of scar.

Unlike unipolar recordings, ablating tissue does not predictably produce a decrease in local bipolar EGM amplitude because the difference between distal and proximal signals may not decrease with ablation. The proximal electrode is farther from the ablated tissue, and therefore, more of the signal it detects could be from healthy, unablated myocardium, and consequently, the difference between proximal and distal signals (the bipolar EGM) could actually increase with ablation.

Another disadvantage when using bipolar EGMs is that the EGM morphology of a single bipolar signal should not be used to determine the direction of wavefront propagation. Rather than using a single bipolar EGM, a comparison of the activation times of multiple bipolar EGMs should be used to determine the direction of wavefront propagation (see **Fig. 4**). Bipolar EGMs are also subject

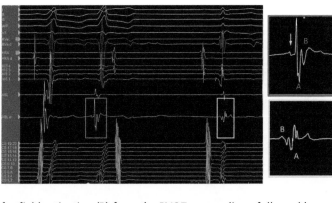

Fig. 3. Signal obtained above the pulmonary valve with a premature ventricular beat (*red box*) and sinus beat (*yellow box*). In the PVC recording signal (*red box, top right*), there is a prepotential (*yellow arrow*) followed by a near-field signal (A) representing local tissue from above the valve and then followed by a far-field signal (B) representing tissue from the RVOT. With the catheter at the same location but instead recording a sinus beat (*yellow box, bottom right*), the order of these signals reverses. There is first an early far-field activation (B) from the RVOT myocardium, followed by near-field activation (A) of the local myocardium above the pulmonary valve.

to signal fractionation (or fragmentation) as a result of a time delay between the signal's detection at each electrode (**Fig. 5**). This can be due to a large electrode spacing or slow signal conduction as a result of an inhomogeneous and highly anisotropic conduction medium (such as dense scar containing sparsely dispersed viable myofibers). The sequential bipolar EGM morphology can be helpful, however, when there is change in polarity of the signal that can be associated with a change in the direction of activation. For example, a change in the sequence of signals across a closely spaced multielectrode catheter occurs when ablation creates successful conduction block in the cavotricuspid isthmus.[8]

ACTIVATION MAPPING

Careful analysis of the basic EGMs with attention to the time of activation of the local region by the arrhythmia wavefront with respect to a reference signal is known as activation mapping, as one is literally mapping *when* an area of myocardium is activated. The activation time for a specific area is cataloged and assigned an isochronal color, with the color red (in the CARTO system) usually indicating "early activation." Later activation times are represented by colors of the visible spectrum toward blue, with purple hues defining sites of very late activation. This process is repeated throughout the myocardium while logging the 3-dimensional (3D) coordinates, a process known as "taking points," and one can begin to construct an anatomic map that is color coded to represent the accrued activation times[9] (**Fig. 6**). In this section, the authors illustrate the fundamentals of activation mapping in relation to the different mechanisms of tachycardia.

Automatic (or Focal) Tachycardia

A focal tachycardia can be very well described with great detail using an activation map, although there are some key practical issues

A   **B**

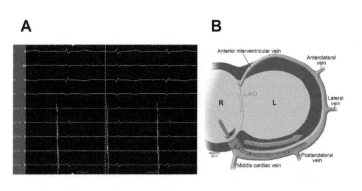

Fig. 4. (*A*) Bipolar EGM recordings from a decapolar catheter inserted into the coronary sinus (CS) measuring wavefront propagation. Direction of propagation can only be determined by comparing the relative timing of EGM signals when using bipolar recordings. In this case, the signal is first detected by the CS (9, 10) bipolar pair that is closest to the CS ostium (time marked by *dashed line* for the center EGM). Each subsequent electrode pair along the CS catheter detects the signal at a later time, indicating the direction of propagation is proximal to distal along the catheter. Concurrent surface ECG recordings are shown at the top (leads I, II, III, and V1). (*B*) CS catheter inserted into the CS and direction of propagation (*orange arrow*) for the signals shown in panel A. L, left; LAO, left anterior oblique view; R, right.

A

B

C

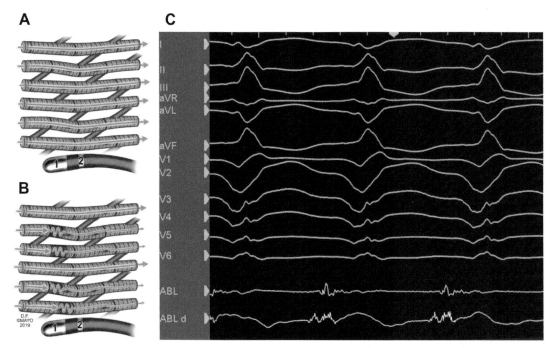

Fig. 5. (*A, B*) Activation wavefront propagating through a normal (*A*) and diseased (*B*) network of myocardial cells. The wavefront is slowed as it travels through diseased tissue, leading to a long delay between detection at each bipolar electrode. (*C*) Example of a highly fragmented middiastolic epicardial signal measured at the distal ablation catheter in a patient with ischemic cardiomyopathy and VT.

that must be addressed in order to create an accurate map.

Choosing a reference electrogram

Often called the "timing reference," this is the fiducial marker used to determine the activation timing that ensures all mapped points are acquired at the same part of the cardiac cycle. This can be any signal so long as it is stable and accurately reflects the cardiac activation at that site. Sites with a multicomponent EGM should be avoided, especially if the reference point is taken on a peak, because the system may accidentally select a different peak with each successive beat.[9] Note

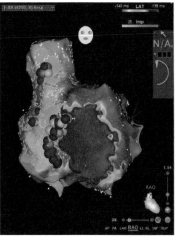
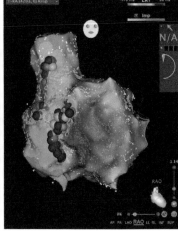

Fig. 6. Three-dimensional electro-anatomical activation map of an atrial flutter wave propagating across the right atrium. In the *left* panel, the window of interest (WOI) is defined from 140 ms before the timing reference point (also called the reference zero point) to 135 ms after the reference point. Anatomical surfaces marked in red indicate local activation times early in the WOI, and surfaces marked in purple indicate local activation late in the WOI. Wavefront propagation is from *red* areas (early) toward blue and purple areas (late). The panel on the right highlights how the apparent activation sequence can change dramatically by adjusting the WOI, in this case changing the WOI to span from 178 ms before the reference zero to 96 ms after the reference zero. Large red markers indicate ablation. (*Courtesy of* Dr. Ammar Killu, Mayo Clinic, Rochester MN.)

that shifting of the reference EGM can change the map appearance quite drastically and should be avoided.[10]

Choosing the window of interest

After establishing an optimal reference, one must next establish an appropriate mapping window that will define the times acquired before and after the reference point. Although the entire signal is continuously recorded, portions of the signal that fall outside the window may not be identified and will not contribute to the activation map. Determining an appropriate window size depends on the specific arrhythmia being mapped. For a focal tachycardia, a true early site of activation is rarely earlier than 50 milliseconds from the onset of the P wave or QRS on the surface ECG. Exceptions do occur, such as when the arrhythmia focus is far from the recording electrodes and there is slow conduction. More complicated is determining the window size for reentrant tachycardias. The window is usually chosen to be nearly the entire tachycardia cycle length. If the window of interest (WOI) is too small, the entire cycle length will not be mapped and 2 different points along the propagation path may inappropriately appear as being activated at the same time. Alternatively, if the WOI is too large (longer than the tachycardia cycle length), a wavefront that has traversed the entire circuit and returned to the original point of recording may appear to be a second (and late) activation at that site. Therefore, similar to the reference point, an improperly chosen WOI can dramatically change the appearance of an activation map (see **Fig. 6**, right panel).

Using unipolar and bipolar signals for electrogram annotation

Bipolar recordings are used for most mapping purposes; however, both types of signals are routinely used to characterize an EGM, and therefore, it is necessary to understand how these signals are annotated. The marker of local activation could be taken at the earliest initial upstroke, the maximum slope of the upstroke or downstroke, or the peak EGM amplitude. The earliest part of the EGM may represent far-field activation, particularly in diseased tissue, and therefore, is not a reliable marker of local activation. This is likely true for both unipolar and bipolar signals. The peak unipolar EGM amplitude in diseased tissue or areas of scar with slow conduction will often have a delay from the onset of local activation, and this can even vary between sites; therefore, peak EGM is not used as an indicator of local activation. However, the *first* peak of the bipolar EGM that is from a near-field source does seem to coincide with local activation, and therefore, marking the first peak of a bipolar EGM is a common technique used to annotate EGMs for activation mapping. For unipolar recordings, it has been determined that the maximum negative slope of the EGM marks the point of activation of the myocardium directly beneath the electrode.[4] This usually occurs near the transition from positive to negative. Also, it may be difficult to determine the exact time of the maximum negative slope due to conduction delay or activation arising from the epicardium or midmyocardium.[11]

Reentrant Tachycardia

The main issue when dealing with reentrant tachycardias is that there is no specific point of arrhythmia generation. In other words, there is no single location of "early" activation, and therefore, the entire macro-reentrant circuit must be mapped to identify its critical isthmus.

Analyzing the entire cycle length

The WOI should be set to capture the arrhythmia cycle length. When only a portion of the cycle length is mapped, there is risk of incompletely defining the anatomic boundaries of the chamber of interest, missing an anatomic variant, mapping in the wrong chamber, or missing a chamber entirely (which can happen in patients with congenital heart disease after surgical correction). Accounting for the entire cycle length may be difficult because of misinterpreting areas of low voltage and fragmented signals as scar and failing to realize that these areas may represent viable myocardium that are part of the arrhythmia circuit. When the entire cycle length cannot be accounted for despite considering these factors, one must consider that the diagnosis is not a reentrant arrhythmia but may actually be an automatic tachycardia.[12]

Mapping the macro-reentrant circuit

Only by mapping the entire cycle length will one be able to correctly visualize the full anatomic extent of a macro-reentrant circuit, looking for the earliest presystolic EGM closest to middiastole, which is usually taken to be the site of origin for a reentrant circuit (although finding a site with continuous diastolic activity or mapping a discrete diastolic pathway is more specific).[13] Assuming this area to be the isthmus of the tachycardia circuit, the authors pace from there at a rate faster than the tachycardia cycle (overdrive pacing) to entrain the tachycardia[14] and prove that the mechanism is due to reentry by careful analysis of EGM morphology, looking for types of fusion (constant vs progressive vs concealed) created by the interaction of orthodromic and antidromic wave-fronts. The tachycardia is then interrogated further through a complex set of pacing maneuvers that include "downstream" pacing from sites that are adjacent to sites of earlier activation and analysis of postpacing intervals. This is known as entrainment mapping,[15,16] and a full discussion of this technique is beyond the scope of this review. However, the interested reader is encouraged to review the articles by Schaeffer and Stevenson,[15] and Kumar and colleagues,[16] for more details. The authors anticipate mapping areas of slow conduction within the circuit and identifying boundaries that are due to the absence of tissue, scar, or electrically inert structures (eg, valves). There are situations, however, when mapping the entire circuit is not possible, such as when (1) the circuit is in another chamber; (2) part of the circuit is in an anatomically excluded site, such as a post-Fontan heart; (3) fragmented signals are annotated as a single point or "location only" point, in which case the duration of the fragmented signal must be subtracted from the duration of tachycardia cycle length for mappable portions of the circuit; and (4) inappropriate diagnosis of scar or missed portions of the circuit that contain key EGMs or slow zones within the circuit.

Micro-Reentrant Tachycardia

Micro-reentry occurs because of local conduction block creating small reentrant circuits, usually associated with areas of myocardial scar. Because of the small size of the reentrant circuit, a micro-reentrant tachycardia can look like a focal tachycardia on initial activation mapping. However, closer inspection of the presumed focus shows EGMs typical of myocardial scar, with low-amplitude signals and signal fractionation.

Defining scar

Accurate mapping of scar can be challenging. EGMs from myocardial scar will have lower voltages, but there is no reliable voltage threshold that can distinguish unexcitable areas of scar from areas interspersed with strands of viable myocardium. Near-field signals as small as 25 to 50 μV that are consistent with each cardiac cycle may be viable (albeit diseased) myocardium and possibly an arrhythmogenic channel. One can try to validate the presence of excitable tissue by pacing at the mapping site, because myocardial capture should not be elicited from an area of true dense fibrous tissue, even with high output pacing of 10 mA or more.[17] During epicardial mapping, areas of fat over the course of coronary arteries can also reduce signal amplitude and be mistaken for scar.

Handling fragmented signals

A multicomponent EGM without isoelectric intervals between components is known as a fragmented signal (see **Fig. 5**C) and can be seen at a site of micro-reentry. These signals can represent near-field activation in an area of very slow conduction (when using a bipolar recording configuration) either within the tachycardia circuit or at bystander sites. Fragmented signals can also arise from the simultaneous detection of local activation and far-field potentials. A specific activation time may be difficult to determine, and therefore, these areas may be initially annotated as "location-only" points.[11] With macro-reentrant tachycardias, defining fragmented signals in this way will essentially remove them from consideration as part of the reentrant circuit and prevent construction of a full map. However, this is less of a problem when dealing with micro-reentry.

Dealing with double potentials

Similar to fragmented signals, double potentials are multicomponent EGMs with 2 distinct peaks separated by an isoelectric interval (**Fig. 7**). They can represent activation on either side of an area of functional conduction block that is at the center of a reentrant circuit, and double potentials have been described in both reentrant atrial[18] and ventricular[19] arrhythmias. There is considerable variation in the morphology of double potentials, depending on catheter orientation and location of the tip with respect to the activation wavefront and position of the line of conduction block. A double potential can also result from a far-field signal that is detected earlier than local activation due to conduction block causing significant delay. As a result, it is not appropriate for an operator to always use the earliest signal when recording a double potential.

In macro-reentry arrhythmias where there is an incomplete line of conduction block (such as after ablation), an ablation gap can be located by careful annotation of multiple double potential EGMs along the line. The interval between components will be widest when the catheter tip is far from the gap and should become progressively shorter as the tip is moved toward it. At the gap itself, one may see a single EGM without multiple components, or possibly a change in morphology to a fractionated EGM. This site should be targeted for ablation if a complete line of conduction block is desired.[11]

SUBSTRATE MAPPING

Some arrhythmias, such as atrial fibrillation (AF), ventricular fibrillation (VF), atrial tachycardia that

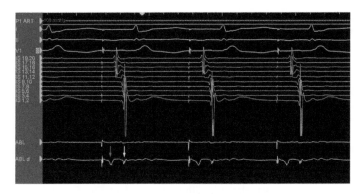

Fig. 7. A double potential recorded at the cavo-tricuspid isthmus with atrial pacing. The red arrow show the first signal recorded at the distal ablation catheter, and the yellow arrow shows a second signal, identified as a double potential due to a nearby area of conduction block. Note the signal from the isthmus catheter proximal electrodes (19, 20) shows a sharp near-field signal with loss of near-field characteristics at electrodes (11, 12) that returns at electrodes (9, 10).

rapidly changes sequence, or even premature ventricular tachycardias (VTs) with changing morphology, are considered "unmappable" using timing of local activation. There are also cases when a tachycardia causes unacceptable hemodynamic instability, and traditional activation mapping techniques cannot be used. In such situations, the authors resort to constructing a map based on voltage amplitudes (**Fig. 8**) and morphology of the measured EGM signals, a technique called voltage mapping or substrate mapping. The authors do this to help differentiate areas of healthy and abnormal, presumably scarred, myocardium, which can be useful in guiding an ablation strategy.

Identifying Abnormal Myocardium

In addition to low voltages (measured peak to peak from a bipolar EGM), there are other EGM features that can be used to help identify areas of abnormal myocardium, including signal fractionation and

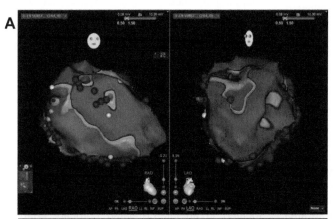

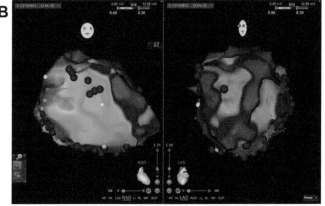

Fig. 8. Substrate (voltage) mapping with 3D EAM software. (*A*) Bipolar map with low-voltage areas identified by red color (bipolar voltage <0.5 mV). Voltages greater than 1.5 mV are marked by purple. (*B*) Unipolar mapping of the same intracardiac activity (voltage thresholds set between 0.6 and 8.3 mV). Although there are similarities, areas of higher and lower voltages are demarcated differently based on the type of recording used to create the voltage map.

late potentials. The authors briefly discuss how these abnormal EGM characteristics are used to create a substrate or voltage map.

Low-amplitude signals

Contiguous areas of abnormal EGMs with amplitudes of less than 0.5 mV have been described as areas of "dense scar" in patients who underwent substrate mapping for VT, with surrounding areas between 0.5 and 1.5 mV marked as a "border zone," which transitioned into normal myocardium.[20] This area of scar can, however, still contain functional myocardial cells that act as conducting channels, and incrementally lowering the voltage threshold on the map can help identify an isthmus. Using unipolar or bipolar EGM voltage to identify areas with low-amplitude signal is relatively straightforward and can be done rapidly (see **Fig. 8**). However, there are several factors that can affect the amplitude of the EGM. As was discussed earlier, the orientation of a bipolar electrode with respect to the propagating wavefront can potentially have a large effect on the amplitude of the recorded signal. The size of the recording electrodes and interelectrode spacing can also affect voltage amplitude as well as the degree of tissue contact and presence of fat. Furthermore, unipolar EGMs are more likely to be contaminated by noise or far-field signals, potentially making the absolute voltage amplitude highly variable. Therefore, voltage amplitude should never be used alone to define a conduction barrier or an area of slow conduction.

Late potentials and fractionated signals

Late potentials are low-amplitude signals that occur after the local EGM and the corresponding ECG wave and represent viable myocardium in an area of scar that is distal to the wavefront breakthrough site through an area of slow conduction. They are indicative of slow conduction through surviving myocardial bundles in an area of scar with downstream viable myocardium and correlate with areas that are potentially conducive to reentrant arrhythmias (**Fig. 9**). Regions with late potentials may contain a critical isthmus, and ablating these areas can close all gaps and exits from slow conduction and prevent reentry. Similar to late potentials, fractionated or fragmented signals also indicate areas of slow conduction with surviving myocardial fibers sparsely dispersed in scar tissue. Fractionation occurs when conduction is so slow that the individual electrodes in a bipolar pair detect the near-field signal from a propagating wavefront at different times (see **Fig. 5**). A late potential is often also fractionated.

Substrate-Guided Ablation Strategies

When they do not have a clear arrhythmia focus or an isthmus to target for ablation, the authors use substrate mapping to identify areas of abnormal myocardium and slow conduction. The rationale for ablating abnormal myocardium originated from the observation that areas of fibrosis identified intraoperatively with local EGMs at the site of VT origin exhibited low-amplitude, fractionated signals.[21,22] Surgical resection of these areas of scarred subendocardium guided by intraoperative mapping resulted in significant decrease in VT burden.[23–25] These areas are characterized by the aforementioned EGM abnormalities, and ablation strategies are usually designed to eliminate the abnormal signals.

Late potential and isthmus ablation

Ablation of low-voltage channels exhibiting isolated late potentials increases the specificity of locating critical VT isthmus sites from 30% to 85%.[26] Late potential ablation has also been shown to be an effective procedural endpoint when combined with VT noninducibility in patients with postmyocardial infarction VT[27] and in high-risk patients with chronic total occlusion located in an infarct-related coronary artery.[28]

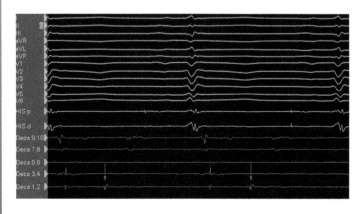

Fig. 9. Late potentials (*red arrows*) detected at electrodes (1, 2) of the decapolar catheter recording in the epicardium of a patient with arrhythmogenic right ventricular cardiomyopathy.

Identification of slow pathways in VT using fragmented potentials has helped identify an isthmus that can then be ablated, a technique called slow zone (or isthmus) ablation.[29,30]

Local abnormal ventricular activity ablation and homogenization

Local abnormal ventricular activity (LAVA) is defined as sharp, high-frequency signals that may be low amplitude and occur *during* or *after* the far-field ventricular EGM when in sinus rhythm but *before* the far-field ventricular EGM during VT. These signals, which are common in scar-related VT, can be fractionated or multicomponent. They are thought to arise from local activation of diseased myocardium. The LAVA ablation approach has a clear endpoint, and it has been shown that ablation procedures ending with complete LAVA elimination yields a 51% to 53% event-free survival rate.[31,32] An extension of the LAVA ablation approach is scar homogenization, whereby an operator extensively ablates throughout the entire scarred regions and border zones using voltage threshold criteria, while looking for any abnormal EGM signals from both the endocardium and the epicardium.[33] Ultimately, the goal in scar homogenization is to ablate such that the measured signal is homogenous in all areas.

Ablation Challenges When Using Substrate Maps

Using an ablation strategy based on a substrate map can be difficult, and at present, there is no consensus on the optimal approach. An operator must be experienced at ablating through scar and will need to be cautious not to miss any areas of myocardium. The extensive area that may require ablation can lead to longer ablation times, especially with the homogenization approach. Operators must also be cautious not to produce coagulum or cause collateral damage. Although mapping late potentials and fragmented signals will usually take less time overall, an operator must be skilled at manipulating the catheter in order to avoid missing an area of tissue. One can also see late potentials at bystander sites that are not part of a reentrant circuit.[34] Also, although fractionated signals are present in AF, they are not yet useful for AF ablation as the authors cannot reliably differentiate AF substrate from bystander.[35] The LAVA ablation is a hybrid approach that avoids the hassle of having to map and then ablate everywhere, as with homogenization, and avoids the need to carefully analyze late potential or fractionated EGM timing and morphology. However, the LAVA ablation approach may miss some conducting channels and reentrant circuits that could potentially cause an ablation failure. Recently, an alternative ablation strategy has been described that uses decrement-evoked potential mapping, whereby areas are targeted for ablation that exhibit late potentials or abnormal EGMs but also display decremental behavior evoked during pacing.[36]

OTHER MAPPING APPROACHES

Aside from substrate mapping and traditional activation mapping, there are other ways to map cardiac activity that are currently in use or being investigated. Focal Impulse and Rotor Modulation is a technique for mapping AF that uses repolarization and conduction dynamics to help identify the core of a rotor (rather than merely the spiral arms) so that it can be ablated. AF is increasingly being recognized as a specific and organized form of functional reentry, and a current strategy is to target the focal impulse of the rotor.[37] A complementary approach, called Shannon Entropy Mapping, uses entropy to quantify the degree of synchronization during AF to help identify the location of rotors (areas of high Shannon Entropy).[38] For VF, current research is looking at the involvement of the His-Purkinje system in the maintenance of VF. This "Purkinje mapping" uses a standard point-to-point mapping technique and may provide insight into the mechanism of VF.[39]

MAPPING SYSTEMS

Electroanatomic mapping (EAM) systems have created a paradigm shift for the electrophysiologist by enabling 3D reconstruction of cardiac anatomy and nonfluoroscopic visualization of mapping and ablation catheters. At present, there are 3 major commercially available systems that rely on magnetic- or impedance-based localization. In this section, the authors describe briefly how these systems work.

CARTO

The first CARTO system was an electromagnetic field-based system only, with the patient in a weak magnetic field (5×10^{-6} T to 5×10^{-5} T), generated by the system. The magnetic field was detected by 3 orthogonal miniature coils embedded in the catheter tip that were used to determine the tip location in space. The present generation of the CARTO system (CARTO 3) integrates this magnetic approach with an impedance-based approach. For this system, 6 patch electrodes are positioned on the patient, 3 on the back and 3 on the chest, and the current produced at a unique frequency from different catheter electrodes is continuously compared with the current produced at each electrode measured at each patch, creating a current ratio unique to each electrode's location. Continuous updates to this system occur with the ability to integrate intracardiac echocardiograph (CARTO Sound), overlap 3D anatomic maps and visualize catheters on prerecorded radiograph images or cine loops (CART-Univu), and integrate images with preacquired computed tomography angiograms or MRI volume data sets (CARTO-Merge).

EnSite NavX

The EnSite NavX involves 3 pairs of surface patches, 10 ECG electrodes, and 1 system reference electrode (usually placed on the patient abdomen), with a reliance on impedance for visualization of catheters. For 3D navigation, 6 patch electrodes create electric fields along 3 orthogonal axes (x, y, and z) with the heart at the center. The patches are placed on the side of the patient (x-axis), the chest and back (y-axis), and the back of the neck and inner left thigh (z-axis). A low-amplitude alternating current is delivered between the electrode pairs and the intracardiac catheters. The electrodes on the catheters measure relative voltages with respect to a reference electrode, and the localization of catheters is based on an impedance gradient in relation to the reference electrode.

Rhythmia

Mapping with this system is a hybrid between magnetic- and impedance-based systems, with mapping performed by a "basket" catheter that contains 64 electrodes (surface area of each electrode is 0.4 mm^2). The location of each electrode is determined by a combination of a magnetic sensor located at the tip of the catheter and impedance sensing of each electrode. The magnetic field is created by a generator positioned under the patient's table (similar to CARTO) and is capable of locating catheters with magnetic sensors, with the impedance location technology used to track catheters that are not equipped with a magnetic sensor. Point acquisition with this basket catheter can be continuous and automated or manual. When continuous and automated, operator-defined criteria for accepting cardiac beats are applied, with the system checking for changes in cycle length, respiratory gating, EGM morphology matching, and automatic rejection of points that do not fit the proposed criteria.

SUMMARY

In this article, the authors have reviewed the basics of cardiac EGM signals and how they can be used to construct a useful cardiac EAM. They have also reviewed some of the ablation strategies that are used in conjunction with cardiac maps. Finally, they have briefly commented on the hardware and software platforms currently in use in the electrophysiology laboratory. Although advances in technology have facilitated the practice of cardiac mapping to identify areas of interest, a solid understanding of the fundamentals of EGM acquisition and annotation is necessary to ensure points are properly mapped and interpreted. Regardless of the complexity of a mapping system, all mapping is done using the basic unipolar and bipolar recording electrode configurations, and there are different factors to consider when choosing the type of EGM for a given scenario. However, once properly annotated, the collection of EGM signals used to construct an accurate map is a powerful tool to help characterize a variety of arrhythmias and design an appropriate plan for ablation.

Fundamentals of Cardiac Mapping: Supplement

Optimizing the Electrogram in the Electrophysiology Laboratory

Creating a successful map is critically dependent on the accurate acquisition of the EGM signals. In practice, these signals often have very small amplitude and coexist in an environment with several interfering signals and noise. Here, the authors briefly review some of the electronic equipment used in a modern EP laboratory and how they attempt to obtain the EGM with high fidelity.

Dealing with Noise in the Electrophysiology Laboratory

Noise is inevitable in recording systems, especially so when recording biopotential signals. These signals are low amplitude (ranging from 25 μV to about 10 mV) and inherently complex and unpredictable. Some of what is interpreted as "noise" may actually be a true biopotential but arising from a different source than what is currently being investigated, such as a far field potential from distant myocardium or detection of an EMG signal from skeletal muscle. Therefore, it is noise in the sense that it is interfering with the recorded signal of interest, but there is no way for the electronic acquisition system to discern which biopotentials are important to us and which are not.

Then there is the contribution of signal noise from the equipment used in the EP laboratory, such as ECM monitoring machines, pulse oximeters, computers with display monitors, and the EAM system itself, all of which are powered with a 120- to 240-V sine wave at a frequency of 50 Hz or 60 Hz. This interferes with the recorded signal of interest and can be difficult to eliminate. However, the fact that the dominant component is usually a distinct sine wave that occurs at a well-defined frequency makes it easier to recognize and filter out. For safety reasons, all medical equipment that is connected to a patient must be separated from earth ground using an isolation transformer to minimize leakage currents that can cause VF. However, there is still some amount of leakage current that will persist despite adequate isolation due to capacitive coupling, and International Organization for Standardization Safety Standards require that this be less than 10 μA for each device that is connected to the patient. This isolation can help reduce some line noise, but noise at the fundamental frequency of 50 Hz or 60 Hz, as well as its harmonics, will persist to some extent. Furthermore, the patient and the numerous intracardiac catheters can act as antennas, which will introduce noise through inductive coupling.

Altogether, noise from various sources will create a measurable voltage of 1 to 3 V_{RMS} (root mean square, a unit used to estimate the average power dissipation of a defined signal or random process such as noise). The goal of the EP system electronics is to amplify and filter the recorded signal while rejecting noise and interfering signals and retaining only the EGM. The best way to reduce noise in the recorded signal is to remove the noise before it is recorded. This can be accomplished through extensive shielding and grounding in the EP laboratory as well as conscientious placement of cables carrying sensitive intracardiac signals and equipment power cables. The walls, ceiling, and floor of an EP laboratory are heavily shielded to reduce the amount of ionizing radiation from radiographs used during fluoroscopy from escaping to the outside, and this will also help reduce electromagnetic interference that arises from outside sources. Power cables coming from an isolation transformer should be kept as far as possible from cables containing signals from recording electrodes. These cables should be separately shielded with a high-density metal braiding that is connected to the system ground (that is "floating" with respect to earth ground) to shunt electromagnetic noise that can couple to these wires. Because all wires can act as antennae that can transmit or receive signals, the orientation of wires with respect to each other should be considered. Maximal coupling occurs between straight, parallel lengths of wire. Therefore, a recording cable should never be placed alongside a power cable, and care should be taken to minimize coiling and bundling of recording cables in order to minimize coupling between those cables.

Signal Frequency Content and Filtering

Before discussing how a signal is acquired in the EP laboratory via electronic amplifiers, it is important to first understand how signals are composed of components at different frequencies and to review how electronic filters can modify those signals. The authors routinely process and visualize signals in the time domain, although it can be helpful to consider the same signals in the frequency domain. It is useful to think of a complex signal, such as an EGM, as a sum of sinusoids, whereby some of these sinusoidal components represent the signal of interest and others are due to noise. The authors design electronic filters to condition a signal before it is acquired. If it is known that biopotential signals contain useful frequency components between 0.05 and 500 Hz, then using a band-pass filter with these cutoff frequencies will help remove unwanted signal components that likely represent only noise. Sometimes, an interfering signal is present that shares some frequency components with the signal of interest. This is the case with 50- to 60-Hz line-related noise. It is not appropriate to use a low-pass or high-pass filter with a cutoff sufficient to reject 50- to 60-Hz components because this would remove too much of the signal of interest. Instead, one can use a notch filter (sometimes called a band-reject filter) that will attenuate signals over a certain range of frequencies and pass all others.

The Instrumentation Amplifier

The pivotal component of the EP laboratory that allows the accurately recorded myocardial biopotentials is the instrumentation amplifier (IA), which is a special type of differential amplifier that is especially suited for the measurement of sensitive signals. This device will amplify the *difference* between 2 signals presented at its inputs. Signal components that are shared at both inputs will be subtracted away and not amplified. If the amplifier inputs are connected to a recording electrode and the circuit ground, then the IA will subtract away common line noise but little else. If, however, the 2 inputs are connected to adjacent bipolar electrodes, there will be much more common signal that will be subtracted out. In reality, the IA cannot perfectly remove all common signal, and some amount will be present at the output. This is described by the Common-Mode Rejection Ratio (CMRR) of the amplifier, defined as the ratio of the "differential gain" to the "common-mode gain." Modern IAs have a CMRR of approximately 100 dB, which translates to a 100,000-fold difference in the magnitude of the signals that are amplified by the IA as compared with those signals that are attenuated by the IA, and this can largely determine the signal-to-noise ratio of the recording system. It is important to note that the CMRR is also a frequency-dependent parameter due to the inherent frequency response of the electronic components and starts to degrade at higher frequencies.[1] Many of the current signal processing systems do not use true IAs but instead subtract the output of 1 channel from another to create a differential output (signal from Distal Electrode 1 − signal from Electrode 2 = Distal Bipolar signal).

The IA circuit gain for differential signals that are amplified is between 100 and 5000, based on amplifier design and user settings. Large gains are sometimes necessary to adequately amplify the extremely small biopotentials. However, the operator must take care not to overgain the amplifier, because there is a limit to the magnitude of the output signal, based on the internal power supply voltage. The dynamic range of the amplifier is defined as the ratio of the largest useful output voltage (defined by the amplifier power supply) divided by the smallest useful output voltage (defined by the signal noise level). It is impossible for the amplifier to output a signal voltage that exceeds its own voltage supply, which can present a problem if the gain is set too high while recording a larger-than-expected signal. In this case, the amplifier will saturate, and signal peaks will be lost. For example, if one is measuring a 3-mV signal and the amplifier gain is set to 5000, the output signal should have a magnitude of 15 V. However, the amplifier supply voltage is usually limited to ± 10 V, and therefore, the portion of the output signal that exceeds this level will simply be cut off. This is known as signal clipping, causing significant signal artifact. Furthermore, when an amplifier is saturated in this way, the amplifier will take time to settle back to baseline before nondistorted signals can be observed at the output. This is known as saturation artifact, and it can prevent the measurement of meaningful signals that may occur immediately after a high amplitude signal, such as a stimulus pulse. It can be particularly troublesome when measuring postpacing intervals during entrainment mapping. When measuring a postpacing EGM signal, it is desirable to artificially clip the signal so that the peak of the high-amplitude stimulation artifact, which may be several orders of magnitude larger than the signals of interest, is not in view, and the operator can focus on those lower-amplitude signals. It should be noted that this is a software setting, and clipping in this way does not produce the same saturation artifact.[2] Caution must be observed when using software clipping to remove large-amplitude signal components, because this may unintentionally mask important parts of the signal and misrepresent the EGM (see figure.).

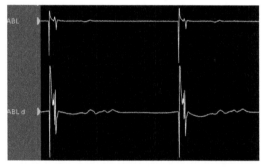

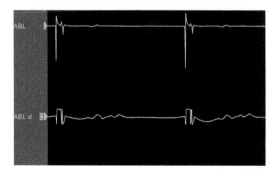

References
[1]Venkatachalam KL, Herbrandson JE, Asirvatham SJ. Signals and Signal Processing for the Electrophysiologist. Circ Arrhythm Electrophysiol 2011;4(6):965–973. doi:10.1161/CIRCEP.111.964304.
[2]Venkatachalam KL, Herbrandson JE, Asirvatham SJ. Signals and Signal Processing for the Electrophysiologist. Circ Arrhythm Electrophysiol 2011;4(6):974–981. doi:10.1161/CIRCEP.111.964973.

ACKNOWLEDGMENTS

The authors acknowledge David Factor for the medical illustrations.

REFERENCES

1. Venkatachalam KL, Herbrandson JE, Asirvatham SJ. Signals and signal processing for the electrophysiologist. Circ Arrhythm Electrophysiol 2011;4(6): 965–73.

2. Ellenbogen KA, Wood MA. Cardiac pacing and ICDs. Hoboken, NJ: John Wiley & Sons; 2011.

3. Wilson FN, Johnston FD, MacLeod AG, et al. Electrocardiograms that represent the potential variations of a single electrode. Am Heart J 1934;9(4): 447–58.

4. Stevenson WG, Soejima K. Recording techniques for clinical electrophysiology. J Cardiovasc Electrophysiol 2005;16(9):1017–22.

5. Venkatachalam KL, Herbrandson JE, Asirvatham SJ. Signals and signal processing for the electrophysiologist. Circ Arrhythm Electrophysiol 2011;4(6): 974–81.

6. Haïssaguerre M, Dartigues JF, Warin JF, et al. Electrogram patterns predictive of successful catheter ablation of accessory pathways. Value of unipolar recording mode. Circulation 1991;84(1):188–202.

7. DeCaprio V, Hurzeler P, Furman S. A comparison of unipolar and bipolar electrograms for cardiac pacemaker sensing. Circulation 1977;56(5):750–5.

8. Tada H, Oral H, Sticherling C, et al. Electrogram polarity and cavotricuspid isthmus block during ablation of typical atrial flutter. J Cardiovasc Electrophysiol 2001;12(4):393–9.

9. Del Carpio Munoz F, Buescher TL, Asirvatham SJ. Three-dimensional mapping of cardiac arrhythmias: what do the colors really mean? Circ Arrhythm Electrophysiol 2010;3(6):e6–11.

10. Deshmukh A, Kapa S, Asirvatham SJ. Electroanatomical mapping for arrhythmias. In: Zipes DP, Jalife J, Stevenson WG, editors. Cardiac electrophysiology: from cell to bedside. Philadelphia, PA: Elsevier Inc.; 2018. p. 574–86.

11. Del Carpio Munoz F, Buescher T, Asirvatham SJ. Teaching points with 3-dimensional mapping of cardiac arrhythmias. Circ Arrhythm Electrophysiol 2011;4(3):e22–5.

12. Del Carpio Munoz F, Buescher TL, Asirvatham SJ. Teaching points with 3-dimensional mapping of cardiac arrhythmia. Circ Arrhythm Electrophysiol 2011; 4(1):e1–3.

13. Issa Z, Miller JM, Zipes DP. Conventional intracardiac mapping techniques. In: Clinical arrhythmology and electrophysiology: a companion to Braunwald's heart disease. Philadelphia, PA: Elsevier Health Sciences; 2019. p. 125–54.

14. Waldo AL, MacLean WAH, Karp RB, et al. Entrainment and interruption of atrial flutter with atrial pacing. Circulation 1977;56(5):737–45.

15. Schaeffer B, Stevenson WG. Entrainment mapping: theoretical considerations and practical implementation. J Cardiovasc Electrophysiol 2018;29(1): 204–13.

16. Kumar S, Tedrow UB, Stevenson WG. Entrainment mapping. Card Electrophysiol Clin 2017;9(1): 55–69.

17. Del Carpio Munoz F, Buescher TL, Asirvatham SJ. Teaching points with 3-dimensional mapping of cardiac arrhythmia. Circ Arrhythm Electrophysiol 2011; 4(6):e72–5.

18. Olshansky B, Okumura K, Henthorn RW, et al. Characterization of double potentials in human atrial flutter. J Am Coll Cardiol 1990;15(4):833–41.

19. Olshansky B, Moreira D, Waldo AL. Characterization of double potentials during ventricular tachycardia. Circulation 1993;87(2):373–81.

20. Marchlinski FE, Callans DJ, Gottlieb CD, et al. Linear ablation lesions for control of unmappable ventricular tachycardia in patients with ischemic and nonischemic cardiomyopathy. Circulation 2000;101(11): 1288–96.

21. Cassidy DM, Vassallo JA, Buxton AE, et al. The value of catheter mapping during sinus rhythm to localize site of origin of ventricular tachycardia. Circulation 1984;69(6):1103–10.

22. Kienzle MG, Miller J, Falcone RA, et al. Intraoperative endocardial mapping during sinus rhythm: relationship to site of origin of ventricular tachycardia. Circulation 1984;70(6):957–65.

23. Josephson ME, Harken AH, Horowitz LN. Endocardial excision: a new surgical technique for the treatment of recurrent ventricular tachycardia. Circulation 1979;60(7):1430–9.

24. Miller JM, Tyson GS, Hargrove WC, et al. Effect of subendocardial resection on sinus rhythm endocardial electrogram abnormalities. Circulation 1995; 91(9):2385–91.

25. Betensky BP, Marchlinski FE. Outcomes of catheter ablation of ventricular tachycardia in the setting of structural heart disease. Curr Cardiol Rep 2016; 18(7):68.

26. Mountantonakis SE, Park RE, Frankel DS, et al. Relationship between voltage map "channels" and the location of critical isthmus sites in patients with post-infarction cardiomyopathy and ventricular tachycardia. J Am Coll Cardiol 2013;61(20): 2088–95.

27. Silberbauer J, Oloriz T, Maccabelli G, et al. Noninducibility and late potential abolition. Circ Arrhythm Electrophysiol 2014;7(3):424–35.

28. Di Marco A, Oloriz Sanjuan T, Paglino G, et al. Late potentials abolition reduces ventricular tachycardia recurrence after ablation especially in higher-risk

patients with a chronic total occlusion in an infarct-related artery. J Cardiovasc Electrophysiol 2018; 29(8):1119–24.

29. Fontaine G, Frank R, Tonet J, et al. Identification of a zone of slow conduction appropriate for VT ablation: theoretical and practical considerations. Pacing Clin Electrophysiol 1989;12(1 Pt 2):262–7.

30. Brunckhorst CB, Delacretaz E, Soejima K, et al. Identification of the ventricular tachycardia isthmus after infarction by pace mapping. Circulation 2004; 110(6):652–9.

31. Jaïs P, Maury P, Khairy P, et al. Elimination of local abnormal ventricular activities: a new end point for substrate modification in patients with scar-related ventricular tachycardia. Circulation 2012;125(18): 2184–96.

32. Sacher F, Lim HS, Derval N, et al. Substrate mapping and ablation for ventricular tachycardia. J Cardiovasc Electrophysiol 2015;26(4):464–71.

33. Di Biase L, Santangeli P, Burkhardt DJ, et al. Endo-epicardial homogenization of the scar versus limited substrate ablation for the treatment of electrical storms in patients with ischemic cardiomyopathy. J Am Coll Cardiol 2012;60(2):132–41.

34. Hood MA, Pogwizd SM, Peirick J, et al. Contribution of myocardium responsible for ventricular tachycardia to abnormalities detected by analysis of signal-averaged ECGs. Circulation 1992;86(6): 1888–901.

35. Caldwell J, Redfearn D. Ablation of complex fractionated atrial electrograms in catheter ablation for AF; where have we been and where are we going? Curr Cardiol Rev 2012;8(4):347–53.

36. Porta-Sánchez A, Jackson N, Lukac P, et al. Multicenter study of ischemic ventricular tachycardia ablation with decrement-evoked potential (DEEP) mapping with extra stimulus. JACC Clin Electrophysiol 2018;4(3):307–15.

37. Waks JW, Josephson ME. Mechanisms of atrial fibrillation—reentry, rotors and reality. Arrhythm Electrophysiol Rev 2014;3(2):90–100.

38. Dharmaprani D, Dykes L, McGavigan AD, et al. Information theory and atrial fibrillation (AF): a review. Front Physiol 2018;9:957.

39. Tri J, Asirvatham R, DeSimone CV, et al. Intramural conduction system gradients and electrogram regularity during ventricular fibrillation. Indian Pacing Electrophysiol J 2018;18(6):195–200.

Cardiac Mapping Systems
Rhythmia, Topera, EnSite Precision, and CARTO

Martin Borlich, MD[a],*, Philipp Sommer, MD, FHRS, FESC, FEHRA[b]

KEYWORDS

- Arrhythmia • High-density mapping • Ablation • Electrophysiology • Mapping systems

KEY POINTS

- Novel cardiac mapping systems nowadays allow providing a safe and highly accurate 3-D reconstruction of cardiac structures as well as a fast and accurate visualization of cardiac arrhythmias.
- In addition, they are increasingly reducing the need for fluoroscopy in these procedures.
- The current state of the art, as well as the presentation of possible uses of individual systems and their limitations, is presented in this article.
- Cardiac mapping systems can significantly contribute to an optimal therapeutic decision making in invasive electrophysiology.
- This article introduces the new developments of Rhythmia, Topera, EnSite Precision, and CARTO systems and provides a look ahead to the future.

INTRODUCTION

The interventional therapy for cardiac arrhythmias is an irreplaceable part of modern cardiological therapy. The development in the field of 3-D mapping systems and catheter technology led to precise 3-D catheter tracking, accurate high-resolution visualization of electroanatomic information, and effective ablation of the underlying substrate. Moreover, the novel cardiac mapping systems contribute significantly to reduction of fluoroscopy time and radiation exposure to avoid stochastic or deterministic radiation risks to both patients and the entire electrophysiology laboratory staff.

RHYTHMIA

The Rhythmia HDx Mapping System (Boston Scientific, Cambridge, Massachusetts) is one of the newest high-resolution 3-D mapping systems, approved in 2013. The system consists of 4 main components: the signal station, the software, the IntellaMap Orion catheter, and the localization system. The signal station provides sophisticated signal processing with advanced filters that results in recording of clear signals with low noise and reduced artifacts. Up to 200 intracardiac channels are supported. It offers an easy connectivity to the IntellaMap Orion as well as other compatible third-party electrophysiology (EP) catheters. Rhythmia

Conflict of Interest Disclosures: M. Borlich receives consultant fees and travel grants from Biosense Webster and grants from Boston Scientific as part of a fellowship. P. Sommer is a member of the Abbott and Biosense Webster physician board and received research funding.
All Authors Declare: The article is original, with no portion under simultaneous consideration for publication elsewhere or previously published. All authors have read and approved the submission.
Authorship: M. Borlich: Article preparation. P. Sommer: Concept and critical review of the article.
^a Heart Center, Segeberger Kliniken (Academic Teaching Hospital of the Universities of Kiel, Lübeck and Hamburg), Am Kurpark 1, Bad Segeberg, Schleswig-Holstein 23795, Germany; ^b Clinic of Electrophysiology, Heart and Diabetes Center NRW, University Hospital of Ruhr-University Bochum, Georgstr. 11, Bad Oeynhausen, Nordrhein-Westfalen 32545, Germany
* Corresponding author.
E-mail address: martin.borlich@segebergerkliniken.de

1877-9182/19/© 2019 Elsevier Inc. All rights reserved.

uses a hybrid tracking technology like CARTO (Biosense Webster, Diamond Bar, California) and EnSite Precision Cardiac Mapping System (Abbott, Chicago, Illinois) combining both impedance-based and magnetic field data. A special electrode is positioned as a patch on a patient's back to serve as a reference electrode. For the creation of high-density maps, the Intella-Map Orion catheter is used (**Fig. 1**). This bidirectional 8.5-French 8-spline basket catheter is designed for rapid collection of clear signals throughout the specific heart chamber. Sixty-four flat low-noise iridium-oxide coated microelectrodes are attached to these splines with an area of 0.4 mm^2 each and a distance of 2.5 mm. Each electrode can be located impedance-based and an additional magnetic field sensor at the catheter tip allows catheter localization with an accuracy of

less than 1 mm in space.[1] The diameter of the 23-mm–long basket-catheter can be varied between 3 mm and 22 mm, allowing adaptation to the respective anatomic conditions. The catheter can be used with both nonsteerable as well as steerable sheaths for better maneuverability. The Rhythmia HDx 0.01-mV noise floor uncovers signals that can not be visualized using standard mapping systems. Low background noise allows very good processing of low-amplitude signals, thus facilitating the discrimination of electrical tissue properties.[2]

During high-density mapping, numerous local electrograms (ECGs) are registered and processed in a short time. For Rhythmia there is no upper limit for the acceptance of point collection. The surface geometry of the heart chamber is created continuously using the location of the

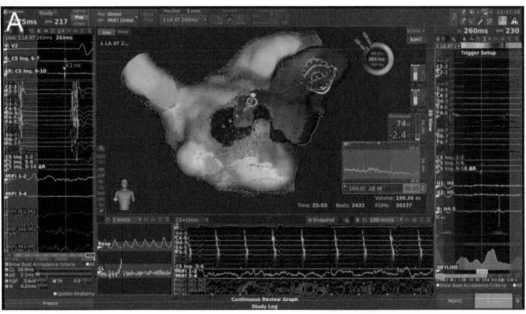

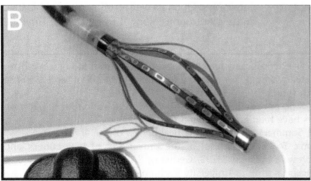

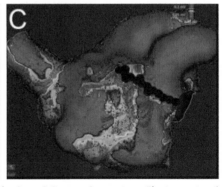

Fig. 1. Rhythmia. Ablation of atypical left atrial flutter using Rhythmia as 3-D mapping system. Electroanatomic reconstruction of the left atrium and LAT map (*A*) was performed with the INTELLAMAP ORION™ Mapping Catheter (Boston Scientific, Cambridge, Massachusetts) (*B*). The corresponding voltage map (*C*) shows low voltage areas of the anterior wall and the ablation line leading to termination of this tachycardia.

outermost electrodes, adapted to respiratory and cardiac cycles. The Rhythmia system offers a very efficient algorithm for automatic annotation. This annotation is based on defined 4 trigger criteria and 7 beat acceptance criteria. Trigger criteria tell the system which ECGs should be analyzed and which ones have to be filtered out. Acceptance criteria ensure efficient discrimination between a specific arrhythmia and other rhythm disturbances.[2] All criteria must be met for inclusion. The criteria described here include signal stability, cycle length, propagation of excitation front, respiratory phase, catheter movement, electrocardiogram (ECG) morphology, accuracy of localization, and ventricular signal overlap. This continuous automatic mapping is very accurate. Mantziari published in 2015 that 99.98% of all points were accurately annotated.[3] To determine the temporal activation, the Rhythmia system combines the acquisition of unipolar and bipolar signals, thus allowing for elimination of far-field signals. ECG timing is based on the maximum negative dV/dt of unipolar ECGs or maximum amplitude of bipolar signals. For fractionated signals, the temporal activation component of surrounding signals is included in the calculation.[4] Nevertheless, there is the possibility of manual annotation. After successful ablation the Rhythmia HDx validation mapping (vMap) feature can generate accurate validation maps in a short time to aid in assessing ablation, detecting gaps and confirming procedural endpoints.

The Rhythmia system with its rapid ultra–high-resolution electroanatomic mapping has proved itself in recent years, and the effectiveness and safety in the treatment of supraventricular and ventricular arrhythmias are well documented.[1,5] Hindricks and colleagues[6] demonstrated recently with the TRUE-HD study that both the rates of ablation-related complications and acute success by using Rhythmia were consistent with the range of reported adverse events for endocardial ablation of arrhythmias in the literature. The acute success rate depends from the type of arrhythmia and ranged from 64% to 96%. In direct comparison with another high-resolution mapping system, CARTO, there is no difference in terms of procedure duration and acute success in pulmonary vein isolation (PVI), only the time required for mapping was marginally longer.[7] There currently are no data available for direct comparison with the EnSite Precision system. The advantages of ultra–high-density mapping for differentiation of electrical tissue properties and the dynamics of ongoing arrhythmias are obvious; it does not seem to matter whether the map is created with an Orion catheter (Boston Scientific, Cambridge,

MA, USA), PentaRay catheter (Biosense Webster, Diamond Bar, CA, USA), or Advisor HD Grid Mapping Catheter, Sensor Enabled (Abbott, Chicago, IL, USA) (St. Jude Medical, Minnesota), catheter of other high-resolution mapping systems.

Unique for the Rhythmia system is the new Directsense technology, which uses the MicroFidelity (MiFi) electrode design of the IntellaNav MiFi open-irrigated ablation catheter to capture and show a local impedance measurement from a local electric field, which is generated at the tip of the catheter to provide a new dimension of data in ultra–high-resolution mapping. It allows the physician to monitor the impact of radiofrequency ablation in real time.[8] This technology differentiates the catheter from the also in 2018 launched IntellaNav ST Open-Irrigated Catheter. In the near future, the IntellaNav StablePoint catheter is expected, a navigation-enabled force-sensing catheter on a total tip cooling platform. Also released in 2018 was the Lumipoint Software Module for Rhythmia HDx, a first-ever suite of tools for automated map analysis, enabling rapid and high-confidence map interpretation.

TOPERA

The Topera Rotor Mapping system (Abbott Laboratories, Austin, Texas) includes the focal impulse and rotor modulation (FIRM) mapping as an interesting novel approach for interventional treatment of atrial fibrillation (AF). Despite promising initial results, the relevance of FIRM-guided ablation of AF remains unclear.

Rotors are considered a special form of reentry mechanism. In theory, as drivers, they could be responsible for the initiation of AF or be involved in its maintenance of AF.[9] The rotors assume a spiral shape revolving around a phase singularity.[10] Rotors can be formed when wavefronts pass over the tissue and interact with functional or anatomic barriers or tissue sections with different conduction properties. These rotors can occur fixed in place or move over the tissue.[11] The data and knowledge about rotors derive from computer models and studies on the hearts of sheeps. Special analyzes showed the existence of highly organized rotational drivers and their potential for the maintenance of AF.[12,13] Later, it also became apparent that the behavior of some K^+ channels also plays an important role in the dynamics of rotors and maintenance of persistent AF due to acceleration of reentrant sources.[14] Mapping and ablation of organized rotors at various atrial sites was initially studied in smaller human studies and could demonstrate long-term maintenance of sinus rhythm after ablation.[15] Nevertheless, later studies did not show stable rotor-like activity in humans during AF or in only a minority of cases.[16] To evaluate FIRM-guided ablation based on the assumption of rotors as drivers of AF in humans, the FIRM studies were initiated and provided us first results from prospective investigations in 2012.

Therefore, the Topera Rotor Mapping system was used, consisting of the RhythmView workstation, which processes and displays electrical rotors, the FIRMap Catheter, and the 64-electrode (distributed among 8 splines) contact mapping basket catheter for collecting intracardiac signals and generating rotor maps on existing geometry being created from a non-Topera 3-D mapping system.[17] Using a phase-mapping algorithm for analysis of repolarization and conduction properties, the software processes intracardiac signals to visualize rotational or focal activity triggering AF, thereby guiding targeted ablation (**Fig. 2**). FIRM filters ensure that far-field signals are filtered out using rate-related repolarization. Likewise, action potential data are used for the phase analysis.[18]

In 2012, Narayan and colleagues[17] published the successful identification of stable rotors or rotational impulses in 47 of 49 patients of a single-center cohort. In the same year, his group published the Conventional ablation for Atrial Fibrillation With or Without Focal Impulse and Rotor Modulation (CONFIRM) trial. In this 2-arm prospective case cohort study, 92 patients were treated either with FIRM-guided ablation and PVI or with PVI alone. Rotors could be identified in 97% of patients. The long-term efficacy after 273 days differed significantly; 82% of patients treated with FIRM-guided ablation plus PVI showed single-procedure freedom from AF compared with 45% in the PVI-only group.[19] Multicenter studies showed similar results in the following years.[20,21] Using a multicenter registry, Miller and colleagues[22] demonstrated in 2014 a single-procedure freedom rate from AF of 80.5% for all patients after 245 days (71.4% freedom from all atrial tachycardias). Rotors were seen in almost every patient.

Along with these early promising data, however, there also was increasing doubt to the effectiveness of FIRM-guided ablation. Benharash and colleagues[23] published in 2015 that FIRM-identified rotor sites did not exhibit quantitative atrial ECG characteristics expected from rotors and did not differ quantitatively from surrounding tissue. Ablation of these sites rarely led to organization or termination of AF. Several prospective multicenter studies in the following years also demonstrated a low success rate of FIRM-guided ablation with high recurrence rates of AF and AT in different observation periods.[24,25] In 2018, a meta analysis

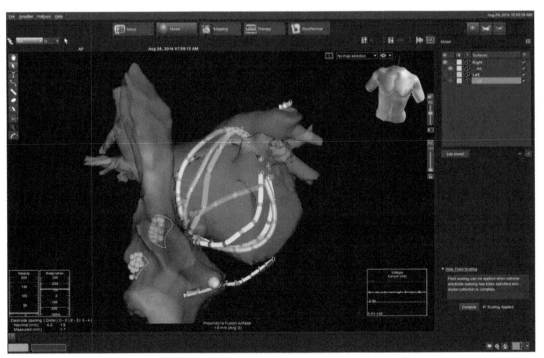

Fig. 2. Topera. FIRM with a 64-electrode basket catheter using Topera Rotor Mapping system and EnSite Precision. 3-D reconstruction of the right and left atrium is seen from an anterior view with splines of the basket catheter and ablated areas of rotors/focal impulses.

of Mohanty and colleagues[26] comparing therapeutic benefit of PVI plus FIRM approach with PVI alone did not show any benefit of this interesting attempt of substrate modification to increase the effectiveness of AF ablation. After a median follow-up of 16 months, the off-antiarrhythmic drugs pooled success rate was 50% in the FIRM plus PVI group and 58% in the PVI group.

These different outcome data may be due to operator-dependent experiences with this novel contact FIRM phase mapping or due to the basket catheter form, which does not achieve total topographic coverage of the heart chamber. Similarly, in some cases, a part of electrodes possibly had not sufficient tissue contact for a complete phase map.

The heterogeneous study situation is currently leading to uncertain evidence for the benefit of FIRM-guided ablation. Currently, no further centers are equipped with the Topera Rotor Mapping system. The ongoing clinical trials (RECONFIRM, REAFFIRM, REDO-FIRM, and SUBSTRATE) have to be awaited to be able to conclusively assess whether this approach represents a useful approach for treatment of cardiac arrhythmias.

EnSite PRECISION

The EnSite Precision has been available since 2016 and uses a hybrid impedance and magnetic field technology to accurately locate diagnostic and ablation catheters within the body. The resolution, accuracy, and stability of this system are much higher compared with the those of predecessors, EnSite NavX and EnSite Velocity. Besides CARTO 3, version 6 plus PentaRay catheter and Rhythmia HDx plus IntellaMap Orion catheter, EnSite Precision with its new HD Grid catheter supports automatic high-resolution mapping. The system consists of the following components: the EnSite Amplifier converts physiologic signals from the patient to digital signals for processing by the workstation, the Field Frame, the display workstation, and 8 surface electrodes (3 transthoracic pairs for 3 orthogonal axes and 2 patient reference sensors). It is, compared with other systems, an open platform with compatibility to almost any EP catheter. The proved EnSite NavX navigation and visualization technology of previous EnSite systems is used for impedance-based catheter tracking. An 8-kHz signal is sent alternately through each of the 3 pairs of surface patches for generating a voltage gradient in all 3 axes of space. Via the electrodes of the used catheter entering this voltage field, the voltage is measured and adjusted to the gradient that is generated by the 8-kHz signal in the X, Y, and Z axes. Additionally, EnSite Precision increases accuracy of less than 1 mm by adding magnetic field–based localization data to refine the impedance-based tracking in real-time. Catheters using this hybrid technology are marked with the addition, "Sensor Enabled." The use of this technology is possible due to an additionally used field frame attached under the catheter table, which generates a weak magnetic field. The magnetic field–based localization data are also used by the EnSite stability monitor to maintain the localization accuracy in case of unexpected changes of the impedance field.[27] With these technical possibilities, a very accurate electroanatomic reconstruction of the respective heart chamber can be created. In addition to a large number of possible catheters, the Advisor™ FL Circular Mapping Catheter is usually used for this purpose as capable circular mapping catheter (**Fig. 3**). Ablation catheters are available without contact force (CF) measurement (FlexAbility) or with this technology (TactiCath Quartz). The sensor-enabled version of TactiCath

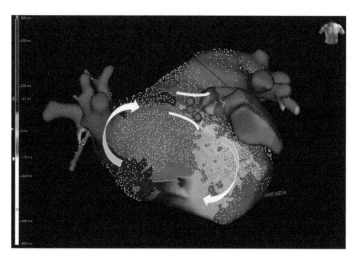

Fig. 3. Precision. LAT map created with EnSite Precision as 3-D mapping system for visualization of left atrial macroreentrent tachycardia. Image integration of MRI data set and fusion with electroanatomic map was performed. Left atrium is shown from an anterior-posterior view. The *white arrows* serve to illustrate the excitation process of this tachycardia. (*From* Sommer P. In times of HD mapping- how much EP do we still need? JACC Clin Electrophysiol 2018 Nov;4(11):1471–1472; with permission.)

CF ablation catheter was already approved in Europe and received Food and Drug Administration approval in the United States in January 2019. This 3.5-mm open-irrigated catheter consists of 6 irrigation holes with 0.4-mm diameter, 1 thermocouple for temperature measurement, and a CF sensor. This triaxial fiberoptic sensor is made up of 3 optical fibers and CF measurement is not influenced by the angle of acting force, leading to high accuracy of CF visualization during ablation.[28] After demonstrating that additional delivery of CF information during ablation correlates with lesion depth and size over time,[29] it could be proved in the following years that ablation with CF measurement offering TactiCath catheter improves outcome.[30,31] Ablation with at least 10 g should be performed for achieving rapid transmurality of the lesion.[31] For better lesion assessment, the EnSite Precision works with several indices providing a feedback about lesion quality. The force–time integral index was tested and presented by Shah and colleagues[29] in 2010 and the relevance of this FTI as independent predictor of outcome after ablation was proved in the touch for catheter ablation (TOCCATA) trial. The combination of several information to a lesion index, which is composed of CF, radiofrequency application duration, and radiofrequency current, has further improved the quality of lesion formation.[32] Therefore, an EnSite CF module was embedded in EnSite systems. The CF technology and the use of lesion assessment tools currently are elementary components of a modern ablation strategy.

In addition to this catheter technology and lesion assessment tools, however, EnSite Precision is able to annotate and visualize arrhythmias quickly and automatically. The system offers automation tools like EnSite AutoMap to reduce mapping time by creating addional maps besides recording anatomic acquisition. The new TurboMap feature can be used to quickly acquire maps of secondary arrhythmias. For creation of high-density maps, the new multipolar mapping catheter, Advisor HD Grid, Sensor Enabled, was developed and released in 2018. This diagnostic catheter allows bipole recording parallel and perpendicular to the splines via 16 electrodes. The catheter has been successfully used endocardially and epicardially. A few case reports have already been published.[33–35]

EnSite Precision also provides image integration tools. By using the EnSite Fusion Registration Module, magnetic resonance imaging (MRI) or computed tomography (CT) images can be fused with electroanatomic maps using fiducial corresponding points. The EnSite Verismo Segmentation Tool allows for segmentation and 3-D reconstruction of cardiac models from 2-D slice-based MRI or CT data.

The system is able to work with nonfluoroscopic catheter tracking systems like MediGuide.

This fact is important because today near-zero fluoroscopy has become a quality standard of interventional treatment of cardiac arrhythmia.[36]

CARTO

The CARTO 3 is a third-generation electroanatomic mapping system from Biosense Webster (Diamond Bar, California) currently available with software version 6. This system works with 3 separate low-level magnetic field (5 T $\times$ 10^{-6} T to 5 T $\times$ 10^{-5} T) emitting coils as part of 1 locator pad, which is fixed under the examination table. Together with 6 body patches, mapping catheters with an embedded magnetic location sensor, a graphic display, and a data processing unit allow the system to create a precise electroanatomic map in real time with high spatial resolution. Compared with other systems, CARTO uses hybrid current-based and magnetic information for catheter tracking and map visualization. The catheter localization is calculated by a triangulation algorithm. The catheter tips move through the 3 magnetic fields generated by the magnetic coils, allowing conclusions to be drawn about the position of the catheter and its orientation.

The accuracy is increased by including the current-based information in the calculation of catheter localization. Therefore, a small current is sent across the catheter electrode and is registered from the 6 body patches. Each electrode emits current at their own unique frequency. A current ratio is established for each coordinate by measuring the current at each point and allows the system to adjust the information received from the magnetic-based data. CARTO can display 6° of freedom (forward/back, up/down, left/right, yaw, pitch, and roll) and color-based visualization of catheter's current position, rotation, deflection, and direction of movement in real time. Artifacts caused by patient movement, cardiac activity, system movement, and respiration are compensated by using the back patches and the locator pad as location reference (body coordinate system). Additional information on breathing through using ACCURESP module can further minimize inaccuracies caused by respiratory artifacts.

For ablation of cardiac arrhythmias with the CARTO system, a variety of catheters is obtainable. These deflectable unidirectional or bidirectional therapeutic catheters are available in 3 sizes—4 mm, 8 mm (solid tips), and 3.5 mm (irrigated tip)—as well as different deflection curves. The surround flow technology, which is available for open-irrigated catheters, allows reduction of fluid for cooling of the catheter tip without trade-offs between signal resolution and power. Numerous diagnostic catheters can be used for derivation of intracardiac signals. Catheters of other manufacturers can be partially used with CARTO with a special connector. A total of 5 catheters can be displayed simultaneously.[27]

The development of numerous modules in recent years has shortened the procedure time, improved clinical outcomes, and reduced need for fluoroscopy.

With the launch of CARTO 3, the fast anatomic mapping became possible. The creation of the 3-D model during continuous movement of the mapping catheter shortened the procedure time and improved map resolution. The CONFIDENSE Mapping Module offers electrophysiologists a complete high-density mapping solution with automated data acquisition. Simultaneous electroanatomic data collection via multielectrode mapping catheters (LASSO or PentaRay) became possible. High-Definition (HD) Coloring, available since a few months, has further improved the interpolation and resolution of high-density maps (Video 1). The 3-D model is generated as a triangular mesh and converted into a grid of congruent cubic voxels (voxelization of a mesh). This Laplacian interpolation for calculation of other voxels and rendering of a high-resolution colored image has further increased the spatial resolution and accuracy. The extended version of CONFIDENSE Mapping Module with a continous pattern-matching filter enables users to selectively capture specific ventricular beats to treat premature ventricular contractions (PVCs) or even challenging ventricular tachycardias (VTs) fast and effectively. Later, the module was extended by Ripple mapping to compensate for inaccuracies in ECG annotation or incorrectly adjusted window of interest. It allows cardiologists to recognize the dominant direction of tachycardia propagation.

With the PaSo Module, the morphology of recorded PVC or part of the tachycardia can be compared with a morphology generated by focal stimulation. It is especially useful in cases with rare PVC or no reinducible tachycardias.

The decisive component for reduction of fluoroscopy was the launch of CartoUnivu. This image integration technology allows physicians to integrate a static fluoroscopy image with the 3-D map after initial registration. Dynamic sequences, such as coronary angiography, also can be integrated. Using CartoUnivu resulted in significantly reduced total fluoroscopy time and mean radiation dose without influencing procedure duration or ablation success rate. Another image integration tool is called Cartomerge. The system can fuse MRI/CT data set with the electroanatomic map and calculate ideal fusion of both models. The recently released CARTOSEG CT Segmentation Module provides a semiautomatic CT segmentation function and speeds up the workflow.[37] Centers with access to intracardiac ultrasound may perform left atrial interventions without need of fluoroscopy. CARTO combines multiple ECG-gated 2-D ultrasound cross-sections from a navigated SOUNDSTAR catheter to generate a 3-D model by using the CARTOSOUND Image Integration Module.[38]

With its built-in algorithm and standard workflow, the CARTOVISITAG Module allows electrophysiologists to focus on the ablation index value combining stability, CF, time, and power and, therefore, improve leasion quality.

Catheters of the Smarttouch series are used for ablation index–guided ablation. This type of 3.5-mm irrigated tip catheter measures the CF via a small precise spring located in the catheter shaft. The CF calculation is based on distance change between the magnetic transmitter coil and 3 location sensors with a known spring constant. Only very lateral acting forces lead to underestimation of CF in Smarttouch catheters.

With this equipment, the CARTO system offers sufficient options for the ablation of all arrhythmias (**Fig. 4**).

Soon, innovations such as COHERENCE Mapping (V7 platform) await us., with CARTO 3, version 7.[39,40] A color-based local activation time (LAT) map combined with direction vectors will revolutionize the presentation of the electrical impulse propagation. For faster detection of ablation targets, the CARTOFINDER 4D LAT Algorithm is being evaluated in patients with persistient AF.[41] CARTOFINDER collects electrical signals from multielectrode catheters like PentaRay or the new multielectrode catheter that is under development.[42–44] The VT tools that will allow the simultaneous acquisition of multiple morphologies in the sense of extended pattern matching also are expected.

On the side of catheter development, the QDOT MICRO catheter will provide further development of lesion formation. The catheter can work with high power and short duration (90 W for 4 seconds), presumably leading to shortening of procedure time. The technology is based on the Smarttouch SF catheter and also contains 56 irrigation holes but a wider tip shell (0.2 mm). Three proximal und 3 distal thermocouples are embedded in the catheter tip, with a distance from outer surface of 75 μm, allowing more

A

B

C

D

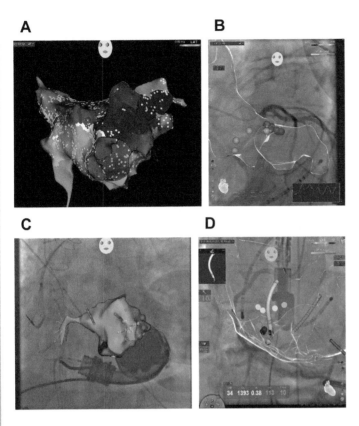

Fig. 4. CARTO. Illustration of using the CARTO3 mapping system for treatment of different arrhythmias. (*A*) LAT map of perimitral flutter with high-definition coloring in left anterior oblique 40° view. (*B*) Ablation of PVC from the LCC with use of CartoUnivu for visualization of sufficient distance to left coronary arteries. (*C*) LAT map and ablation of VT in a patient with left ventricular assist device. (*D*) Ablation of premature ventricular complex with epicardial origin. Right coronary artery angiography was integrated via CartoUnivu and helped to maintain a sufficient distance from this vessel during ablation. HD, high-definition; LCC, left coronary cusp.

accurate temperature measurement from the parts of the catheter tip in direct contact with cardiac tissue. An additional 3 microelectrodes with an surface area of 0.06 mm² each are embedded in the tip of the distal electrode.[45–47] The catheter can operate in temperature-controlled or temperature-limited mode. A special generator will be used that is capable of delivering high power and process temperature data several times per second (nGEN RF generator, Biosense Webster). The CARTO Vizigo bidirectional guiding sheath, which was released in 2018, can be visualized during ablation procedures on the map so there is no need for fluoroscopy to locate the catheter. The upgrade to CARTO 4 is expected in a few years. The new system possibly will be equipped with its own EP recording system.

SUMMARY

The modern 3-D mapping techniques and current catheter technology allow increasing accuracy and automation of electroanatomic reconstruction, annotation of intracardiac signals, and high quality of lesion formation. This increases ablation success with high safety for patients, while at the same time reducing the need of fluoroscopy. Intensive research in the field of invasive EP and

rapid adoption into innovative technologies have made this treatment method indispensable in cardiology in recent years and should further encourage making interventional therapy even faster, safer, and more successful.

ACKNOWLEDGMENTS

We thank Professor Christian Meyer from the University Hospital Hamburg for providing us illustrations of the Rhythmia system. We also thank Sebastian Riedel from Biosense Webster for careful reading of the CARTO section and the technical counseling.

SUPPLEMENTARY DATA

Supplementary data related to this article can be found online at https://doi.org/10.1016/j.ccep.2019.05.006.

REFERENCES

1. Sohns C, Saguner AM, Lemes C, et al. First clinical experience using a novel high-resolution electroanatomical mapping system for left atrial ablation procedures. Clin Res Cardiol 2016;105(12):992–1002.
2. Ellermann C, Frommeyer G, Eckardt L. High-resolution 3D mapping: opportunities and limitations of the

Rhythmia™ mapping system. Herzschrittmacherther Elektrophysiol 2018;29(3):284–92 [in German].

3. Mantziari L, Butcher C, Kontogeorgis A, et al. Utility of a novel rapid high-resolution mapping system in the catheter ablation of arrhythmias: an initial human experience of mapping the atria and the left ventricle. JACC Clin Electrophysiol 2015;1(5): 411–20.

4. Nakagawa H, Ikeda A, Sharma T, et al. Rapid high resolution electroanatomical mapping: evaluation of a new system in a canine atrial linear lesion model. Circ Arrhythm Electrophysiol 2012;5(2):417–24.

5. Viswanathan K, Mantziari L, Butcher C, et al. Evaluation of a novel high-resolution mapping system for catheter ablation of ventricular arrhythmias. Heart Rhythm 2017;14(2):176–83.

6. Hindricks G, Weiner S, Jais P, et al. Safety and acute effectiveness of the 3D RHYTHMIA mapping system for ablation of arrhythmias: results of the TRUE-HD study. EP Europace 2018;20(suppl_1):i101.

7. Rottner L, Metzner A, Ouyang F, et al. Direct comparison of point-by-point and rapid ultra-high-resolution electroanatomical mapping in patients scheduled for ablation of atrial fibrillation. J Cardiovasc Electrophysiol 2017;28(3):289–97.

8. Sulkin MS, Laughner JI, Hilbert S, et al. Novel measure of local impedance predicts catheter-tissue contact and lesion formation. Circ Arrhythm Electrophysiol 2018;11(4):e005831.

9. Vaquero M, Calvo D, Jalife J. Cardiac fibrillation: from ion channels to rotors in the human heart. Heart Rhythm 2008;5(6):872–9.

10. Wann D, Waks JW, Kramer DB. Clinical and regulatory considerations for novel electrophysiology mapping systems: lessons from FIRM. Pacing Clin Electrophysiol 2018;41(12):1669–80.

11. Waks JW, Josephson ME. Mechanisms of atrial fibrillation - reentry, rotors and reality. Arrhythm Electrophysiol Rev 2014;3(2):90–100.

12. Berenfeld O. Ionic and substrate mechanism of atrial fibrillation: rotors and the exitación frequency approach. Arch Cardiol Mex 2010;80(4):301–14.

13. Mansour M, Mandapati R, Berenfeld O, et al. Left-to-right gradient of atrial frequencies during acute atrial fibrillation in the isolated sheep heart. Circulation 2001;103(21):2631–6.

14. Atienza F, Almendral J, Moreno J, et al. Activation of inward rectifier potassium channels accelerates atrial fibrillation in humans: evidence for a reentrant mechanism. Circulation 2006;114(23): 2434–42.

15. Atienza F, Almendral J, Jalife J, et al. Real-time dominant frequency mapping and ablation of dominant frequency sites in atrial fibrillation with left-to-right frequency gradients predicts long-term maintenance of sinus rhythm. Heart Rhythm 2009; 6(1):33–40.

16. Lee S, Sahadevan J, Khrestian CM, et al. Simultaneous biatrial high-density (510-512 electrodes) epicardial mapping of persistent and long-standing persistent atrial fibrillation in patients: new insights into the mechanism of its maintenance. Circulation 2015;132(22):2108–17.

17. Narayan SM, Krummen DE, Rappel WJ. Clinical mapping approach to diagnose electrical rotors and focal impulse sources for human atrial fibrillation. J Cardiovasc Electrophysiol 2012;23(5): 447–54.

18. Maury P, Monteil B, Marty L, et al. Three-dimensional mapping in the electrophysiological laboratory. Arch Cardiovasc Dis 2018;111(6–7):456–64.

19. Narayan SM, Krummen DE, Shivkumar K, et al. Treatment of atrial fibrillation by the ablation of localized sources: CONFIRM (conventional ablation for atrial fibrillation with or without focal impulse and rotor modulation) trial. J Am Coll Cardiol 2012; 60(7):628–36.

20. Shivkumar K, Ellenbogen KA, Hummel JD, et al. Acute termination of human atrial fibrillation by identification and catheter ablation of localized rotors and sources: first multicenter experience of focal impulse and rotor modulation (FIRM) ablation. J Cardiovasc Electrophysiol 2012;23(12): 1277–85.

21. Narayan SM, Baykaner T, Clopton P, et al. Ablation of rotor and focal sources reduces late recurrence of atrial fibrillation compared with trigger ablation alone: extended follow-up of the CONFIRM trial (Conventional Ablation for Atrial Fibrillation with or without Focal Impulse and Rotor Modulation). J Am Coll Cardiol 2014;63(17):1761–8.

22. Miller JM, Kowal RC, Swarup V, et al. Initial independent outcomes from focal impulse and rotor modulation ablation for atrial fibrillation: multicenter FIRM registry. J Cardiovasc Electrophysiol 2014;25(9): 921–9.

23. Benharash P, Buch E, Frank P, et al. Quantitative analysis of localized sources identified by focal impulse and rotor modulation mapping in atrial fibrillation. Circ Arrhythm Electrophysiol 2015;8(3):554–61.

24. Gianni C, Mohanty S, Di Biase L, et al. Acute and early outcomes of focal impulse and rotor modulation (FIRM)-guided rotors-only ablation in patients with nonparoxysmal atrial fibrillation. Heart Rhythm 2016;13(4):830–5.

25. Mohanty S, Gianni C, Mohanty P, et al. Impact of rotor ablation in nonparoxysmal atrial fibrillation patients: results from the randomized OASIS trial. J Am Coll Cardiol 2016;68(3):274–82.

26. Mohanty S, Mohanty P, Trivedi C, et al. Long-term outcome of pulmonary vein isolation with and without focal impulse and rotor modulation mapping: insights from a meta-analysis. Circ Arrhythm Electrophysiol 2018;11(3):e005789.

27. Borlich M, Iden L, Kuhnhardt K, et al. 3D mapping for PVI- geometry, image integration and incorporation of contact force into work flow. J Atr Fibrillation 2018;10(6):1795.

28. Bourier F, Gianni C, Dare M, et al. Fiberoptic contact-force sensing electrophysiological catheters: how precise is the technology? J Cardiovasc Electrophysiol 2017;28(1):109–14.

29. Shah DC, Lambert H, Nakagawa H, et al. Area under the real-time contact force curve (force-time integral) predicts radiofrequency lesion size in an in vitro contractile model. J Cardiovasc Electrophysiol 2010;21(9):1038–43.

30. Reddy VY, Dukkipati SR, Neuzil P, et al. Randomized, controlled trial of the safety and effectiveness of a contact force-sensing irrigated catheter for ablation of paroxysmal atrial fibrillation: results of the TactiCath contact force ablation catheter study for atrial fibrillation (TOCCASTAR) study. Circulation 2015;132(10):907–15.

31. Kautzner J, Neuzil P, Lambert H, et al. EFFICAS II: optimization of catheter contact force improves outcome of pulmonary vein isolation for paroxysmal atrial fibrillation. Europace 2015;17(8):1229–35.

32. Neuzil P, Reddy VY, Kautzner J, et al. Electrical reconnection after pulmonary vein isolation is contingent on contact force during initial treatment: results from the EFFICAS I study. Circ Arrhythm Electrophysiol 2013;6(2):327–33.

33. Chow A, Khan F, Behar J, et al. 74Early experience using the adivsor HD grid to map atrial fibrillation. EP Europace 2018;20(suppl_4):iv33–4.

34. Sultan A, Steven D, Plenge T, et al. First endocardial mapping of the left ventricle using the AdvisorTM HD Grid Catheter in a patient with a mitral valve clip. Eur Heart J 2018;39(31):2911.

35. Bellmann B, Lüker J, Steven D, et al. First epicardial mapping of the left ventricle using the Advisor ™ HD Grid catheter. J Interv Card Electrophysiol 2018; 53(1):103–4.

36. Sommer P, Bertagnolli L, Kircher S, et al. Safety profile of near-zero fluoroscopy atrial fibrillation ablation with non-fluoroscopic catheter visualization: experience from 1000 consecutive procedures. Europace 2018;20(12):1952–8.

37. Imanli H, Bhatty S, Jeudy J, et al. Validation of a novel CARTOSEG™ segmentation module software for contrast-enhanced computed tomography-guided radiofrequency ablation in patients with atrial fibrillation. Pacing Clin Electrophysiol 2017;40(11): 1206–12.

38. den Uijl DW, Tops LF, Tolosana JM, et al. Real-time integration of intracardiac echocardiography and multislice computed tomography to guide radiofrequency catheter ablation for atrial fibrillation. Heart Rhythm 2008;5(10):1403–10.

39. Anter E, Duytschaever M, Shen C, et al. Activation mapping with integration of vector and velocity information improves the ability to identify the mechanism and location of complex scar-related atrial tachycardias. Circ Arrhythm Electrophysiol 2018; 11(8):e006536.

40. Bertagnolli L, Torri F, Richter S, et al. [Three-dimensional mapping : special aspects and new features of CARTO®]. Herzschrittmacherther Elektrophysiol 2018;29(3):259–63.

41. Honarbakhsh S, Schilling RJ, Providencia R, et al. Automated detection of repetitive focal activations in persistent atrial fibrillation: validation of a novel detection algorithm and application through panoramic and sequential mapping. J Cardiovasc Electrophysiol 2019;30(1):58–66.

42. Honarbakhsh S, Hunter RJ, Dhillon G, et al. Validation of a novel mapping system and utility for mapping complex atrial tachycardias. J Cardiovasc Electrophysiol 2018;29(3):395–403.

43. Verma A, Sarkozy A, Skanes A, et al. Characterization and significance of localized sources identified by a novel automated algorithm during mapping of human persistent atrial fibrillation. J Cardiovasc Electrophysiol 2018;29(11):1480–8.

44. Daoud EG, Zeidan Z, Hummel JD, et al. Identification of repetitive activation patterns using novel computational analysis of multielectrode recordings during atrial fibrillation and flutter in humans. JACC Clin Electrophysiol 2017;3(3):207–16.

45. Rozen G, Ptaszek L, Zilberman I, et al. Prediction of radiofrequency ablation lesion formation using a novel temperature sensing technology incorporated in a force sensing catheter. Heart Rhythm 2017; 14(2):248–54.

46. Barkagan M, Contreras-Valdes FM, Leshem E, et al. High-power and short-duration ablation for pulmonary vein isolation: safety, efficacy, and long-term durability. J Cardiovasc Electrophysiol 2018;29(9): 1287–96.

47. Leshem E, Tschabrunn CM, Jang J, et al. High-resolution mapping of ventricular scar: evaluation of a novel integrated multielectrode mapping and ablation catheter. JACC Clin Electrophysiol 2017;3(3): 220–31.

Noninvasive Mapping and Electrocardiographic Imaging in Atrial and Ventricular Arrhythmias (CardioInsight)

Ghassen Cheniti, MD[a,b,*], Stephane Puyo, PhD[b], Claire A. Martin, MD[a,b], Antonio Frontera, MD[a,b], Konstantinos Vlachos, MD[a,b], Masateru Takigawa, MD[a,b], Felix Bourier, MD[a,b], Takeshi Kitamura, MD[a,b], Anna Lam, MD[a,b], Carole Dumas-Pommier, PhD[a], Xavier Pillois, PhD[a], Thomas Pambrun, MD[a,b], Josselin Duchateau, MD[a,b], Nicolas Klotz, MD[a,b], Arnaud Denis, MD[a,b], Nicolas Derval, MD[a,b], Hubert Cochet, MD[b,c], Frederic Sacher, MD[a,b], Remi Dubois, PhD[b], Pierre Jais, MD[a,b], Meleze Hocini, MD[a,b], Michel Haissaguerre, MD[a,b]

KEYWORDS

• ECGI • Electrocardiographic imaging • Noninvasive mapping • Arrhythmias • Ablation

KEY POINTS

- Electrocardiographic imaging aims to noninvasively characterize cardiac electrical activity using signals collected from the torso to reconstruct epicardial potentials.
- Signals recorded by the system and included in the calculation should be checked manually to avoid errors related to automatic processing.
- Signals of good quality and high amplitude provide maps with the highest accuracy.
- Reentry is confirmed in the presence of local activation covering all the arrhythmia cycle length.
- Focal breakthroughs demonstrate a QS pattern associated to centrifugal activation; these mechanisms are typically unstable and transient.
- Electrocardiographic imaging offers a unique opportunity to better understand the mechanism of cardiac arrhythmias and to guide ablation.

INTRODUCTION

Electrocardiographic imaging (ECGI) is a mapping technique aiming to noninvasively characterize cardiac electrical activity. This approach uses signals collected from the torso to reconstruct epicardial potentials. Its efficacy has been demonstrated in a wide variety of clinical scenarios ranging from the mapping of premature ventricular complexes (PVCs) and accessory pathways (APs) to the mapping of complex arrhythmias including atrial and ventricular fibrillation (VF).[1,2] This approach allows guidance of catheter ablation and offers a unique

[a] Cardiac electrophysiology department, Hôpital Haut-Lévêque, 1 Magellan Avenue, Bordeaux, Pessac 33600, France; [b] Electrophysiology and Heart Modeling Institute (LIRYC), Bordeaux University, avenue Haut Leveque, Pessac 33600, France; [c] Department of Cardiovascular Imaging, Hôpital Haut-Lévêque, 1 Magellan Avenue, Bordeaux, Pessac 33600, France
* Corresponding author.
E-mail address: ghassen.chniti@gmail.com

Card Electrophysiol Clin 11 (2019) 459–471
https://doi.org/10.1016/j.ccep.2019.05.004
1877-9182/19/© 2019 Elsevier Inc. All rights reserved.

opportunity to better understand the mechanism of cardiac arrhythmias.

We review in this article the basics of ECGI, the different fields where it has proven efficient, and finally discuss the limitations of this approach.

PRINCIPLES OF NONINVASIVE MAPPING

Research related to noninvasive mapping commenced several decades ago, involving purely analytical studies,[3–5] torso tank[6–10] and large animal models,[11–13] followed by application in humans.[14–16] Mathematically, ECGI solves the inverse problem of electrocardiography that aims to locate on the epicardium the source of a signal recorded on the torso.[17–19]

Briefly, a 252-electrode vest is applied to the patient's torso and connected to the system (ECVue, Cardioinsight Technologies Inc, Cleveland, OH). A high-resolution noncontrast computed tomography scan is then performed, allowing the definition of cardiac anatomy and the position of each electrode on the torso. Atrial and/or ventricular

geometry are then reconstructed to obtain a three-dimensional mesh. This model serves for the projection of unipolar signals represented by virtual nodes of the epicardial surface. The collected signals are post processed using mathematical reconstruction algorithms[20,21] to create different maps, including activation maps, voltage maps, isopotential maps, and phase maps.

Activation maps are computed using intrinsic deflection-based methods from unipolar electrograms (maximal dV/dT).

Phase is calculated at each node using a dedicated Hilbert transform. The system uses reconstructed signals to calculate the phase of each signal ranging between $-\pi$ and π. The intersection between the depolarization and the repolarization isolines defines phase singularities.[22] Phase mapping allows identification of focal breakthrough, where activation starts from a discrete point and has a centrifugal spread, and reentry, where a wavefront rotates on itself within a localized area.

ECGI uses a standardized workflow (**Fig. 1**) where each step is critical for the following ones.

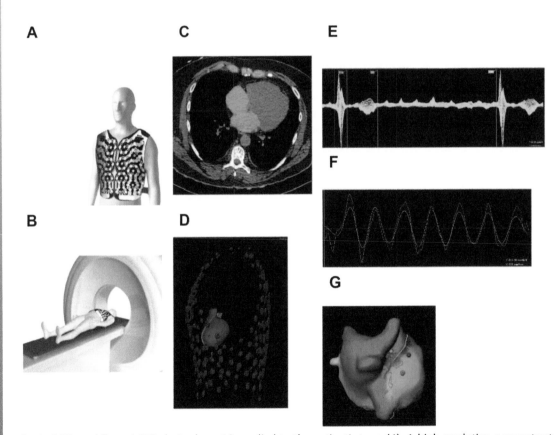

Fig. 1. ECGI workflow. A 252-electrode vest is applied to the patient's torso (*A*). A high-resolution noncontrast computed tomography scan is then performed (*B*), allowing the definition of cardiac anatomy (*C*) and the position of each electrode on the torso (*D*). The collected signals are post processed using mathematical reconstruction algorithms (*E*, *F*) and projected on the cardiac surface (*G*).

It is essential to ensure optimal workflow to acquire accurate results.

ATRIAL ARRHYTHMIAS
Atrial Fibrillation

Recent research has demonstrated that atrial fibrillation (AF) is mainly driven by localized sources, including focal and anatomic or functional reentries.[23] These sources are typically unstable and dynamic, which dramatically affects the results of point-by-point mapping.

Particularities of noninvasive mapping during atrial fibrillation

Atrial signals are of lower amplitude compared with ventricular signals. During AF, they are collected between the end of the T wave and the beginning of QRS. Pauses exceeding 1000 milliseconds are included in the analysis. The number of windows can be chosen at operator discretion. This analysis can be performed before the procedure. Intravenous diltiazem is infused in patients with rapid ventricular rates, in the absence of left ventricular dysfunction. Cumulative maps are used to locate the areas of focal breakthrough and reentrant drivers.

Results of noninvasive mapping

Cuculich and colleagues[24] first used ECGI to evaluate the mechanisms and complexity of AF in 26 patients. The authors analyzed paroxysmal and persistent AF episodes. The spatial accuracy for determining different pacing sites was 6 ± 4 mm. Multiple wavelets (defined as contiguous areas of epicardial activation lasting ≥ 5 milliseconds) were the most predominant pattern, representing 92% of fibrillatory activity. Rotor activity was present in 15% of cases, only in patients with nonparoxysmal AF. The authors defined a complexity index as the sum of the number of wavelets and focal activities and showed an increased complexity correlating with duration of AF (**Fig. 2**).

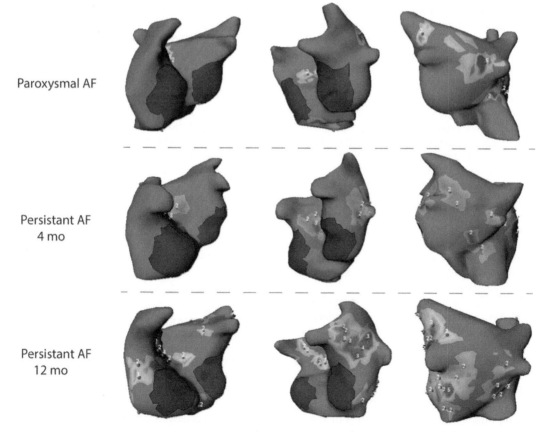

Fig. 2. Phase maps showing areas of reentrant activities in patients with different AF durations. The maps show and increase in the number of areas with rotational activities and the number of rotations associated to AF duration. (From Cheniti G, Vlachos K, Pambrun T, Hooks D, Frontera A, Takigawa M, et al. Atrial Fibrillation Mechanisms and Implications for Catheter Ablation. Front Physiol. 2018;9:1458; with permission.)

Data from our laboratory[15] reported the results of 103 patients with persistent AF (PsAF). Analysis of cumulative windows of 9 ± 1 seconds of AF was performed using phase mapping. Focal and reentrant activities were the main mechanisms identified by ECGI. AF complexity increased with AF duration, being driven by 2 to 3 regions during the first months and becoming biatrial in PsAF of longer duration. Reentrant drivers were located in the pulmonary vein antra and surrounding structures, the left atrial appendage and septum in nearly all the cases. Focal breakthroughs arose predominantly from the pulmonary vein ostia and left and right appendages.

In the prospective AFACART study,[25] ECGI was used to guide ablation in 118 patients with PsAF lasting less than 1 year. Reentrant activities were recorded in all patients and were more frequently located around the pulmonary veins, at the anterior interatrial groove and the posterior and inferior left atrium. Focal breakthroughs were mapped in 95% of the cases and were more commonly located in the pulmonary veins and both appendages. Ablation strategy consisted in targeting driver areas identified by ECGI, followed by pulmonary vein isolation and finally by linear ablation if the AF persisted. Driver-only ablation resulted in AF termination in 64% of cases after a mean radiofrequency time of 46 ± 26 minutes; additional pulmonary vein isolation and left atrial lines increased the success rate to 72%.

Lim and colleagues[26] prospectively recruited 105 consecutive patients referred for ablation of PsAF, including 32 patients in sinus rhythm, 45 patients with an AF duration of less than 12 months, and 28 patients in AF for more than 12 months. Phase mapping was used to characterize the AF complexity in each group. AF complexity significantly increased between the different groups, as attested by an increase in the number of reentries and focal activities and the number of regions harboring reentrant activities. ECGI-guided AF termination was 70%, being lowest in patients with the longest AF duration.

The effects of antiarrhythmic drugs were assessed in a group of 13 patients who underwent ablation for PsAF.[27] ECGI recordings were acquired before and after infusion of flecainide. Flecainide infusion reduced the number of regions that hosted reentrant activity (from 7 to 4 regions; $P<.001$). Importantly, AF terminated to sinus rhythm in 11 cases, involving targeting the regions remaining after flecainide infusion in 9 of the 11 cases. This result suggests that antiarrhythmic drugs select more stable and important regions that sustain AF. Similarly, amiodarone was used in patients with structural heart disease and PsAF, and resulted in AF termination with a shorter duration of radiofrequency.[28] In our practice, an antiarrhythmic drug is used before ablation for PsAF to limit the effects of the electrical remodeling.

Atrial Tachycardia

- ECGI can locate the source of focal atrial tachycardias (ATs). Wang and colleagues[29] successfully used ECGI to locate the origin of a left focal AT close to the septum. The site was confirmed by invasive mapping by recording diastolic potentials 58 milliseconds before the onset of the P wave. Local ablation terminated the tachycardia. Several more cases have reported the usefulness of ECGI in patients with focal ATs.[30]
- In addition, ECGI can also help to characterize macroreentrant AT. Wang and colleagues[31] used ECGI to characterize an atypical flutter that developed in a patient with a previous Cox maze surgical procedure.
- Shah and colleagues[32] performed a multicenter, prospective study to evaluate ECGI in 52 patients who presented with spontaneous or post-AF ablation ATs. ECGI correctly identified the mechanism of AT in 92% of the cases, including 85% of macroreentries and 100% of focal ATs. For macroreentrant AT, ECGI was most accurate in diagnosing peritricuspid and roof-dependent flutters; however, only 20% of perimitral flutters were identified successfully.
- In a recent study (HRS abstract C-AB32-04), Kitamura and colleagues[33] mapped 7 AT using high-density mapping (Rhythmia, Boston Scientific, Marlborough, MA) and ECGI. Activation mapping identified 2 focal ATs, 1 localized reentry, and 4 macroreentries. ECGI correctly identified the mechanism of AT in 6 of 7 ATs. Accuracy was greatest for focal ATs (**Fig. 3**).

VENTRICULAR ARRHYTHMIAS
Ventricular Fibrillation

VF is a major a cause of sudden death that may result from a range of cardiac diseases. Patients who survive after sudden cardiac death (SCD) remain at high risk of VF recurrence and of implantable cardioverter defibrillator shocks. Identifying the VF triggers and substrate and the sources that maintain VF offers a unique opportunity to better understand this fatal arrhythmia and prevent its recurrence.

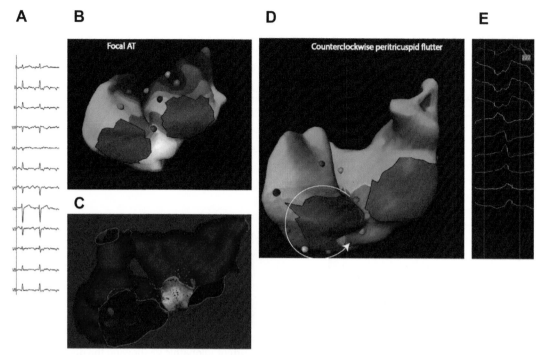

Fig. 3. (*A*) On the left, a patient with a focal AT originating from the ostium of the coronary sinus. The tachycardia is accurately diagnosed by ECGI (*B*) and confirmed by high-density invasive mapping (*C*). (*D*) On the right, a patient with a counterclockwise peritricuspid atrial flutter. Signals around the tricuspid annulus cover all the tachycardia cycle length (*E*).

Particularities of mapping during ventricular fibrillation

Ventricular signals have a higher amplitude than atrial signals. In our experience, signals recorded during VF are frequently of good quality, allowing accurate post processing. We perform a separate analysis for each VF episode. This process includes systematic mapping of spontaneous PVCs initiating VF, the definition of areas with abnormal epicardial signals during sinus rhythm, and the analysis of each VF episode using windows of different durations chosen at operator discretion. All abnormal signals and areas of interest identified by the system are checked during extensive biventricular and epicardial invasive mapping.

Mapping and ablation of idiopathic ventricular fibrillation

In a recent study, Haissaguerre and colleagues[16] demonstrated that almost two-thirds of patients with idiopathic VF have subclinical localized structural alterations. The authors evaluated 24 patients (mean age of 29 years) who survived idiopathic VF. They characterized VF drivers during the initial 5 seconds of spontaneous or induced VF. In addition, they performed high-density endocardial and epicardial biventricular mapping during sinus rhythm to identify subclinical substrates focusing on VF driver areas. A decapolar catheter was used to map the endocardium of the right and left ventricles, while 20-pole catheters with a 2-mm interelectrode spacing (Pentaray, Biosense, Webster, CA; Lasso, Biosense) were used for biventricular epicardial mapping.

A total of 19 VF episodes were analyzed. The mean VF cycle length was 183 ± 23 milliseconds including 28 ± 3 VF cycles. A mean of 2.8 ± 0.7 activities (including focal and reentrant activities) were recorded per cycle, being reentrant in 87% and focal in 13%.

A dominant ventricle, hosting more than 50% of activities, was identified in 9 patients and the rest demonstrated biventricular distribution of the fibrillatory activities (**Fig. 4**). Abnormal electrograms lasting 70 milliseconds or more and 3 or more spikes were seen in 15 of 24 patients (62.5%). These electrograms were predominantly located on the epicardium of the right ventricle (RV); they were arranged in a confluent pattern and covered a limited surface area (13 ± 6 cm^2), representing 5 ± 3% of the total ventricular surface area. They colocated with the driver regions in 76% of cases (*P*<.001; **Fig. 5**). The 9 patients without structural

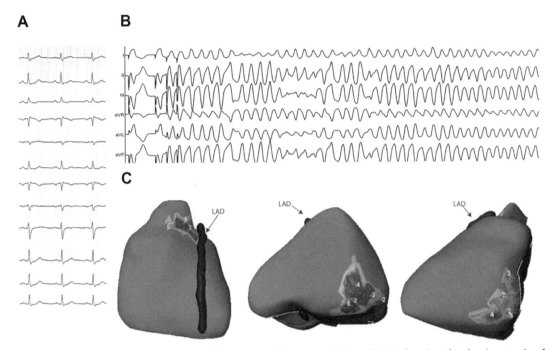

Fig. 4. Noninvasive mapping in a 59-year-old woman with recurrent idiopathic VF showing the dominant role of the left ventricle. (*A*) Normal 12-lead ECG. (*B*) VF induced by programmed ventricular stimulation from the right ventricle (RV). (*C*) Phase mapping identifies a cluster of reentrant activity located at the inferobasal left ventricular wall. This area was consistently identified in 2 episodes of VF and was targeted by endocardial ablation with a good outcome. LAD, left anterior descending. (*Reprinted by permission of Edizioni Minerva Medica from: Minerva Cardioangiologica 2018;66(1):75–82.*)

alterations had a high incidence of Purkinje triggers (7/9).

J wave syndromes

J wave syndromes include early repolarization syndrome (ERS) and Brugada syndrome (BS). Both conditions are associated with a higher vulnerability to ventricular arrhythmias and SCD and can coexist in the same patient.

Early repolarization syndrome ERS is defined as an ER pattern[34] (J point elevation of ≥1 mm in 2 contiguous inferior and/or lateral leads of a 12-lead ECG) and (1) a patient who has survived an SCD or (2) an SCD with a negative autopsy and medical chart review with a previous ECG. Nademanee and associates[36,37] (HRS 2018) performed high-density biventricular endocardial and epicardial mapping in 31 patients with ERS and a history of frequent VF episodes (between 2 and 150 VFs). The ER pattern was present in the inferolateral leads in 8 patients and only in the inferior leads in 23 patients. A Brugada pattern was also present in 23 patients. The authors identified low-voltage areas with fractionated signals in 22 of the 23 patients with BS

and ER patterns. These signals were epicardial and were recorded on the right ventricular outflow tract (RVOT) and inferior RV, and colocalized with VF drivers identified by ECGI. Ablation targeting abnormal areas was performed in this group, although patients without structural alterations underwent ablation of Purkinje triggers. Ablation prevented VF induction in 81% of the cases and was associated with VF freedom in 90% of cases after a median follow-up of 37 months.

This study allowed the identification of 2 mechanisms underlying the J wave syndromes.[35] The first one consists of delayed depolarization of the inferior RV that is predominantly found in the presence of concomitant BS and ERS. The second mechanism is a repolarization abnormality, either delayed repolarization (24%) or early repolarization (76%), that is mainly encountered in the absence of BS.

Brugada syndrome Nademanee and colleagues[36,37] first described the presence of epicardial substrate located on the RVOT. The authors recorded areas with low voltage, involving fragmented late potentials

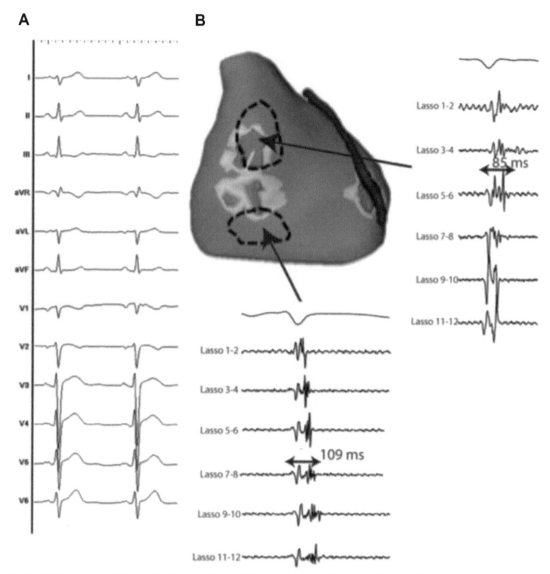

Fig. 5. (*A*) Phase map of the initial 5seconds of an idiopathic VF in a 37-year-old man. (*B*) The map shows areas of rotational activities on the anterior and lateral RV. (*C*) Epicardial signals acquired by high-density invasive mapping show fragmented and prolonged electrograms close to the driver site. (From Cheniti G, Vlachos K, Meo M, Puyo S, Thompson N, Denis A, et al. Mapping and Ablation of Idiopathic Ventricular Fibrillation. Frontiers in cardiovascular medicine. 2018;5:123; with permission.)

(96 ± 47 milliseconds beyond QRS) with long duration (132 ± 48 milliseconds) in 9 symptomatic patients with type 1 BS. Zhang and colleagues[38] used ECGI in 25 patients to characterize the substrate underlying BS in 25 patients with BS. The authors recorded delayed activation of the RVOT, where unipolar signals were fractionated and had a lower amplitude. In a recent study, Hocini and colleagues[47] (HRS 2017) analyzed VF drivers during 34 VF episodes that were recorded in 25 patients with BS. The mean number of VF episodes before ablation was 9 ± 10. The RV was dominant during the initial phase of VF in 76% of cases. VF drivers were mainly represented by focal breakthrough and figure of 8 reentries. RV drivers were predominant for 4.6 ± 3.2 seconds, after which VF drivers become biventricular. Endocardial and epicardial mapping recorded abnormal potentials located at the RVOT and the anterior RV in 17 cases. Ablation of the substrate was associated with VF freedom in 15 of 17 patients after 14 months of follow-up.

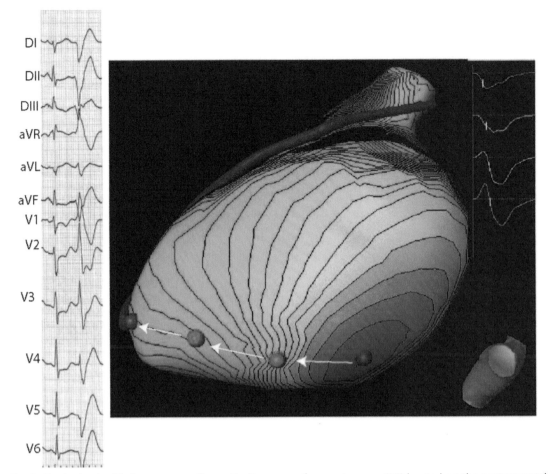

Fig. 6. Twelve-lead with the corresponding activation map of a spontaneous PVC located on the posteroseptal wall of the left ventricle.

Premature Ventricular Complexes and Ventricular Tachycardia

- ECGI has proven to be efficient in locating the origin of PVCs.[39,40] This role is particularly useful in patients with infrequent or transient PVCs and allows optimal scheduling of the procedure (**Figs. 6** and **7**)
- Cakulev and colleagues[40] used ECGi in 27 patients, including 10 patients with PVCs and 1 patient with focal VT. ECGI correctly located the origin of the arrhythmia in 9 of 11 cases and resulted in arrhythmia suppression in 2 patients who underwent ECGI-guided ablation alone in the absence of spontaneous PVCs during the case.
- Intini and colleagues[41] first used ECGI to guide diagnosis and therapy for focal VT in a young athlete. ECGI was used before the invasive procedure and correctly identified the origin of the VT that arose from a left ventricular apical diverticulum. Local unipolar signals at the site of origin showed a QS pattern consistent with an epicardial exit.
- Jamil-Copley and colleagues[39] recruited 24 patients with outflow tract PVCs. ECGI correctly identified the origin of the PVCs in 23 of 24 patients (RVOT = 18; LV outflow tract = 8) and sublocalized the origin of the PVCs in all cases.

Substrate Characterization in Patients with Adult Congenital Heart Diseases

Patients with adult congenital heart disease are at risk of atrial and ventricular arrhythmias. The complex anatomy and substrate in such patients represents a limitation to invasive mapping. Ernst and colleagues[42] used ECGI in 14 patients with adult congenital heart disease (mean age of 37 ± 18 years) to document clinical arrhythmia,

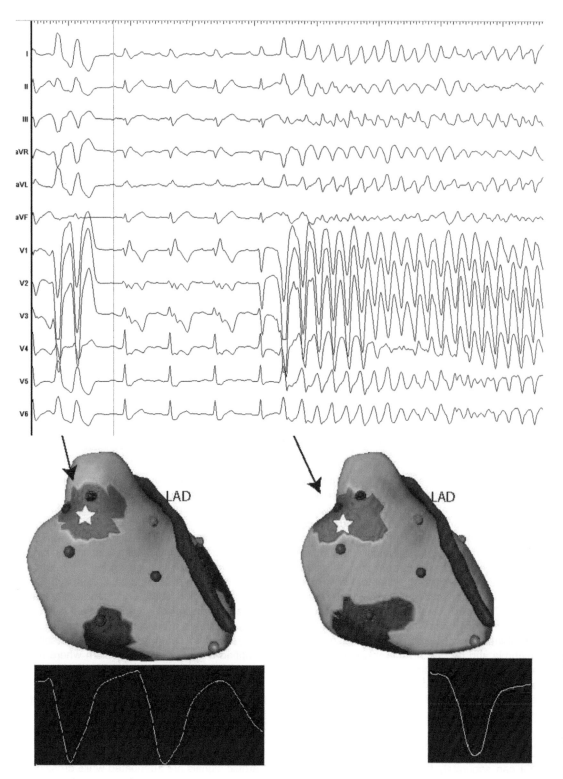

Fig. 7. Twelve-lead ECG and activation maps of spontaneous PVC in a 30-year-old man. PVCs. The PVC initiating the VF has a similar morphology (*right*) as the previous PVC (*left*) with subtle changes in the precordial leads (V2–V3). The PVC initiating the VF is located at the anterobasal RV (*white star*) that was targeted by ablation. LAD, left anterior descending.

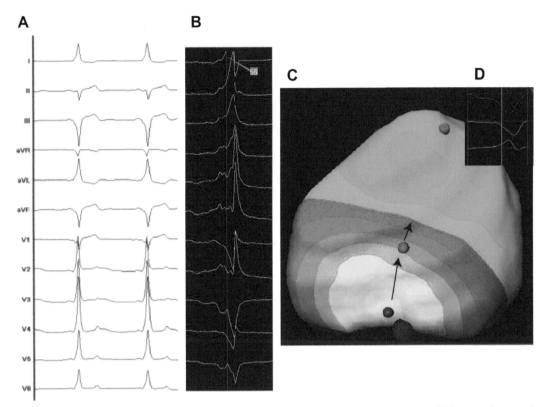

Fig. 8. Twelve-lead ECG (*A*) showing a posteroseptal pathway. Mapping of the delta wave (*B*) locates the ventricular insertion at the base of the interventricular septum (*C*). Local signals show a QS pattern with an early local activation (*D*).

inducible or spontaneously occurring, before invasive ablation. The underlying structural disease ranged from left atrial isomerism to tricuspid atresia with Fontan operation, aortic coarctation, and atrial switch for d-transposition of the great vessels. The majority of the patients had at least 1 failed sequential electrophysiologic study. ECGI correctly identified the chamber of origin in all cases, being the atria in 6 cases and the ventricles in 7 cases. One patient was excluded because no arrhythmia was recorded. ECGI facilitated ablation by showing the mechanism of the arrhythmia and by guiding the ablation. This role was particularly interesting in patients with multiple arrhythmias and a complex anatomy. After a median follow-up of 18 months, 64% of the patients remained in sinus rhythm.

Ventricular Preexcitation

ECGI can accurately locate APs (**Fig. 8**). Ghosh and colleagues[43] used ECGI to map 14 patients with Wolff–Parkinson–White syndrome. All AP locations were correctly identified by ECGI, corresponding with the site of successful ablation. AP were left lateral in 5 cases, posteroseptal in 4

case, right posteroseptal in 2 cases, mid septal in 1 case, right posterior in 1 case, and epicardial within a coronary sinus diverticulum in 1 case. Ghosh and colleagues[44] also reported successful AP ablation guided by ECGI in patients with structural heard disease, including congenital heart disease with univentricular heart, hypertrophic cardiomyopathy,[45] and Ebstein anomaly.[46]

Data from our laboratory[47] reported a patient with a right malignant AP and multiple failed ablation procedures. The combination of ECGI and high-resolution computed tomography scanning identified a right atrial diverticulum where the AP was located and facilitated catheter ablation.

LIMITATIONS OF ELECTROCARDIOGRAPHIC IMAGING

Noninvasive mapping has some limitations that should be considered to obtain optimal results. Cardiac signals are attenuated while crossing the thorax, leading to a blurred vision by the recording electrode on the torso. Subsequently, the recorded signals by each electrode on the torso represent the average of multiple signals. ECGI solves the inverse problem in electrocardiography,[48,49] but this

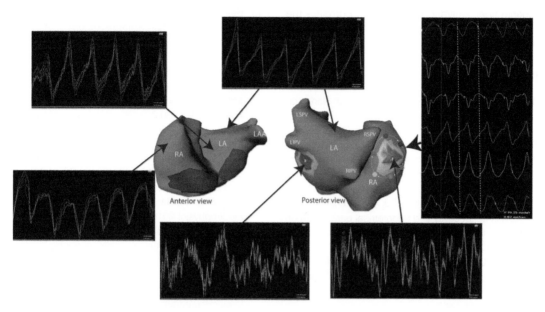

Fig. 9. Electrograms at the sites of reentrant activities show complex activities while signals in the remaining atria are organized. Right atrial signals are checked manually, confirming the presence of a local reentry with signals covering all AF cycle lengths. LA, left atrium; LAA, left atrial appendage; LIPV, left inferior pulmonary vein; LSPV, left superior pulmonary vein; RA, right atrium; RIPV, right inferior pulmonary vein; RSPV, right superior pulmonary vein. (From Cheniti G, Vlachos K, Pambrun T, Hooks D, Frontera A, Takigawa M, et al. Atrial Fibrillation Mechanisms and Implications for Catheter Ablation. Front Physiol. 2018;9:1458; with permission.)

process may lead to even small errors in the signals measured on the torso (measurement noise, electrode position, etc), resulting in very large errors in the reconstruction of the epicardial signals.

Performing activation mapping may have limitations that are demonstrated in a recent study performed by Duchateau and colleagues.[50] The authors evaluated the accuracy of activation maps acquired by automatic processing of the system in 55 patients and compared them with epicardial maps collected in the same patients. They concluded that the correlation between ECGI and invasive epicardial mapping was poor, as attested by the recording of fewer epicardial breakthroughs and the creation of false epicardial lines of block in areas of low voltages. Remapping, performed manually thereafter, successfully identified the epicardial breakthroughs with a mean of more than 2 breakthroughs per patient. In addition, areas with low voltage and septal signals represent a major limitation of this mapping technique and should be analyzed with caution. However, the correlation between ECGI and invasive mapping was good in patients with a wide QRS, either paced or owing to bundle branch block. This technique can therefore be used for better selection of candidates for cardiac resynchronization therapy.[51]

Phase mapping have some limitations.[52,53] First, this technique uses reconstructed signals, which should be of good quality for better calculation. The presence of noise may induce some errors during the reconstruction. Reentrant activities identified by the system do not preclude the presence of a rotor, as has been electrophysiologically described by optical mapping.[54] It identifies areas of complex activity surrounded by signal covering all the arrhythmia cycle length, suggesting the presence of a reentrant activity without specifying its mechanism (**Fig. 9**). To overcome these problems, local signals are checked manually to demonstrate the presence of a QS pattern for focal breakthrough and the presence of signals covering all the arrhythmia cycle length for reentrant activities.

SUMMARY

ECGI is a noninvasive mapping technique that has been proven efficient in treating and understanding the mechanisms of a wide variety of atrial and ventricular arrhythmias. An optimal workflow is mandatory to obtain optimal results. Signals recorded by the system and included in the calculation should be checked manually to avoid some errors related to automatic processing. Signals of good quality and high amplitude provide maps with the greatest accuracy. Further research aiming to record signals of high quality, better understand cardiac activation (eg, septal activation,

Purkinje fiber activation), and better correlate the maps with the underlying mechanism can improve the accuracy of ECGI.

REFERENCES

1. Shah A, Hocini M, Haissaguerre M, et al. Non-invasive mapping of cardiac arrhythmias. Curr Cardiol Rep 2015;17(8):60.

2. Frontera A, Cheniti G, Martin CA, et al. Frontiers in non-invasive cardiac mapping: future implications for arrhythmia treatment. Minerva Cardioangiol 2018;66(1):75–82.

3. Rudy Y, Plonsey R, Liebman J. The effects of variations in conductivity and geometrical parameters on the electrocardiogram, using an eccentric spheres model. Circ Res 1979;44(1):104–11.

4. Figuera C, Suarez-Gutierrez V, Hernandez-Romero I, et al. Regularization techniques for ECG imaging during atrial fibrillation: a computational study. Front Physiol 2016;7:466.

5. Svehlikova J, Teplan M, Tysler M. Geometrical constraint of sources in noninvasive localization of premature ventricular contractions. J Electrocardiol 2018;51(3):370–7.

6. Oster HS, Taccardi B, Lux RL, et al. Noninvasive electrocardiographic imaging: reconstruction of epicardial potentials, electrograms, and isochrones and localization of single and multiple electrocardiac events. Circulation 1997;96(3):1012–24.

7. Oster HS, Taccardi B, Lux RL, et al. Electrocardiographic imaging: noninvasive characterization of intramural myocardial activation from inverse-reconstructed epicardial potentials and electrograms. Circulation 1998;97(15):1496–507.

8. Shome S, Macleod R, editors. Simultaneous high-resolution electrical imaging of endocardial, epicardial and torso-tank surfaces under varying cardiac metabolic load and coronary flow. Berlin: Springer Berlin Heidelberg; 2007.

9. Ramanathan C, Rudy Y. Electrocardiographic imaging: II. Effect of torso inhomogeneities on noninvasive reconstruction of epicardial potentials, electrograms, and isochrones. J Cardiovasc Electrophysiol 2001;12(2):241–52.

10. Bear LR, Huntjens PR, Walton RD, et al. Cardiac electrical dyssynchrony is accurately detected by noninvasive electrocardiographic imaging. Heart Rhythm 2018;15(7):1058–69.

11. Liu C, Eggen MD, Swingen CM, et al. Noninvasive mapping of transmural potentials during activation in swine hearts from body surface electrocardiograms. IEEE Trans Med Imaging 2012;31(9):1777–85.

12. Cluitmans MJM, Bonizzi P, Karel JMH, et al. In vivo validation of electrocardiographic imaging. JACC Clin Electrophysiol 2017;3(3):232–42.

13. Bear LR, LeGrice IJ, Sands GB, et al. How accurate is inverse electrocardiographic mapping? A systematic in vivo evaluation. Circ Arrhythm Electrophysiol 2018;11(5):e006108.

14. Ghanem RN, Jia P, Ramanathan C, et al. Noninvasive electrocardiographic imaging (ECGI): comparison to intraoperative mapping in patients. Heart Rhythm 2005;2(4):339–54.

15. Haissaguerre M, Hocini M, Denis A, et al. Driver domains in persistent atrial fibrillation. Circulation 2014; 130(7):530–8.

16. Haissaguerre M, Hocini M, Cheniti G, et al. Localized structural alterations underlying a subset of unexplained sudden cardiac death. Circ Arrhythm Electrophysiol 2018;11(7):e006120.

17. Cluitmans M, Brooks DH, MacLeod R, et al. Validation and opportunities of electrocardiographic imaging: from technical achievements to clinical applications. Front Physiol 2018;9:1305.

18. Rudy Y, Messinger-Rapport BJ. The inverse problem in electrocardiography: solutions in terms of epicardial potentials. Crit Rev Biomed Eng 1988;16(3): 215–68.

19. Barr RC, Ramsey M 3rd, Spach MS. Relating epicardial to body surface potential distributions by means of transfer coefficients based on geometry measurements. IEEE Trans Biomed Eng 1977; 24(1):1–11.

20. Messinger-Rapport BJ, Rudy Y. The inverse problem in electrocardiography: a model study of the effects of geometry and conductivity parameters on the reconstruction of epicardial potentials. IEEE Trans Biomed Eng 1986;33(7):667–76.

21. Ramanathan C, Ghanem RN, Jia P, et al. Noninvasive electrocardiographic imaging for cardiac electrophysiology and arrhythmia. Nat Med 2004;10(4): 422–8.

22. Gray RA, Pertsov AM, Jalife J. Spatial and temporal organization during cardiac fibrillation. Nature 1998; 392(6671):75–8.

23. Cheniti G, Vlachos K, Pambrun T, et al. Atrial fibrillation mechanisms and implications for catheter ablation. Front Physiol 2018;9:1458.

24. Cuculich PS, Wang Y, Lindsay BD, et al. Noninvasive characterization of epicardial activation in humans with diverse atrial fibrillation patterns. Circulation 2010;122(14):1364–72.

25. Knecht S, Sohal M, Deisenhofer I, et al. Multicentre evaluation of non-invasive biatrial mapping for persistent atrial fibrillation ablation: the AFACART study. Europace 2017;19(8):1302–9.

26. Lim HS, Hocini M, Dubois R, et al. Complexity and distribution of drivers in relation to duration of persistent atrial fibrillation. J Am Coll Cardiol 2017;69(10): 1257–69.

27. Amraoui S, Pomier C, Sacher F, et al. 209-05: does flecainide pre-treatment helps to identify the most

important players? EP Europace 2016;18(suppl_1): i141–i.

28. Cheniti G, Takigawa M, Denis A, et al. 216-28: electrophysiological effects of amiodarone in patients with persistent atrial fibrillation. EP Europace 2016; 18(suppl_1). i148-i.

29. Wang Y, Cuculich PS, Woodard PK, et al. Focal atrial tachycardia after pulmonary vein isolation: noninvasive mapping with electrocardiographic imaging (ECGI). Heart Rhythm 2007;4(8):1081–4.

30. Yamashita S, Hooks DA, Cheniti G, et al. High-density contact and noninvasive mapping of focal atrial tachycardia: evidence of dual endocardial exits from an epicardial focus. Pacing Clin Electrophysiol 2018;41(6):666–8.

31. Wang Y, Schuessler RB, Damiano RJ, et al. Noninvasive electrocardiographic imaging (ECGI) of scar-related atypical atrial flutter. Heart Rhythm 2007; 4(12):1565–7.

32. Shah AJ, Hocini M, Xhaet O, et al. Validation of novel 3-dimensional electrocardiographic mapping of atrial tachycardias by invasive mapping and ablation: a multicenter study. J Am Coll Cardiol 2013; 62(10):889–97.

33. Kitamura T, Takigawa M, Martin R, et al. C-AB32-04. Validation of body surface mapping of atrial tachycardia by novel high density mapping. Heart Rhythm 2017;14(Suppl 5):S79–80.

34. Bourier F, Denis A, Cheniti G, et al. Early repolarization syndrome: diagnostic and therapeutic approach. Front Cardiovasc Med 2018;5:169.

35. Haissaguerre M, Nademanee K, Hocini M, et al. Depolarization versus repolarization abnormality underlying inferolateral J-wave syndromes: new concepts in sudden cardiac death with apparently normal hearts. Heart Rhythm 2019;16(5):781–90.

36. Nademanee K, Veerakul G, Chandanamattha P, et al. Prevention of ventricular fibrillation episodes in Brugada syndrome by catheter ablation over the anterior right ventricular outflow tract epicardium. Circulation 2011;123(12):1270–9.

37. Nademanee K, Hocini M, Haissaguerre M. Epicardial substrate ablation for Brugada syndrome. Heart Rhythm 2017;14(3):457–61.

38. Zhang J, Sacher F, Hoffmayer K, et al. Cardiac electrophysiological substrate underlying the ECG phenotype and electrogram abnormalities in Brugada syndrome patients. Circulation 2015;131(22):1950–9.

39. Jamil-Copley S, Bokan R, Kojodjojo P, et al. Noninvasive electrocardiographic mapping to guide ablation of outflow tract ventricular arrhythmias. Heart Rhythm 2014;11(4):587–94.

40. Cakulev I, Sahadevan J, Arruda M, et al. Confirmation of novel noninvasive high-density electrocardiographic mapping with electrophysiology study:

implications for therapy. Circ Arrhythm Electrophysiol 2013;6(1):68–75.

41. Intini A, Goldstein RN, Jia P, et al. Electrocardiographic imaging (ECGI), a novel diagnostic modality used for mapping of focal left ventricular tachycardia in a young athlete. Heart Rhythm 2005; 2(11):1250–2.

42. Ernst S, Saenen J, Rydman R, et al. Utility of noninvasive arrhythmia mapping in patients with adult congenital heart disease. Card Electrophysiol Clin 2015;7(1):117–23.

43. Ghosh S, Rhee EK, Avari JN, et al. Cardiac memory in patients with Wolff-Parkinson-White syndrome: noninvasive imaging of activation and repolarization before and after catheter ablation. Circulation 2008; 118(9):907–15.

44. Ghosh S, Avari JN, Rhee EK, et al. Noninvasive electrocardiographic imaging (ECGI) of a univentricular heart with Wolff-Parkinson-White syndrome. Heart Rhythm 2008;5(4):605–8.

45. Ghosh S, Avari JN, Rhee EK, et al. Hypertrophic cardiomyopathy with preexcitation: insights from noninvasive electrocardiographic imaging (ECGI) and catheter mapping. J Cardiovasc Electrophysiol 2008;19(11):1215–7.

46. Ghosh S, Avari JN, Rhee EK, et al. Noninvasive electrocardiographic imaging (ECGI) of epicardial activation before and after catheter ablation of the accessory pathway in a patient with Ebstein anomaly. Heart Rhythm 2008;5(6):857–60.

47. Hocini M, Shah AJ, Cochet H, et al. Noninvasive electrocardiomapping facilitates previously failed ablation of right appendage diverticulum associated life-threatening accessory pathway. J Cardiovasc Electrophysiol 2013;24(5):583–5.

48. Rudy Y. Noninvasive electrocardiographic imaging of arrhythmogenic substrates in humans. Circ Res 2013;112(5):863–74.

49. Tikhonov AN, Arsenin VY. On the solution of ill-posed problems. New York: John Wiley and Sons; 1977.

50. Duchateau J, Sacher F, Pambrun T, et al. Performance and limitations of noninvasive cardiac activation mapping. Heart Rhythm 2019;16(3):435–42.

51. Ploux S, Lumens J, Whinnett Z, et al. Noninvasive electrocardiographic mapping to improve patient selection for cardiac resynchronization therapy: beyond QRS duration and left bundle branch block morphology. J Am Coll Cardiol 2013;61(24):2435–43.

52. Umapathy K, Nair K, Masse S, et al. Phase mapping of cardiac fibrillation. Circ Arrhythm Electrophysiol 2010;3(1):105–14.

53. Nair K, Umapathy K, Farid T, et al. Intramural activation during early human ventricular fibrillation. Circ Arrhythm Electrophysiol 2011;4(5):692–703.

54. Pandit SV, Jalife J. Rotors and the dynamics of cardiac fibrillation. Circ Res 2013;112(5):849–62.

Contact Force and Ablation Index

Sohaib A. Virk, BMed, MD[a], Richard G. Bennett, MBBS[b], Ivana Trivic, BSc[a],
Timothy Campbell, BSc[a], Saurabh Kumar, MBBS, PhD[a],*

KEYWORDS

• Contact force • Radiofrequency ablation • Arrhythmias • Atrial fibrillation • Ablation index

KEY POINTS

- During radiofrequency ablation, the contact force (CF) exerted by the catheter on cardiac tissue is a key determinant of lesion quality and ablation efficacy.
- Excessive CF is associated with major complications, whereas insufficient CF increases the risk of electrical reconnection and arrhythmia recurrence.
- As traditional surrogate markers do not reliably correlate with actual CF, CF-sensing catheters have been developed that can directly measure CF in real-time.
- Randomized controlled trial data suggest the use of CF-sensing catheters does not reduce procedural durations, fluoroscopy exposure, incidence of procedural complications, or long-term arrhythmia recurrence.
- Further research is warranted to assess the clinical utility of novel markers of lesion quality such as ablation index, which incorporate CF with other ablation parameters.

INTRODUCTION

Radiofrequency ablation (RFA) has become an increasingly established treatment option for atrial and ventricular arrhythmias. The success of RFA is predicated on the formation of durable transmural lesions that maintain bidirectional conduction block between ablated sites and surrounding cardiac tissue. Despite improvements in ablation technologies and devices, long-term success rates for RFA remain suboptimal due to late recovery of ablated tissue. This limitation of contemporary RFA is best exemplified by the paradigm of pulmonary vein isolation (PVI) for atrial fibrillation (AF). Although electrical isolation of the pulmonary veins can almost always be achieved by the end of the procedure, late reconnection of at least one pulmonary vein occurs in up to 70% of cases

and this phenomenon is the primary driver of AF recurrence.[1] Consequently, following a single RFA procedure, freedom from AF is only seen in 54.1% and 41.8% of patients with paroxysmal and persistent AF, respectively, at long-term (≥3 year) follow-up.[2] Even in arrhythmias with more clearly elucidated mechanisms such as cavotricuspid isthmus–dependent atrial flutter, late recurrence of conduction is observed in up to one-fifth of patients, suggesting suboptimal lesion formation with contemporary RFA technologies.[3] Furthermore, in arrhythmias with more complex substrates such as ventricular tachycardia (VT) ablation, recurrence of VT can occur during follow-up in up to 50% of patients despite achievement of noninducibility at procedure end.[4]

Durable lesions form during RFA when irreversible tissue destruction occurs due to sufficiently

Disclosure Statement: The authors have nothing to disclose.
[a] Department of Cardiology, Westmead Hospital, Westmead Applied Research Centre, University of Sydney, Sydney, Australia; [b] Bristol Heart Institute, Bristol Royal Infirmary, Bristol, UK
* Corresponding author. Westmead Applied Research Centre, University of Sydney, Hawkesbury Road, Westmead, Sydney, New South Wales 2145, Australia.
E-mail address: saurabh.kumar@health.nsw.gov.au

1877-9182/19/© 2019 Elsevier Inc. All rights reserved.

high levels of thermal energy being directed at the target ablation site. Lesion size can thus be increased by using higher power to achieve greater electrode-tissue temperatures, increasing the duration of radiofrequency application, or by optimizing the contact force (CF) exerted by the catheter tip on cardiac tissue.[5] Catheter stability is also critical in maintaining efficiency of heat transfer, and instability has been shown to be strongly predictive of decreased lesion size.[6] Catheter stability is itself affected by several dynamics, including cardiac rhythm and the degree of cardiac or respiratory motion. Furthermore, even with the use of identical ablation settings, lesion sizes vary across different regions of the atria and ventricles, suggesting local tissue thickness and architecture also have a significant influence on lesion formation.[7]

CF, in particular, has been increasingly recognized as one of the most critical determinants of lesion quality during ablation. In recent years, efforts to optimize lesion formation and ablation efficacy have focused on the use of CF-sensing (CFS) technologies capable of providing real-time monitoring of catheter-tissue contact. This article reviews the role of CF in lesion formation, evaluates the evidence for use of emerging CF-sensing technologies, and explores potential avenues for optimizing CF data to improve clinical outcomes.

CONTACT FORCE AS A DETERMINANT OF LESION QUALITY

Preclinical studies have consistently shown that greater catheter tip-tissue contact leads to increased lesion size and higher frequency of transmural lesions during RFA.[8] Pooled data from animal studies show that lesion size increases linearly with CF for values less than 10g but that this correlation plateaus once CF exceeds 10 g, suggesting diminished gains at higher CF. This was further reinforced by a study of porcine models in which increasing CF beyond 20 g did not provide any further increase in lesion size or transmurality but resulted in greater degree of tissue edema on cardiac MRI.[9] Other studies using electrogram markers of transmurality have found an average CF greater than 16 g to be predictive of durable lesion formation.[10]

In the clinical realm, the multi-center EFFICAS I study showed CF to be a significant predictor of PV reconnection at 3 months following RFA for paroxysmal AF.[11] Median CF achieved during ablation was significantly higher in PV segments that remained isolated on repeat electrophysiology study compared with those displaying reconnection (19.5 g vs 15.5 g; $P = .02$). Based

on this data, a CF target of 20 g was derived and tested in a subsequent prospective trial, EFFICAS II.[12] Application of this CF target of 20 g improved the rate of PV isolation at 3 months from 72% in EFFICAS I to 85% in EFFICAS II ($P = .037$). Larger trials of patients with paroxysmal AF have demonstrated that the average CF achieved during RFA is also predictive of longer-term recurrence. In the multi-centre TOCCASTAR trial, AF recurrence at 12 months was 58.1% when CF was mostly greater than 10 g during ablation, compared with 75.9% when CF was predominantly less than 10g ($P < .001$).[13] Likewise, in a retrospective analysis of the TOCATTA trial, recurrence of AF was observed at 1 year in all cases in which average CF during ablation was less than 10g, but only 47% of cases in which average CF was 10 to 20 g and 20% of cases in which average CF was greater than 20 g ($P = .01$).[14] Conversely, in the SMART AF trial, the highest freedom from AF occurred within a tight CF range of 6.5 to 10.3 g, suggesting a U-shaped rather than a linear relationship between average CF and recurrence of AF.[15] This relationship may also be region specific, with studies showing higher CF is required to maintain electrical isolation in anterior and roof segments of the left atrium and lower CF being sufficient for ablation of posteroinferior pulmonary vein segments.[16]

Excessively high CF values have been associated with the occurrence of steam pops, perforations, thrombus formation, and increased risk of injuries to extracardiac structures such as the esophagus and phrenic nerve.[5] In one study of porcine models, the incidence of steam pops was only 3% when CF was 2 g but increased significantly to 17% when CF was 20g and to 37% when CF was raised to 60g.[17] In another preclinical study, there were no steam pops observed when ablation was performed at moderate power settings until CF exceeded 40 g.[18] Perforations have been induced in preclinical models at CF values as low as 38 g.[19] However, in clinical studies such as the TOCATTA trial, CF has often been seen to exceed 100g without associated perforation.[14] As such, the precise CF threshold beyond which the risk of complications is significantly increased remains unclear. This uncertainty is reflected in the most recent Heart Rhythm Society Consensus Document, which makes a class IIa recommendation for a "minimum targeted CF of 5 to 10 g" but does not inform a definitive upper limit.[20]

ASSESSMENT OF CONTACT FORCE

Traditionally, catheter tip-tissue contact was indirectly gauged by operators using surrogate measures such as tactile feedback, visual assessment of catheter motion, baseline electrogram amplitude, and impedance. However, these markers have been shown to be poor predictors of the actual CF exerted during ablation.[18,21] The use of traditional surrogate measures alone is associated with considerable intra- and interoperator variability, even amongst experienced electrophysiologists.[22] Furthermore, when relying on indirect markers of CF, operators often fail to detect excessively high CF and routinely overestimate CF at common regions of electrical reconnection, such as the ridge between the left atrial appendage and left pulmonary vein.

To address these limitations, CFS catheters have been developed that allow direct measurement of CF and provide operators with continuous real-time feedback to guide ablation. There are currently 2 major commercially available CFS catheters: the fibreoptic-based TactiCath (St Jude Medical Inc., St Paul, MN, USA) and the electromagnetic sensing ThermoCool SmartTouch (Biosense Webster Inc., Diamond Bar, CA, USA). Both catheters have been shown to be highly accurate and sensitive, providing CF measurements within an error margin of ~1g.[23,24]

The TactiCath catheter contains 3 optical fibers located between the electrodes of the catheter and its elastic polymer tip. The catheter tip undergoes microdeformations as it comes into contact with cardiac tissue, causing changes in the wavelength of infrared light transmitted by the optical fibers that are proportional to the magnitude of CF being applied.

The ThermoCool SmartTouch catheter has an ablation tip electrode that is mounted on a precision spring, which permits a small amount of deflection on contact with cardiac tissue. Magnetic sensor coils at the proximal end of the spring measure this deflection, which correlates with the CF being exerted by the catheter tip. The SmartTouch catheter can be integrated with the CARTO 3 (Biosense Webster Inc.) electroanatomic navigation system, allowing graphical and numerical displays of CF on the CARTO 3 screen in real-time.

IMPACT OF CONTACT-FORCE SENSING CATHETERS ON CLINICAL OUTCOMES: AN APPRAISAL OF THE EVIDENCE

Nonrandomized studies comparing CF-sensing catheters with standard catheters have largely reported promising results. In these observational studies, the use of CF-sensing catheters to guide AF ablation is associated with significantly shorter total procedure times, reduced ablation durations, and lower fluoroscopy exposure.[25–27] In one retrospective study including greater than 400 patients with AF, the incidence of major procedural complications (primarily cardiac tamponade) was significantly lower when PVI was performed with CF-sensing catheters.[28] Several observational studies have also found the use of CF-sensing catheters to increase rates of acute PV isolation and improve freedom from AF at long-term follow-up.[26,29,30]

Data from randomized controlled trials (RCTs) have not been as encouraging (**Table 1**).[13,31–36] To date, no RCT assessing the use of CFS catheters has been able to demonstrate a significant reduction in the incidence of major procedural complications or recurrence of AF at long-term follow-up. Although individual RCTs may have been underpowered to detect small differences in clinical endpoints, a recent meta-analysis of 9 RCTs (including > patients) confirmed the lack of improvement in either safety or efficacy of AF ablation using CF-sensing technologies.[37] Furthermore, data from current RCTs also suggest the use of CF-sensing catheters does not significantly shorten procedural durations or reduce fluoroscopy exposure. These negative findings were similar for patients with paroxysmal or persistent AF and also consistent regardless of whether the TactiCath or ThermoCool SmartTouch CFS catheters were used.

The discrepancies in findings by study design indicate the benefits of CF-guided ablation demonstrated in early observational reports may largely reflect inherent biases and confounders in these studies. Potential confounders include lack of blinding during outcome assessment, inconsistencies in follow-up, significant imbalances in baseline clinical characteristics, and differences in the use of image integration and mapping systems between CF- and non-CF–guided groups. Also, as CF-sensing catheters have only recently been introduced in many institutions, results of observational studies using noncontemporaneous control groups are likely to be influenced by significant temporal bias.

OPTIMIZING CONTACT FORCE DATA TO IMPROVE OUTCOMES

Although the availability of real-time CF data has not been shown to improve outcomes, this does not contradict the evidence demonstrating CF to be a significant determinant of lesion quality during ablation. Rather, the negative findings of current trials indicate deficiencies in how the data obtained from CF-sensing catheters is interpreted and applied. Of note, in several trials, the use of CFS catheters actually resulted in reduced CF

Table 1
Summary of randomized controlled trials assessing impact of contact force-sensing catheters on safety and efficacy of radiofrequency ablation of atrial fibrillation

| Study | Sample Size | AF Type (%) | | CFS Catheter | Target CF Range | Summary of Findings |
		Paroxysmal	Persistent			
Borregaard et al,[31] 2017	50	84	16	ThermoCool SmartTouch	10–40 g	At 12 mo, recurrence of AF not significantly different for CF-guided vs conventional ablation (36% vs 52%, $P = .2$). No significant difference in total procedure, RF ablation, or fluoroscopy durations. No major complications in either group.
Conti et al,[32] 2018	128	100	0	Thermocool SmartTouch	10–20 g	At 12 mo, single procedure freedom from AF similar for CF-guided vs conventional ablation (60% vs 63%; $P = $ NS). No significant difference in total procedure, RF ablation, or fluoroscopy durations. No major complications in either group.
Kimura et al,[33] 2014	38	74	26	Thermocool SmartTouch	10–20 g	At 6 mo, freedom from AF not significantly different for CF-guided vs conventional ablation (95% vs 84%; $P = .34$). Total procedure duration (59 vs 96 min; $P = .001$) significantly shorter in CF-guided ablation arm but fluoroscopy times not significantly different (9 vs 22 min; $P = $ NS). No major complications in either group.
Nakamura et al,[34] 2015	120	67	33	Thermocool SmartTouch	20 g	At 12 mo, freedom from AF similar for CF-guided vs conventional ablation (90% vs 88%; $P = .6$). Total procedure duration (50 vs 56 min; $P = .02$) significantly shorter in CF-guided ablation arm. Incidence of major complications not significantly different (5% in CF group vs 2% in non-CF group; $P = .3$).
Pedrote et al,[35] 2016	50	100	0	Thermocool SmartTouch	>10 g	At 12 mo, freedom from AF similar for CF-guided vs conventional ablation (84% vs 75%, $P = .4$). Total procedure (140 vs 158 min; $P = .04$) and fluoroscopy (21 vs 25 min; $P = .04$) durations significantly shorter in CF-guided ablation arm, but RF ablation times similar. No major complications in either group.

(continued on next page)

Table 1 (*continued*)						
		AF Type (%)			**Target CF**	
Study	**Sample Size**	**Paroxysmal**	**Persistent**	**CFS Catheter**	**Range**	**Summary of Findings**
Reddy et al,[13] 2015	295	100	0	TactiCath	NR	At 12 mo, freedom from AF similar for CF-guided vs conventional ablation (78% vs 81%; $P = .7$). Fluoroscopy (27 vs 23 min; $P = .04$) and RF ablation (47 vs 53 min; $P = .02$) durations significantly longer in CF-guided ablation arm. Incidence of major complications not significantly different (2% in CF group vs 1% in non-CF group; $P = NS$).
Ullah et al,[36] 2016	117	100	0	Thermocool SmartTouch	5–40 g	At 12 mo, freedom from AF similar for CF-guided vs conventional ablation (49% vs 52%; $P = .9$). No significant difference in total procedure, RF ablation, or fluoroscopy durations. Incidence of major complications not significantly different (3% in CF group vs 5% in non-CF group; $P = .7$).

Abbreviations: NR, not reported; NS, not significant; RF, radiofrequency.

variability during ablation and greater proportion of time spent within the target CF range, but this did not lead to improved freedom from AF.[33,34,36] The discordance between improved ability to titrate CF and lack of improved efficacy may reflect the absence of a clearly defined optimal CF value, and this is reflected in the broad spectrum of CF targets used in current RCTs, ranging from as low as 5 g to as high as 40 g. Furthermore, as CF is only one of several factors that determine lesion quality during ablation, it is likely that the optimal use of CF data is in combination with other ablation parameters such as RF duration and power.

Force-Time Integral

Force-time integral (FTI) is a marker of lesion quality that represents the product of CF and ablation duration. As such, FTI not only takes into account the catheter-tissue contact but also the period of time for which this is applied, thereby providing a measure of the spatiotemporal stability of contact. Retrospective analysis of clinical trials has found greater FTI values are associated with higher incidence of acute PV isolation.[32] Some prospective studies suggest FTI-guided ablation may also reduce the incidence of late PV reconnection, compared with CF-guided ablation, but these results have not been consistently reproduced.[12] As a marker of lesion quality, FTI has 2 fundamental limitations. Firstly, the actual interplay between CF and RF duration is dynamic and their relative contributions to lesion formation are more complex than the simple multiplication implied in the FTI formula. Secondly, FTI completely omits the role of power, which is a modifiable ablation parameter and critical determinant of lesion size.

Ablation Index

Ablation index (AI) is a novel marker of lesion quality that overcomes the deficiencies of FTI by incorporating CF, RF duration, and power in a weighted logarithmic formula. AI has been shown to be an extremely robust measure of lesion size in preclinical studies, predicting lesion depth with great precision.[5] In clinical studies, AI values have been shown to be a stronger and more significant predictor of PV reconnection than CF.[38] Initial prospective studies assessing the efficacy of ablation guided by AI targets have produced promising results. In one study of 40 patients with persistent AF undergoing AI-guided ablation, maintenance of sinus rhythm was seen in 95% of cases at 12 months.[39] Furthermore, in a propensity-matched analysis of 178 patients with paroxysmal AF, AI-guided ablation was found to be superior to CF-guided ablation in reducing the incidence of acute PV reconnection, major procedural complications, and recurrence of AF at 12 months.[38] Although these results are promising, the impact of AI-guided ablation on clinical outcomes has yet to be assessed in randomized trials.

SUMMARY

During radiofrequency ablation, catheter tip-tissue CF is a key determinant of lesion quality and ablation efficacy. Although CF-sensing catheters have been developed with the ability to accurately measure CF in real-time, their use has not been shown to improve the safety or efficacy of ablation in RCTs. Current trials of CF-guided ablation have been limited by poorly defined CF targets, and further research is warranted to provide consensus regarding the optimal CF parameters for ablation. AI is a promising marker of lesion quality that incorporates CF, power, and RF duration. Although observational data suggest AI-guided ablation may improve clinical outcomes, this remains to be evaluated in randomized trials.

REFERENCES

1. Kuck KH, Hoffmann BA, Ernst S, et al. Impact of complete versus incomplete circumferential lines around the pulmonary veins during catheter ablation of paroxysmal atrial fibrillation: results from the gap-atrial fibrillation-german atrial fibrillation competence network 1 trial. Circ Arrhythm Electrophysiol 2016; 9(1):e003337.
2. Ganesan AN, Shipp NJ, Brooks AG, et al. Long-term outcomes of catheter ablation of atrial fibrillation: a systematic review and meta-analysis. J Am Heart Assoc 2013;2(2):e004549.
3. Sawhney N, Anand K, Robertson CE, et al. Recovery of mitral isthmus conduction leads to the development of macro-reentrant tachycardia after left atrial linear ablation for atrial fibrillation. Circ Arrhythm Electrophysiol 2011;4(6):832–7.
4. Mallidi J, Nadkarni GN, Berger RD, et al. Meta-analysis of catheter ablation as an adjunct to medical therapy for treatment of ventricular tachycardia in patients with structural heart disease. Heart Rhythm 2011;8(4):503–10.
5. Ariyarathna N, Kumar S, Thomas SP, et al. Role of contact force sensing in catheter ablation of cardiac arrhythmias: evolution or history repeating itself? JACC Clin Electrophysiol 2018;4(6):707–23.
6. Shah DC, Lambert H, Nakagawa H, et al. Area under the real-time contact force curve (force-time integral) predicts radiofrequency lesion size in an in vitro contractile model. J Cardiovasc Electrophysiol 2010;21(9):1038–43.
7. Kistler PM, Ho SY, Rajappan K, et al. Electrophysiologic and anatomic characterization of sites resistant to electrical isolation during circumferential pulmonary vein ablation for atrial fibrillation: a prospective study. J Cardiovasc Electrophysiol 2007;18(12):1282–8.
8. Okumura Y, Johnson SB, Bunch TJ, et al. A systematical analysis of in vivo contact forces on virtual catheter tip/tissue surface contact during cardiac mapping and intervention. J Cardiovasc Electrophysiol 2008;19(6):632–40.
9. Williams SE, Harrison J, Chubb H, et al. The effect of contact force in atrial radiofrequency ablation: electroanatomical, cardiovascular magnetic resonance, and histological assessment in a chronic porcine model. JACC Clin Electrophysiol 2015; 1(5):421–31.
10. Kumar S, Chan M, Lee J, et al. Catheter-tissue contact force determines atrial electrogram characteristics before and lesion efficacy after antral pulmonary vein isolation in humans. J Cardiovasc Electrophysiol 2014;25(2):122–9.
11. Neuzil P, Reddy VY, Kautzner J, et al. Electrical reconnection after pulmonary vein isolation is contingent on contact force during initial treatment: results from the EFFICAS I study. Circ Arrhythm Electrophysiol 2013;6(2):327–33.
12. Kautzner J, Neuzil P, Lambert H, et al. EFFICAS II: optimization of catheter contact force improves outcome of pulmonary vein isolation for paroxysmal atrial fibrillation. Europace 2015;17(8):1229–35.
13. Reddy VY, Dukkipati SR, Neuzil P, et al. Randomized, controlled trial of the safety and effectiveness of a contact force-sensing irrigated catheter for ablation of paroxysmal atrial fibrillation: results of the TactiCath contact force ablation catheter study for atrial fibrillation (TOCCASTAR) study. Circulation 2015;132(10):907–15.
14. Reddy VY, Shah D, Kautzner J, et al. The relationship between contact force and clinical outcome during radiofrequency catheter ablation of atrial fibrillation in the TOCCATA study. Heart Rhythm 2012;9(11):1789–95.
15. Reddy VY, Pollak S, Lindsay BD, et al. Relationship between catheter stability and 12-month success after pulmonary vein isolation: a subanalysis of the SMART-AF trial. JACC Clin Electrophysiol 2016; 2(6):691–9.

16. Sotomi Y, Kikkawa T, Inoue K, et al. Regional difference of optimal contact force to prevent acute pulmonary vein reconnection during radiofrequency catheter ablation for atrial fibrillation. J Cardiovasc Electrophysiol 2014;25(9):941–7.

17. Thiagalingam A, D'Avila A, Foley L, et al. Importance of catheter contact force during irrigated radiofrequency ablation: evaluation in a porcine ex vivo model using a force-sensing catheter. J Cardiovasc Electrophysiol 2010;21(7):806–11.

18. Ikeda A, Nakagawa H, Lambert H, et al. Relationship between catheter contact force and radiofrequency lesion size and incidence of steam pop in the beating canine heart: electrogram amplitude, impedance, and electrode temperature are poor predictors of electrode-tissue contact force and lesion size. Circ Arrhythm Electrophysiol 2014;7(6): 1174–80.

19. Quallich SG, Van Heel M, Iaizzo PA. Optimal contact forces to minimize cardiac perforations before, during, and/or after radiofrequency or cryothermal ablations. Heart Rhythm 2015;12(2):291–6.

20. Calkins H, Hindricks G, Cappato R, et al. 2017 HRS/EHRA/ECAS/APHRS/SOLAECE expert consensus statement on catheter and surgical ablation of atrial fibrillation. Heart Rhythm 2017;14(10):e275–444.

21. Nakagawa H, Kautzner J, Natale A, et al. Locations of high contact force during left atrial mapping in atrial fibrillation patients: electrogram amplitude and impedance are poor predictors of electrode-tissue contact force for ablation of atrial fibrillation. Circ Arrhythm Electrophysiol 2013;6(4):746–53.

22. Kuck KH, Reddy VY, Schmidt B, et al. A novel radiofrequency ablation catheter using contact force sensing: toccata study. Heart Rhythm 2012;9(1): 18–23.

23. Bourier F, Gianni C, Dare M, et al. Fiberoptic contact-force sensing electrophysiological catheters: how precise is the technology? J Cardiovasc Electrophysiol 2017;28(1):109–14.

24. Bourier F, Hessling G, Ammar-Busch S, et al. Electromagnetic contact-force sensing electrophysiological catheters: how accurate is the technology? J Cardiovasc Electrophysiol 2016;27(3):347–50.

25. Itoh T, Kimura M, Tomita H, et al. Reduced residual conduction gaps and favourable outcome in contact force-guided circumferential pulmonary vein isolation. Europace 2016;18(4):531–7.

26. Nair GM, Yeo C, MacDonald Z, et al. Three-year outcomes and reconnection patterns after initial contact force guided pulmonary vein isolation for paroxysmal atrial fibrillation. J Cardiovasc Electrophysiol 2017;28(9):984–93.

27. Sigmund E, Puererfellner H, Derndorfer M, et al. Optimizing radiofrequency ablation of paroxysmal and persistent atrial fibrillation by direct catheter force measurement-a case-matched comparison in 198 patients. Pacing Clin Electrophysiol 2015; 38(2):201–8.

28. Akca F, Janse P, Theuns DA, et al. A prospective study on safety of catheter ablation procedures: contact force guided ablation could reduce the risk of cardiac perforation. Int J Cardiol 2015;179:441–8.

29. Deubner N, Greiss H, Akkaya E, et al. Clinical experience with contact-force and flexible-tip ablation catheter designs. J Interv Card Electrophysiol 2016;47(1):75–82.

30. Hussein AA, Barakat AF, Saliba WI, et al. Persistent atrial fibrillation ablation with or without contact force sensing. J Cardiovasc Electrophysiol 2017;28(5): 483–8.

31. Borregaard R, Jensen HK, Tofig BJ, et al. Is the knowledge of contact force beneficial in pulmonary vein antrum isolation? Scand Cardiovasc J 2017; 51(3):129–37.

32. Conti S, Weerasooriya R, Novak P, et al. Contact force sensing for ablation of persistent atrial fibrillation: a randomized, multicenter trial. Heart Rhythm 2018;15(2):201–8.

33. Kimura M, Sasaki S, Owada S, et al. Comparison of lesion formation between contact force-guided and non-guided circumferential pulmonary vein isolation: a prospective, randomized study. Heart Rhythm 2014;11(6):984–91.

34. Nakamura K, Naito S, Sasaki T, et al. Randomized comparison of contact force-guided versus conventional circumferential pulmonary vein isolation of atrial fibrillation: prevalence, characteristics, and predictors of electrical reconnections and clinical outcomes. J Interv Card Electrophysiol 2015;44(3):235–45.

35. Pedrote A, Arana-Rueda E, Arce-Leon A, et al. Impact of contact force monitoring in acute pulmonary vein isolation using an anatomic approach. A randomized study. Pacing Clin Electrophysiol 2016;39(4):361–9.

36. Ullah W, McLean A, Tayebjee MH, et al. Randomized trial comparing pulmonary vein isolation using the SmartTouch catheter with or without real-time contact force data. Heart Rhythm 2016;13(9):1761–7.

37. Virk SA, Ariyaratnam J, Bennett RG, et al. Updated systematic review and meta-analysis of the impact of contact force sensing on the safety and efficacy of atrial fibrillation ablation: discrepancy between observational studies and randomized control trial data. Europace 2019;21(2):239–49.

38. Hussein A, Das M, Chaturvedi V, et al. Prospective use of Ablation Index targets improves clinical outcomes following ablation for atrial fibrillation. J Cardiovasc Electrophysiol 2017;28(9):1037–47.

39. Hussein A, Das M, Riva S, et al. Use of ablation index-guided ablation results in high rates of durable pulmonary vein isolation and freedom from arrhythmia in persistent atrial fibrillation patients. Circ Arrhythm Electrophysiol 2018;11(9):e006576.

Noninvasive Cardioablation

Marwan M. Refaat, MD, FHRS, FESC, FRCP[a],[*],[1], Patrick Zakka, MD[b],[1], Bassem Youssef, MD[c], Youssef H. Zeidan, MD, PhD[c], Fadi Geara, MD, PhD[c], Amin Al-Ahmad, MD[d]

KEYWORDS

- Radioablation • Ablation • Cardiac ablation • Noninvasive • Arrhythmia • Atrial fibrillation
- Ventricular tachycardia

KEY POINTS

- Stereotactic body radiotherapy uses the principle of 3-dimensional localization of a target to deliver a high dose of radiation to a precise location.
- The aim of this technique is to ablate tissue noninvasively.
- Because of its high precision and target conformity, it can deliver a high dose of radiation to a specific area in a tissue without significantly affecting nearby tissues.
- It is being actively studied, and even used in therapy for atrial fibrillation and ventricular tachycardia.

INTRODUCTION

Stereotactic radiosurgery (SRS) uses the principle of 3-dimensional localization of a target to deliver a high dose of radiation to a precise location. The aim of this technique is to ablate tissue noninvasively. Because of its high precision, it can deliver a high dose of radiation to a specific area in a tissue without significantly affecting nearby tissue. Stereotactic body radiotherapy (SBRT) was first introduced in the early 1950s, using a system known as Gamma Knife, where a spherical dose of radiation from a multitude of Cobalt sources focused on a target volume of tissue in the brain, with the main limitation that it could not be used for targets outside the head.[1] Later, in the mid-1980s, "linear accelerator"–based radiosurgery

was introduced. These systems used X rays instead of the gamma rays, which were used in the Gamma Knife system. A stereotactic frame is used to create 3-dimensional coordinates of a specific tissue location where radiation would be delivered. This system initially required the frame to be fitted onto the skull of a patient. In the 1990s, CyberKnife was developed and allowed submillimeter accuracy, but more importantly later became able to be used for extracranial targets.[2]

SBRT uses high-dose radiation (usually 25–30 Gy) delivered to a target tissue point causing local tissue destruction, likely from double-strand breaks in DNA causing apoptosis and vascular damage resulting in ischemia. Unlike standard catheter ablation procedures (radiofrequency ablation, cryoablation), which produce immediate

---

Disclosures: None.

Funding Sources: None.

[a] Cardiovascular Fellowship Program, Department of Internal Medicine, Cardiology Division, Cardiac Electrophysiology Section, American University of Beirut Faculty of Medicine and Medical Center (AUBMC), PO Box 11-0236, Riad El-Solh, Beirut 1107 2020, Lebanon; [b] Department of Internal Medicine, Emory University Hospital, 550 Peachtree Street Northeast, Atlanta, GA 30308, USA; [c] Department of Radiation Oncology, American University of Beirut Medical Center, PO Box 11-0236, Riad El-Solh, Beirut 1107 2020, Lebanon; [d] Texas Cardiac Arrhythmia Institute, St David's Medical Center, 919 East 32nd Street, Austin, TX 78705, USA

[1] Authors contributed equally to this article.

* Corresponding author. Department of Biochemistry and Molecular Genetics, American University of Beirut Faculty of Medicine and Medical Center (AUBMC), PO Box 11-0236, Riad El-Solh, Beirut 1107 2020, Lebanon.

E-mail addresses: mr48@aub.edu.lb; marwanrefaat@alumni.harvard.edu

Card Electrophysiol Clin 11 (2019) 481–485

https://doi.org/10.1016/j.ccep.2019.05.008
1877-9182/19/© 2019 Elsevier Inc. All rights reserved.

results, SBRT can take up to months to show results.

Recently, SBRT has been used on the heart to create cardiac lesions with the aim to ablate cardiac arrhythmias noninvasively. This review discusses how SBRT has progressed in the treatment of cardiac arrhythmia.

STEREOTACTIC BODY RADIOTHERAPY ON THE HEART

The potential of success of SBRT relies mainly on its noninvasive nature. For drug-refractory arrhythmias, cardiac ablation can be an effective strategy but is not always successful because of complications secondary to the invasive nature of the procedure and the substrate that is either not easily ablated or not accessible from a percutaneous approach. Bipolar ablation may be unable to deliver enough energy to the intended target to ablate. Sympathectomy and stellate ganglion block are not always effective and could have neuroautonomic side effects.[3] A challenge to radiation therapy is to adjust for cardiac motion from both respiration and the cardiac cycle. Techniques have been developed to compensate for respiratory motion, and to track the location of the target throughout both the cardiac and the respiratory cycle and create an internal target volume; such as, for instance, the use of a 4-dimensional computed tomography (**Box 1**).

Feasibility studies of radiation ablation on the heart were initially done on a swine model. Targets included were the cavotricuspid isthmus, atrioventricular (AV) node, pulmonary vein-left atrial junction, or left atrial appendage. The dose of radiation used in this study was 25 Gy. The ablation was successful in producing bidirectional cavotricuspid isthmus block and AV nodal block. Pulmonary vein–left atrial junction and left atrial appendage also significantly decreased in voltage. Electrophysiologic (EP) effects were seen at approximately 90 days after ablation. Histologic specimens of ablated tissue showed vacuoles, fibrosis, and calcification. Surrounding tissues did not show any damage from radiation.[4]

A group of researchers who have initially brought forth data on radiation ablation using isolated Langendorff-perfused beating heart preparations also demonstrated that ablation can cause permanent interruption of impulse propagation in different locations in the heart. Lehmann and colleagues[5] studied 17 swine and targeted the AV node, right superior pulmonary vein, left atrial junction, and free-wall left ventricle. Three different doses of radiation were used (25, 40, and 55 Gy). Dose dependency was seen because 25 Gy

> **Box 1**
> **Steps followed in noninvasive ablation of ventricular tachycardia**
>
> 1. Anatomic scar imaging (MRI)
> 2. Nuclear imaging (Thallium-201 single-photon emission computed tomography, Rubidium-82 PET)
> 3. EP mapping: 3-dimensional electroanatomical catheter-derived map or electrocardiogram (ECG) imaging map
> 4. Creation a clinical target volume identifying arrhythmogenic scar substrate
> 5. Imaging fiducial marker for respiratory tracking: existing ICD lead or insertion of a temporary pacing wire
> 6. Creation an internal target volume with respiratory motion compensation and with cardiac motion compensation during phases of the cardiac cycle (systole and diastole)
> 7. Development of a radiation treatment plan targeting the scar
> 8. Positioning, simulation with imaging, and aligning of the patient
> 9. Treatment with a single fraction ablative dose of x-ray radiation energy of 25 Gy on the targeted area from a linear accelerator in a shielded room
> 10. Monitor patient with ECG via a closed-circuit TV

produced subtle fibrotic changes, whereas 40 and 55 Gy produced significant fibrotic response. No damage was seen in surrounding tissues, and there was no change in left ventricular ejection fraction after 6 months of follow-up. No skin reaction was seen at the entry point of the radiation beam. In all targets, they were successfully able to produce interruptions in cardiac impulse propagation resulting in EP change.

Linear accelerator-based SRS was tested in vivo in AV node ablation in an intact swine model. SRS doses ranging from 35 to 40 Gy were delivered by a linear accelerator to the AV node. All pigs had disturbances of AV conduction with progressive transition into complete heart block. Macroscopic inspection did not reveal damage to the myocardium, and pigs had preserved systolic function on echocardiography. Immunostaining revealed fibrosis in the target region of the AV node, whereas no fibrosis was detected in the nontargeted regions.[6,7] In a study by Lehman and colleagues[8] in 2017, AV nodal ablation was successfully achieved in 6 out of 7 irradiated swine in dose groups of 25,

40, 50, and 55 Gy, and no short-term side effects were observed. Histologic studies did show in-field beam effects outside of the target volume, but no damage was observed in tissues of the esophagus, trachea, or phrenic nerves.

STEREOTACTIC BODY RADIOTHERAPY AND VENTRICULAR TACHYCARDIA

The origin of ventricular arrhythmia often occurs in areas of myocardial scar. During routine invasive cardiac ablations, areas of scar can be identified during catheter mapping using electroanatomic mapping systems, where scars are noted as low-voltage regions. This information is used when choosing targets for SBRT. Because the growing interest is to noninvasively ablate substrate, noninvasive techniques can be used to identify myocardial scars (computed tomography or echo-cardiography, nuclear perfusion imaging, PET, or contrast-enhanced MRI).[9] In addition, noninvasive electroanatomic mapping with electrocardio-graphic imaging can identify location and depth of ventricular tachycardia (VT) origin in patients.[10,11]

SBRT for cardiac arrhythmia is now termed stereotactic arrhythmia radioablation (STAR). Loo and colleagues[12] reported the first in-human treatment of cardiac arrhythmia using STAR. In the patient with myocardial scar, a dose of 33 Gy targeted the center of the scar, with a dose falloff to 25 Gy at the border of the scar that is thought to be the origin of the VT. Significant decrease in VT burden was seen in this patient after the proced-ure. The patient did have recurrent VT 9 months af-ter STAR treatment, so it was thought that the transient reduction in VT may have been because of underdosing of radiation. Cvek and col-leagues[13] used the CyberKnife SRS on a patient

with malignant VT, and after the 120-day follow-up period, there were no more episodes of malig-nant arrhythmia detected.

Robinson and colleagues[14] conducted SBRT on 19 patients who had both drug and routine ablation refractory VT. A single treatment dose of 25 Gy was used. Endpoints included reported median number of VT episodes in the 6 months before ablation compared with the 6 months after ablation, which were reduced from 119 to 3. Implantable cardioverter-defibrillator (ICD) shocks were also reduced from 4 to 0, and antitachycardia pacing therapies were reduced from 81 to 3.5. The 2 pa-tients with premature ventricular contraction (PVC)-induced cardiomyopathy had their PVC burden significantly reduced. Overall survival at 1 year was 72% (3 deaths were related to recurrent VT).

Cuculich and colleagues[15] published a study on 5 patients with refractory VT (failed 2 antiarrhythmic drugs and had at least 1 traditional invasive ablation or contraindication to ablation). Patients received a single 25-Gy dose of radiation to target tissue. The procedure results in a significant decrease in VT burden with a strong short-term safety profile.

EP-guided noninvasive cardiac radioablation (ENCORE) was used for VT and myocardial perfor-mance assessed after the procedure. Global myocardial function was preserved after a year, with some cases of actual improvement in left ventricular ejection fraction likely because of decreased burden of VT.[16] Noninvasive electrophysiology-guided cardiac radioablation in the phase 1/2 ENCORE-VT trial of 19 patients was associated with markedly reduced ventricular arrhythmia burden with modest short-term risks, reduction in antiarrhythmic drug use, and improve-ment in quality of life.[14] **Table 1** summarizes studies of SBRT in VT management.

Table 1
Summary of stereotactic body radiotherapy studies in ventricular tachycardia and atrial fibrillation

Arrhythmia	Author	Target	Dose, Gy	Endpoint
VT	Cvek et al[13]	Scar in a patient	25	No episode after 120 d
VT	Loo et al,[12] 2015	Scar in a patient	33 (center), 25 (border)	Decrease in VT burden, recurrence in 9 mo
VT	Cuculich et al,[15] 2017	5 patients	25	Decrease in VT burden
VT	Robinson et al,[14] 2019	19 patients	25	Decreased median number of VT episodes in 6 mo
AF	Bode et al,[18] 2015	8 mini-pigs	22.5–40	Complete pulmonary vein isolation with 40 Gy
AF	Zei et al,[19] 2018	17 canines/2 swine	25–35	Pulmonary vein isolation (partial effect with 15–20 Gy)

STEREOTACTIC BODY RADIOTHERAPY AND ATRIAL FIBRILLATION

Feasibility studies are being performed for the treatment of atrial fibrillation (AF) by targeting pulmonary vein tissue using SBRT. Before this was possible, it was important to prove that doses of radiation targeting the pulmonary veins did not affect ventricular tissue and result in scarring that will ultimately promote arrhythmia. Gardner and Weidlich[17] demonstrated that dose of radiation that is received in the ventricles when targeting radiation to the pulmonary veins was below the standard acceptable threshold for heart dose in single fraction spine treatments.

Bode and colleagues[18] isolated pulmonary veins by stereotactic radioablation in a study on 8 mini-pigs delivering circumferential doses of 22.5 to 40 Gy to the target vein antrum. Complete block of atrioventricular electrical conduction occurred in the 40-Gy treatment group, and histology confirmed that transmural scarring occurred throughout the entire target circumference, leading to pulmonary vein isolation.

Zei and colleagues[19] assessed the safety and efficacy of SBRT in targeting pulmonary vein antral tissues in experimental models (17 adult canines and 2 adult swine) using 4 different treatment doses (15, 20, 25, and 35 Gy). Treatment effects were seen in all treated pulmonary veins in the 35- and 25-Gy groups. Partial effects were seen in the 2 lower-dose treatment groups. Two animals underwent histopathologic study, where there was evidence of circumferential transmural scar at the pulmonary vein ablation sites without damage to surrounding structures.

Cardiac stereotactic radioablation has great potential for therapy in AF and has been portrayed to be more cost-effective than current treatment options for AF.[20] **Table 1** summarizes studies of SBRT in AF.

ADVERSE EVENTS REPORTED WITH CARDIAC STEREOTACTIC BODY RADIOTHERAPY

Complications that have been reported with SBRT on the heart include pericarditis, pericardial effusions, and radiation pneumonitis.[14] Fatigue and hypotension that required change in antihypertensive regimen have also been reported. Collateral damage to surrounding tissues has not been consistently seen (no papillary muscle dysfunction or new conduction abnormalities). Radiation ablation has also not been shown to have significant effect on ICDs. Long-term effects are still unclear not only because of this technique being novel but also because radiation ablation has been mainly used as palliative therapy in patients who have poor long-term survival rates.

SUMMARY

SBRT for cardiac ablation is being shown to be both effective and relatively safe as a noninvasive technique for refractory arrhythmia. It is especially useful in patients in which direct catheter-based approaches are not possible because of inaccessible substrate. Patients who either fail or cannot undergo endocardial/epicardial ablations generally do not have other promising options. Cardiac SBRT could address most of these limitations. This new modality has its limitations, including the lack of long-term efficacy/safety data and delayed effect. Although SBRT takes months to have an effect, there may be some unknown early effects with VT episodes stopping within days of therapy. It is still not used as an early therapeutic option and is still being used when other modalities fail. Although stereotactic radioablation is currently heavily being studied in arrhythmia, there may be potential applicability to other cardiac conditions, such as ablating tissue in hypertrophic cardiomyopathy (left ventricular outflow obstruction).

REFERENCES

1. Leksell L. An historical vignette. Radiosurgery: baseline and trends. New York: Raven Press; 1992. p. 257–61.
2. Kurup G. CyberKnife: a new paradigm in radiotherapy. J Med Phys 2010;35(2):63–4.
3. Zei P, Mak R. Noninvasive stereotactic radioablation for ventricular tachycardia: ENCORTE-VT (EP-guided noninvasive cardiac radioablation): is the sequel as good as the original? Circulation 2019; 139(3):322–4.
4. Sharma A, Wong D, Weidlich G, et al. Noninvasive stereotactic radiosurgery (CyberHeart) for creation of lesions in the atrium. Heart Rhythm 2010;7(6): 802–10.
5. Lehmann HI, Graeff C, Simoniello P, et al. Feasibility study on cardiac arrhythmia ablation using high-energy heavy ion beams. Sci Rep 2016;6:38895.
6. Refaat MM, Ballout JA, Zakka P, et al. Swine atrioventricular node ablation using stereotactic radiosurgery: methods and in vivo feasibility investigation for catheter-free ablation for cardiac arrhythmias. J Am Heart Assoc 2017;6(11) [pii: e007193].
7. Ramia P, Hilal L, Geara FB, et al. Stereotactic radiosurgery for atrioventricular node ablation in swine: a study on efficacy and dosimetric evaluation of

organs at risk. Int J Radiat Oncol Biol Phys 2018; 102(3):e435.

8. Lehman HI, Deisher AJ, Takami M, et al. External arrhythmia ablation using photon beams. Ablation of the atrioventricular junction in an intact animal model. Circ Arrhythm Electrophysiol 2017;10(4): e004304.

9. John RM, Shinohara ET, Price M, et al. Radiotherapy for ablation of ventricular tachycardia: assessing collateral dosing. Comput Biol Med 2018;102: 376–80.

10. Wang Y, Cuculich PS, Zhang J, et al. Noninvasive electroanatomic mapping of human ventricular arrhythmias with electrocardiographic imaging. Sci Transl Med 2011;3(98):98ra84.

11. Zhang J, Cooper DH, Desouza KA, et al. Electrophysiologic scar substrate in relation to VT: noninvasive high-resolution mapping and risk assessment with ECGI. Pacing Clin Electrophysiol 2016;39(8): 781–91.

12. Loo BW Jr, Soltys SG, Wang L, et al. Stereotactic ablative radiotherapy for the treatment of refractory cardiac ventricular arrhythmia. Circ Arrhythm Electrophysiol 2015;8(3):748–50.

13. Cvek J, Neuwirth R, Knybel K, et al. Cardiac radiosurgery for malignant ventricular tachycardia. Cereus 2014;6(7):e190.

14. Robinson CG, Samson PP, Moore KMS, et al. Phase I/II trial of electrophysiology-guided noninvasive cardiac radioablation for ventricular tachycardia. Circulation 2019;139(3):313–21.

15. Cuculich PS, Schill MR, Kashani R, et al. Noninvasive cardiac radiation for ablation of ventricular tachycardia. N Engl J Med 2017;377(24):2325–36.

16. Cuculich P, Kashani R, Mutic S, et al. Myocardial performance after EP-guided noninvasive cardiac radioablation (ENCORE) for ventricular tachycardia (VT). Int J Radiat Oncol Biol Phys 2017;99(2S): e511–2.

17. Gardner EA, Weidlich GA. Analysis of dose distribution in the heart for radiosurgical ablation of atrial fibrillation. Cureus 2016;8(7):e703.

18. Bode F, Blanck O, Gebhard M, et al. Pulmonary vein isolation by radiosurgery: implications for noninvasive treatment of atrial fibrillation. Europace 2015;17(12):1868–74.

19. Zei PC, Wong D, Gardner E, et al. Safety and efficacy of stereotactic radioablation targeting pulmonary vein tissues in an experimental model. Heart Rhythm 2018;15(9):1420–7.

20. Bhatt N, Turakhia M, Fogarty T. Cost-effectiveness of cardiac radiosurgery for atrial fibrillation: implications for reducing health care morbidity, utilization, and costs. Cureus 2016;8:e720.

Radiofrequency Balloon Devices for Atrial Fibrillation Ablation

Carola Gianni, MD, PhD[a], Qiong Chen, MD[a,b], Domenico Della Rocca, MD[a],
Uğur Canpolat, MD[a,c], Hüseyin Ayhan, MD[a,d], Bryan MacDonald, MD[a],
Sanghamitra Mohanty, MD[a,e], Chintan Trivedi, MD[a],
Andrea Natale, MD[a,e,f,g,h,i], Amin Al-Ahmad, MD[a],*

KEYWORDS

- Radiofrequency • Balloon-based ablation • Atrial fibrillation • Pulmonary vein isolation

KEY POINTS

- Radiofrequency catheter ablation for pulmonary vein isolation is a challenging procedure, because maneuvering the catheter to obtain effective lesions is technically complex and time consuming.
- To overcome this, balloon-based ablation systems have been developed, which can quickly and easily isolate the pulmonary veins in a single-shot fashion.
- Radiofrequency energy is the latest emerging technology used by balloon-based devices and is an alternative option to cryoenergy or laser for single-shot pulmonary vein isolation.

INTRODUCTION

Isolation of the pulmonary veins (PVs) and their antra is the cornerstone of treatment of paroxysmal atrial fibrillation (AF). This is usually performed using a radiofrequency (RF) ablation catheter in combination with 3D electroanatomic mapping (EAM) systems to create continuous, circumferential, point-by-point lesions around the PV antra. Despite technology advancements (most notably, contact force sensing), RF catheter ablation remains a challenging procedure, because maneuvering the catheter to obtain effective lesions is technically complex and time consuming. For this reason, balloon-based

ablation systems have been developed that can quickly and easily isolate the PVs (single-shot), with outcomes comparable with point-by-point RF catheter ablation in the paroxysmal AF population.[1,2] In this review, we discuss 3 balloon-based devices that use RF to obtain permanent lesions, a relatively emerging technology, which may pose as a safe and effective alternative option to cryoenergy or laser for single-shot PV isolation.

THE SATAKE HotBalloon

The Satake HotBalloon ablation system (Toray Industries, Tokyo, Japan) is comprised of a 13F balloon catheter, a 13F deflectable transseptal

Disclosure: A. Natale and A. Al-Ahmad received honoraria from Toray Industries, Apama Medical, Boston Scientific, and Biosense Webster.
[a] Texas Cardiac Arrhythmia Institute, St. David's Medical Center, 3000 N. IH-35, Suite 720, Austin, TX 78705, USA; [b] Department of Cardiopulmonary Function Test, Henan Provincial People's Hospital, People's Hospital of Zhengzhou University, China; [c] Arrhythmia and Electrophysiology Unit, Department of Cardiology, Hacettepe University, Ankara, Turkey; [d] Department of Cardiology, Faculty of Medicine, Yıldırım Beyazıt University, Ankara, Turkey; [e] Dell Medical School, University of Texas, Austin, TX, USA; [f] Department of Biomedical Engineering, University of Texas, Austin, TX, USA; [g] Interventional Electrophysiology, Scripps Clinic, La Jolla, CA, USA; [h] MetroHealth Medical Center, Case Western Reserve University School of Medicine, Cleveland, OH, USA; [i] Division of Cardiology, Stanford University, Stanford, CA, USA
* Corresponding author.
E-mail address: aalahmadmd@gmail.com

1877-9182/19/© 2019 Elsevier Inc. All rights reserved.

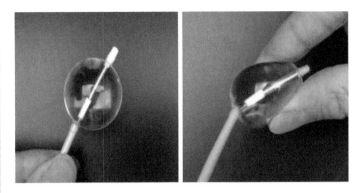

Fig. 1. Satake HotBalloon. (*Courtesy of* Toray Industries, Tokyo, Japan.)

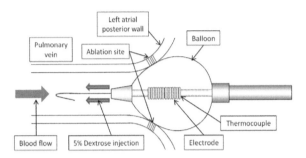

sheath, and a dedicated RF generator with a mixing pump. The balloon is made of a polyurethane membrane, which is highly compliant and can be inflated to 20 to 35 mm in diameter with 10 to 20 mL of a mix of 1:1 saline and iodinated contrast (to ease fluoroscopic visualization), thus easily adapting to different PV anatomies (**Fig. 1**). The balloon can be heated by delivering an RF current between a coil electrode mounted inside the balloon and 4 cutaneous patches positioned on

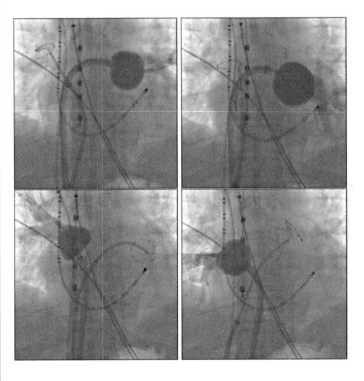

Fig. 2. Pulmonary vein isolation with the Satake HotBallloon. Fluorscopic visualization of the balloon positioned in the left (*top*) and right (*bottom*) pulmonary veins. (*Courtesy of* Toray Industries, Tokyo, Japan.)

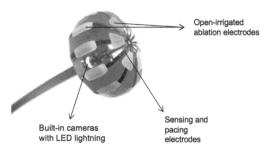

Fig. 3. Luminize RF balloon. (*Courtesy of* Boston Scientific, Inc, Marlborough, MA; with permission.)

the patient's back, and the mixing pump agitates the inner fluid to maintain uniform heating inside the balloon. Power (max 150 W) is delivered in a temperature-controlled fashion, to reach a target balloon temperature of 65°C to 75°C. The resulting capacitive-type heating of the fluid inside the balloon is transferred to the tissue in contact with the balloon surface resulting in permanent, homogeneous, circumferential lesions.[3,4]

The balloon can be manipulated within the left atrium via the steerable sheath and an over-the-wire technique (**Fig. 2**). A separate circular mapping catheter is needed to assess the efficacy of PV isolation. Once the balloon is positioned along one of the PV antra, it is inflated until proper sealing confirmed with intracardiac echocardiography and/or contrast injection. The balloon is then heated for 2 to 3 minutes, which can be repeated if residual PV potentials are observed after the first RF application.[5] In addition to PV, posterior wall isolation has been proven to be feasible by dragging the balloon along the roof and inferior aspect of the PVs.[6] Because the temperature on the surface of the balloon is uniform, heating of surrounding structures (ie, esophagus or phrenic nerve) cannot be prevented. Therefore, cooling of the esophagus is performed according to luminal esophageal temperatures via injection of iced saline, and phrenic nerve pacing is performed during ablation of the septal PVs.[7] Of note, PV stenosis is not an

uncommon complication: indeed, given its compliance profile, the balloon can be wedged too deep into the vein, usually as a result of underinflation because of inadequate filling (<10 mL).[8]

Several clinical studies have been performed with the Satake HotBalloon, which showed feasibility and safety, and led to its approval for clinical use in Japan.[5,6,9] Lesions are durable, and although less wide than those obtained with cryoballoon ablation, outcomes are comparable and superior to a strategy of rhythm control with antiarrhythmic drugs in the paroxysmal AF population.[8,10]

THE LUMINIZE RADIOFREQUENCY BALLOON

The Luminize RF balloon ablation system (Boston Scientific, Marlborough, MA, USA; formerly, Apama Medical) is comprised of a 12.5F steerable (bidirectional) balloon catheter, 13.5F steerable sheath, and dedicated multichannel generator. The RF balloon is a 28-mm compliant balloon with 12 equatorial and 6 forward-facing irrigated electrodes wrapped on its extremity (**Fig. 3**). This design allows not only to ablate, but also to sense using microelectrodes and pace using the RF electrodes eliminating the need for a separate diagnostic catheter. The catheter also incorporates built-in cameras with LED lightning to provide real-time visualization of tissue-electrode contact. RF energy is delivered through each electrode separately in bipolar or unipolar fashion, which allows for quick circumferential as well as focal ablation, as needed.

The balloon is manipulated in the left atrium via the steerable sheath and an over-the-wire technique. The efficacy of PV isolation is assessed. Once the balloon is positioned along one of the PV antra, tissue-electrode contact is confirmed via direct visualization and individual electrode impedance readings, showing an adequate change in impedance (>20%) (**Fig. 4**). To isolate the veins, RF energy is delivered through the equatorial electrodes in a bipolar fashion at 6 to 10

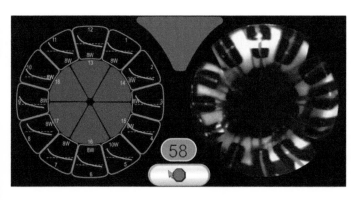

Fig. 4. Tissue-electrode contact assessment via individual electrode impedance readings (*left*) and direct camera visualization (*right*).

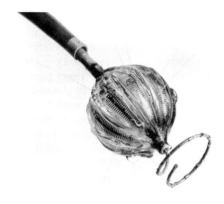

Fig. 5. Heliostar RF balloon. (*Courtesy of* Biosense Webster, Irvine, CA; with permission.)

Watts for up to 60 seconds with irrigation of normal saline at 30 mL/min. Of note, if needed, RF can be tailored at PV breakthrough sites as well as limited in areas of esophageal and phrenic nerve proximity (which is easily assessed with pacing from the balloon electrodes themselves), thus improving safety. In addition to PV isolation, it is possible to perform additional ablation using the forward-facing electrodes (bipolar or unipolar ablation), thus addressing extra-PV targets, as needed.

Clinical data for the Luminize RF balloon are scarce: the recently presented early outcomes from the feasibility study AF-FICIENT 1 have demonstrated a high rate of acute PV isolation with no serious adverse events.[11] Long-term clinical follow-up is ongoing, and a US trial comparing the RF Luminize balloon versus catheter ablation is planned to help clarify the role of this technology to treat patients with paroxysmal AF and proceed with Food and Drug Administration (FDA)/conformité Européenne (CE) approval.

THE HELIOSTAR RADIOFREQUENCY BALLOON

The Heliostar RF balloon ablation system (Biosense Webster, Irvine, CA, USA) is comprised of a 13.5F RF balloon catheter, a 3F circular mapping catheter (Frontera; 15, 20, and 25 mm), a 13.5F steerable sheath and dedicated multichannel generator. The RF balloon is a 28-mm compliant balloon with 10 irrigated, flexible, gold-plated electrodes that encompass the distal end of the

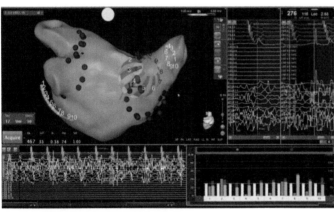

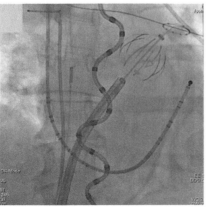

Fig. 6. PV isolation performed with the Heliostar RF balloon. Carto (*top*) and fluoroscopic (*bottom*) visualization. (*Courtesy of* Biosense Webster, Irvine, CA.)

Table 1
Comparison of radiofrequency balloon technologies

	Balloon Compliance	Over the Wire	Built-In Camera	Contrast Injection	Pacing	Sensing	EAM System Integration	RF Delivery	Non-PV Ablation
Satake HotBalloon	+++	Yes	No	Yes	No	Planned	No	RF to heat saline	Yes, with manipulation
Luminize	+	Yes	Yes	No	Yes	Yes	Planned	Unipolar or bipolar	Yes, with dedicated electrodes
Heliostar	++	Yes (CMC/wire)	No	Yes	Yes	Yes	Yes	Unipolar	Yes, with manipulation

Abbreviations: CMC, circular mapping catheter; EAM, electroanatomic mapping; PV, pulmonary vein; RF, radiofrequency.

Table 2
Approval status for radiofrequency balloon technologies

	Japan	Europe	United States
Satake HotBalloon (Toray)	Approved	Not approved	Not approved FDA-IDE trial planned
Luminize (Boston Scientific)	Not approved	Not approved CE mark trial started	Not approved FDA-IDE trial planned
Heliostar (Biosense Webster)	Not approved	Not approved CE mark trial started	Not approved FDA-IDE trial started

Abbreviations: CE, conformité Européenne (European conformity); FDA-IDE, Food and Drug Administration investigational device exemption.

balloon (**Fig. 5**), each with an integrated thermistor to monitor temperature. The balloon and circular mapping catheters are equipped with sensors to allow magnet-based visualization on the Carto 3 EAM system, and 3 electrodes (1, 4, and 7) are marked to easily compare fluoroscopy with Carto (**Fig. 6**). All electrodes can ablate, sense, and pace; however, to accurately detect time to isolation, a separate circular mapping catheter (different diameters for variably sized PVs) is provided, which is also used for balloon manipulation instead of a wire. RF energy is delivered through each electrode independently in a unipolar fashion, which allows for quick, single-shot circumferential (all electrodes) as well as segmental (selected electrode/s) ablation.

The balloon is manipulated in the left atrium via the steerable sheath and an over-the-wire or over-the-catheter technique. Both the circular mapping catheter and balloon can be visualized on Carto and used for fast anatomic mapping (see **Fig. 6**); in addition, the circular mapping catheter can be used for electroanatomic mapping point acquisition, but this is not possible from the electrodes of the RF balloon (too large electrodes). Once the balloon is positioned along one of the PV antra, the balloon is inflated (the degree of which can be displayed on Carto), and proper sealing is confirmed with contrast injection. In addition, via fluoroscopy and Carto, the posterior facing electrodes are identified and marked on the RF generator (see **Fig. 6**). To isolate the veins, RF energy is delivered in a temperature-controlled fashion (max power 15 W, max temperature 55°C) for up to 60 seconds with irrigation of normal saline at 35 mL/min; to prevent esophageal injury, RF energy is turned off after a maximum of 20 seconds in the posterior electrodes. During ablation of the septal PVs, phrenic nerve pacing from the superior vena cava is performed to prevent its injury. Extra-PV ablation is possible with dragging and tailored RF application.

There are still few clinical data available for the Heliostar RF balloon: the feasibility study RADIANCE has shown an efficient and effective acute PV isolation in all patients enrolled, but before CE and FDA approval are granted, long-term outcomes as well direct comparison with other established technologies are pending.[12]

SUMMARY

RF balloon-based ablation systems are promising technologies, which might help improve outcomes when performing PV isolation. The available devices carry different advantages and limitations (**Table 1**): most importantly, as with any balloon-based ablation, there is an interplay between compliance and maneuverability, which affects safety and effectiveness of a single-shot PV isolation. Therefore, the clinical efficacy of RF balloons is still under investigation (**Table 2**), and although the rate of acute PV isolation is high, few data are available on the chronic durability of RF balloon lesions as well as long-term clinical outcomes. Finally, ability to perform non-PV ablation is also an important aspect and might limit their use in patients with nonparoxysmal AF, in whom more widespread, noncircumferential ablation is needed.

REFERENCES

1. Dukkipati SR, Cuoco F, Kutinsky I, et al. Pulmonary vein isolation using the visually guided laser balloon a prospective, multicenter, and randomized comparison to standard radiofrequency ablation. J Am Coll Cardiol 2015;66(12):1350–60.

2. Kuck K-H, Brugada J, Fürnkranz A, et al. Cryoballoon or radiofrequency ablation for paroxysmal atrial fibrillation. N Engl J Med 2016;374(23): 2235–45.

3. Tanaka K, Satake S, Saito S, et al. A new radiofrequency thermal balloon catheter for pulmonary

vein isolation. J Am Coll Cardiol 2001;38(7): 2079–86.

4. Evonich RF, Nori DM, Haines DE. Efficacy of pulmonary vein isolation with a novel hot balloon ablation catheter. J Interv Card Electrophysiol 2012;34(1): 29–36.

5. Satake S, Tanaka K, Saito S, et al. Usefulness of a new radiofrequency thermal balloon catheter for pulmonary vein isolation: a new device for treatment of atrial fibrillation. J Cardiovasc Electrophysiol 2003; 14(6):609–15.

6. Sohara H, Takeda H, Ueno H, et al. Feasibility of the radiofrequency hot balloon catheter for isolation of the posterior left atrium and pulmonary veins for the treatment of atrial fibrillation. Circ Arrhythm Electrophysiol 2009;2(3):225–32.

7. Sohara H, Satake S, Takeda H, et al. Prevalence of esophageal ulceration after atrial fibrillation ablation with the hot balloon ablation catheter: what is the value of esophageal cooling? J Cardiovasc Electrophysiol 2014;25(7):686–92.

8. Sohara H, Ohe T, Okumura K, et al. HotBalloon ablation of the pulmonary veins for paroxysmal AF: a multicenter randomized trial in Japan. J Am Coll Cardiol 2016;68(25):2747–57.

9. Yamaguchi Y, Sohara H, Takeda H, et al. Long-term results of radiofrequency hot balloon ablation in patients with paroxysmal atrial fibrillation: safety and rhythm outcomes. J Cardiovasc Electrophysiol 2015;26(12):1298–306.

10. Nagashima K, Okumura Y, Watanabe I, et al. Hot balloon versus cryoballoon ablation for atrial fibrillation: lesion characteristics and middle-term outcomes. Circ Arrhythm Electrophysiol 2018;11(5). https://doi.org/10.1161/CIRCEP.117.005861.

11. Al-Ahmad A, Aidietis A, Daly M, et al. Assessment of the safety and performance of a novel RF balloon catheter system to isolate pulmonary veins: results of the multicenter AF-FICIENT 1 trial. In: European Heart Rhythm Association Scientific Sessions. Lisbon, Portugal, 2019.

12. Reddy VY, Schilling RJ, Grimaldi M, et al. PV isolation with a novel multielectrode radiofrequency balloon catheter that allows directionally-tailored energy delivery (RADIANCE): a multicenter first-in-man experience. Heart Rhythm 2017;14(6):949–50.

Optical Mapping

Omer Berenfeld, PhD[a], Igor Efimov, PhD[b],*

KEYWORDS

- Optical mapping • Ventricular fibrillation • Atrial fibrillation • Arrhythmia

KEY POINTS

- Optical mapping of electrical activity in the heart is based on voltage-sensitive and lipophilic fluorescence dyes.
- Optical signals recorded from cardiac cells correlate well with their transmembrane potentials.
- High spatiotemporal resolution, wide field mapping, and high sensitivity to transmembrane potential enable detailed characterization of action potential initiation and propagation.
- Optical mapping is used to study complex patterns of excitation propagation, including propagation across the sinoatrial and atrioventricular nodes and during atrial and ventricular arrhythmias.
- Optical mapping is used to study the role of reentrant activity in atrial and ventricular fibrillation.

INTRODUCTION

The abnormal spread of electrical waves of excitation across the heart, known as arrhythmia, can be detrimental to its function. Atrial fibrillation (AF) is the most common sustained cardiac arrhythmia.[1] It affects more than 2.5 million Americans and 5 million Europeans and is a major cause of embolic stroke.[2–4] Globally there were an estimated 33.3 million prevalent cases of AF in 2015.[5] The current understanding of and therapy for AF are inadequate[6]; antiarrhythmic drugs perform poorly, making ablation, with controversial success rate and long-term effects, the preferred therapy.[7–9] Ventricular tachycardia (VT) and ventricular fibrillation (VF) cause sudden cardiac death, which remains a major cause of mortality and morbidity, accounting for up to 20% of all deaths in the United States.[10,11] Despite numerous advances in diagnosis of, prevention of, and therapy for VT/VF, available antiarrhythmic drugs failed so far to reduce mortality. Implantable cardioverter defibrillators are the main therapy for VT/VF, with 90,000 implanted annually.[12]

Accurate characterization of the spread of electrical excitation is critical for understanding the mechanisms responsible for both normal cardiac rhythm and for initiation and maintenance of arrhythmias. Although much has been learned regarding the ionic basis of the cardiac action potential using intracellular microelectrodes, single cell impalements cannot be practically used to simultaneously record action potentials from hundreds of recording sites. Also, mapping cardiac activation and repolarization can be based on surface unipolar and bipolar electrograms measured with arrays of electrodes[13,14] but interpretation of data in some cases is ambiguous.[13,15] For instance, activation sequences were difficult to interpret during rapid synchronous depolarization as after electric shock application and during slowly changing, low-level depolarization, as in ischemia. Repolarization time measured by extracellular electrodes often does not coincide with the actual repolarization at the recording site.[15,16] Electrical mapping is particularly challenging during fibrillation with its complex patterns of activation and repolarization.[17]

Funded by: NIHHYB Grant number(s): R01HL141470; R21EB023106 NIHMS-ID: 1528775.
[a] Department of Internal Medicine (Cardiology), Center for Arrhythmia Research, University of Michigan, 7300 Medical Science Building, 1301 Catherine Street, Ann Arbor, MI 48109, USA; [b] Department of Biomedical Engineering, The George Washington University, 800 22nd Street Northwest, 5000 Science and Engineering Hall, Washington, DC 20052, USA
* Corresponding author.
E-mail address: irefimov@gmail.com

An alternative approach for mapping the electrical activation of large areas of the heart is offered by optical methods. Optical methods of recordings transmembrane potential in excitable cells using chemical probes sensitive to electrical field was conceived by Larry Cohen and developed in 1960 to 1970s, first in neurons[18,19] and then in cardiac preparations.[20] Subsequently, other molecular probes were developed or endogenous fluorophores were used to image intracellular calcium, nicotinamide adenine dinucleotide, and mitochondrial inner membrane potential, and so forth (most recently reviewed by Cathey and colleagues).[21] The method for measuring the transmembrane potential consists of using fluorescent probes designed to regulate their photon absorbance and emittance by electric field. In addition, these probes are designed to include a lipophilic tail, which binds to lipid membrane to make the fluorescence sensitive to the local electric field across the cell membrane. Current probes and sensors permit high spatiotemporal resolution over wide areas. An array of probes and sensors is currently available for the range spanning from the UV, through the visible and to near-infrared, which are most suitable for deep tissue penetration. The purpose of this article is to discuss various applications of optical mapping to characterize the electrical excitation of the heart with high fidelity and high spatiotemporal resolution. The article focuses on describing the electrical activation patterns mostly relevant to arrhythmia and for which optical mapping offers a unique advantage over other electrical mapping approaches.

MAPPING EXCITATION IMPULSES, ROTORS, AND WAVE PROPAGATION

The earliest development of voltage-sensitive dyes started with merocyanine molecules, which exhibited 1% fractional changes in fluorescence in cardiac tissue.[20,22,23] As shown in **Fig. 1**A, action potentials recorded by Salama and Morad through the fluorescence changes of that potentiometric dye were validated against action potentials simultaneously recorded with intracellular microelectrode. The fluorescence or optical action potentials were recorded from frog ventricular tissue stained with merocyanine 540 from a 2-mm diameter excitation spot and compared with microelectrode recording from one of the cells excited by the incident light beam. The signals obtained with 2 techniques show excellent correlation of signal morphology. Optical signals were easily recorded from different regions of the heart by simply displacing the optical paths. **Fig. 1**B

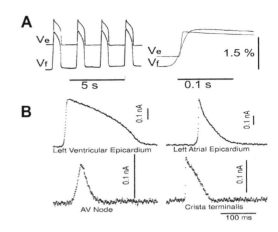

Fig. 1. Optical signals of cardiac action potentials. (*A*) Simultaneous fluorescent (Vf) and microelectrode (Ve) recordings of action potentials in the frog heart stained with merocyanine 540. Recordings show a faithful reproduction of transmembrane potential by the fluorescence signals. Upstroke of optical action potential typically is slower than that of the microelectrode, due to spatial averaging of a propagating wavefront. (*B*) Optical recording of action potentials from different regions of the heart stained with di-4-ANEPPS: ventricular and atrial working myocardium, AV node, and crista terminalis. (*From* Efimov IR, Nikolski VP, Salama G. Optical imaging of the heart. Circ Res 2004;95:21-33; with permission.)

shows examples of optical action potentials from different regions of atrial and ventricular rabbit myocardium. In the intact heart during sinus rhythm, epicardial optical activation times are also are in excellent correlation, with activation times obtained with surface electrical recordings.[24,25] The distinct optical action potential morphologies, however, enable assessment of the distribution of its upstroke velocity and duration across the heart, which are not attainable in extracellular potentials commonly recorded with electrodes and catheters in the clinic. Optical action potentials are processed and analyzed to reconstruct dynamic patterns of activation and repolarization. **Fig. 2** illustrates standard methods of measuring activation time (see **Fig. 2**A), repolarization time (see **Fig. 2**B), and action potential duration, with corresponding maps and conduction velocity maps (see **Fig. 2**C).[26] More advanced methods are required for analysis of complex patterns of reentrant arrhythmias, when detection of activation and repolarization is more challenging.

The work of Davidenko and colleagues[27] used optical mapping to demonstrate functional reentry in cardiac tissue and set the stage for an extensive research on its mechanism and role in atrial

A

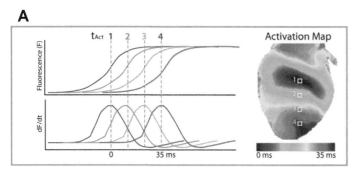

B

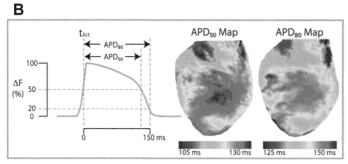

C

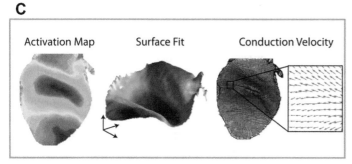

Fig. 2. Methods for optical mapping of activation, repolarization, and action potential duration. (*A*) Optical action potential upstrokes are differentiated and dV/dt_{max} is calculated to determine activation time at each recording site. Map of activation is reconstructed based on these activation times. (*B*) Repolarization time is measured at 50% or 80% of repolarization to the resting potential, which determines action potential duration at corresponding percentage of repolarization: APD_{50} or APD_{80}. (*C*) conduction velocity analysis. Data are taken from the activation map (left) to fit onto a smoothed surface (middle). The surface was smoothed with a 5×5 Gaussian kernel. Local conduction vectors are then calculated from the smoothed activation surface with the magnitudes of local conduction velocity represented by the length of the arrows and the directions of activation represented by the directions of the arrows. (*From* Laughner JI, Ng FS, Sulkin MS, Arthur RM, Efimov IR. Processing and analysis of cardiac optical mapping data obtained with potentiometric dyes. American journal of physiology Heart and circulatory physiology 2012;303:H753-65; with permission.)

and VF. In their study, Davidenko and colleagues[28] consistently initiated sustained spiral-wave activity (also known as functional reentry or rotor) in thin (20-mm × 20-mm × 0.5-mm) slices of sheep and dog epicardial muscle by cross-field stimulation.[29,30] A full revolution of a clockwise-rotating spiral and the pattern of local activation are shown in **Fig. 3**A. The rotation period (183 ms ± 68 ms) was 1.39-times longer than the refractory period; the tip of the spiral has a pronounced curvature, and, as a result of the anisotropic properties of epicardial ventricular muscle,[31] wave propagation in the long axis of the cells was 3.9-times ± 2.2-times faster than in the transverse direction, which resulted in an elliptical spiral shape. Spiral waves are considered stationary when the tip of the spiral, which circulates around the core, follows a closed circular or elliptical trajectory and the periodicity is preserved everywhere outside the core.[32] To determine whether the low-voltage activity in the core was solely produced by tissue

discontinuities or was functionally determined, the spatial voltage distribution in the preparation during spiral wave activity (**Fig. 3**B) was compared with that during planar wave propagation (**Fig. 3**C). Frame-stack plots were obtained sequentially from narrow rectangular sections across the core's center (see **Fig. 3**A [*red line*]). The amplitude of fluorescence (depolarization) of 50 superimposed frames taken from the same section is shown at the bottom of **Fig. 3**B, C. The amplitude was lower in the core's center than in the periphery (*red arrow*). In addition, the minimum value was higher, thus indicating that the core region never reached full repolarization. Signals of normal amplitude were recorded in the same region of tissue during planar wave propagation (see **Fig. 3**C). Although the region contained a small artery, activity was uniform throughout the segment, which demonstrated that the differences in fluorescence associated with spiral wave activity are determined by functional differences between the core

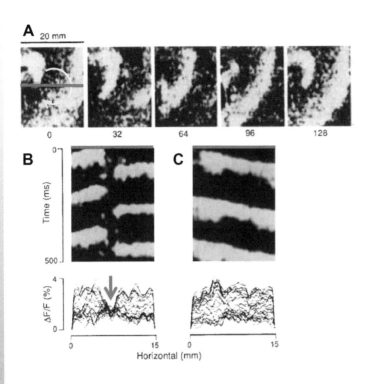

Fig. 3. Mapping rotors in cardiac tissue. (A) Clockwise-rotating spiral wave in canine epicardial muscle. (White) Maximal depolarization; (black) resting potential; numbers, time in ms. (B) (Top left) Time-space plot F(x t) of cross-section through center of the core of a stationary spiral wave. (Bottom) Superimposed traces of ΔFIF; 50 frames (approximately 6 rotating cycles) in the same region as in (C). (Top right) F(x t) ΔFIF plots obtained 10 minutes later from the same section as in right panel during planar wave propagation. (From Davidenko JM, Pertsov AV, Salomonsz R, Baxter W, Jalife J. Stationary and drifting spiral waves of excitation in isolated cardiac muscle. Nature 1992;355:349-51; with permission.)

and the periphery of the spiral wave. In 14 episodes of stationary spiral waves, the core amplitude was 25% ± 17% of the absolute maximum amplitude. So far, optical mapping is the only available method enabling such detailed characterization of the voltage at the core of the reentry.

The curvature of the action potential wavefront and its anisotropic propagation play a major role in the formation of the functional reentry (rotor) and the core, seen in **Fig. 3**. The effect of the wavefront curvature and the tissue anisotropy on propagation was studied by determining the characteristics of propagation through isthmuses of varying widths using optical mapping of 2-D thin slices of sheep epicardial tissue.[33] The spatial resolution in those optical mapping studies depended on the size of the image and was typically between 50 μm and 100 μm per pixel. An example of longitudinal propagation through an isthmus in a thin sheet of epicardial muscle is presented in **Figs. 4** and **5**.[33] The leftmost frame on the top row shows the real image of the tissue to illustrate the 2 cuts produced horizontally across the fibers in the middle of the preparation. The additional 5 frames show images of the dye fluorescence (white) taken once every 16 milliseconds (ms) during propagation of a planar wave initiated at the top border of the preparation (proximal side of the isthmus) at a basic cycle length of 500 ms. On reaching the isthmus, the planar wavefront was diffracted to an elliptical wavefront that evidenced the fiber

orientation: the velocity was much faster in the longitudinal direction of propagation than orthogonally (propagation in the direction of the cuts). The electrical activity emerging from the isthmus

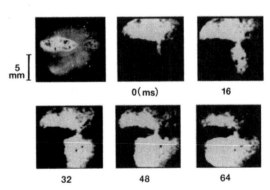

Fig. 4. Propagation of an action potential wave through an isthmus. Video frames of experiment in a sheep epicardial preparation showing longitudinal propagation through a 1.09-mm wide isthmus. A planar wave front, initiated at the top of the preparation at a basic cycle length of 500 milliseconds, propagated downward through the isthmus. The first frame (top left) is an image of the preparation. Subsequent frames show the electrical activity every 16 milliseconds. Depolarized tissue is shown in white, and resting tissue is shown in black. (From Cabo C, Pertsov AM, Baxter WT, Davidenko JM, Gray RA, Jalife J. Wave-front curvature as a cause of slow conduction and block in isolated cardiac muscle. CircRes 1994;75:1014-28; with permission.)

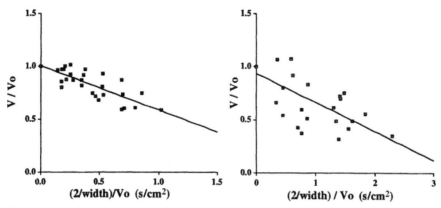

Fig. 5. Conduction velocity and curvature of an action potential wave. Graphs showing normalized conduction velocity as a function of the width of the isthmus in experiments as shown in Figure 4. Left, summary of the results of seven experiments during longitudinal propagation through the isthmus. Right, summary of the results of six experiments during transverse propagation through the isthmus. V indicates velocity; V_o, the velocity of a planar wave. (From Cabo C, Pertsov AM, Baxter WT, Davidenko JM, Gray RA, Jalife J. Wave-front curvature as a cause of slow conduction and block in isolated cardiac muscle. CircRes 1994;75:1014-28; with permission.)

was similar to that which would be initiated by a point source.

The velocity of the waves crossing the isthmus was calculated as the spatial distance between the last isochrone before the isthmus and the first isochrone after the isthmus, which was divided by the time between isochrones and averaged over 3 consecutive beats.[33] The velocity (V) of propagation through the isthmus with a width (w) was modeled as $V/V_0 = 1-D[(2/w)/V_0$, where V_0 is the plane wave velocity and D is a diffusion factor. **Fig. 5** summarizes the results of experiments for longitudinal (*left*) and transverse (*right*) propagation at a basic cycle length of 500 ms. The results were well-fitted by a straight line (correlation coefficient 0.8), having a slope of 0.41 cm²/s and of 0.27 cm²/s for the longitudinal and transverse conductions, respectively. The fact that the velocity of propagation after passing the isthmus decreased as the isthmus was narrowed strongly suggests that (as in the computer simulations) the slowing of conduction was caused by the increased wavefront curvature imposed by the narrowing isthmus and explained by a reduction in the source-to-sink areas ratio of excitation spread.[34]

MAPPING ELECTRICAL STIMULATION

Electrical stimulation and defibrillation have become indispensable therapies for both bradyarrhymias and tachyarrhythmias. Traditional electrode-based methods, however, do not allow investigation of cellular excitation induced by electrical stimulation due to the overwhelming artifacts produced by the stimuli or shocks. Optical mapping is immune to these artifacts and therefore it

has become key technology in studying pacing and defibrillation. Using the bidomain computer model, Sepulveda and colleagues[35] predicted the existence of areas of hyperpolarization and depolarization adjacent to the electrode during unipolar stimulation of the tissue. These areas were termed virtual electrode polarizations (VEPs). For a point-size cathodal stimulus, the transmembrane potential (V_m) distribution pattern had a central depolarized virtual cathode (VC) region with a characteristic dog-bone shape and 2 elongated hyperpolarized virtual anode (VA) regions on the sides that were parallel to the direction of the fibers. In the linear bidomain model, for the opposite polarity of the stimulus, the VEP pattern was symmetrically reversed. Bipolar stimuli create VEP patterns, which superimpose VC and VA patterns. **Fig. 6** shows 6 different VEP patterns predicted by a bidomain model for anodal and cathodal unipolar stimulation and for bipolar stimulation when electrodes are positioned along or across the fiber orientation.[36]

The dog-bone VEP pattern induced by point stimulation was experimentally confirmed by optical mapping.[37–39] This virtual electrode phenomenon resulted in the formulation of a unified theory of stimulation and suggested solutions to the old puzzles of break-excitation and anodal stimulation.[39,40] The concept of activating function generalized VEP theory to electric fields of any geometric configuration.[41] In particular, strong electric shocks applied during defibrillation also induce areas of adjacent positive and negative polarization, which can be considered VEPs.[42] This concept allowed the explanation of shock-induced arrhythmias and defibrillation

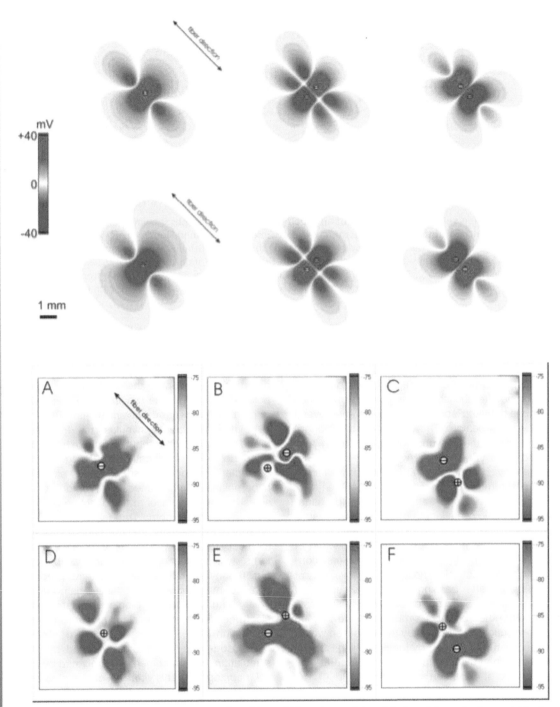

Fig. 6. Virtual electrodes polarizations predicted by a bidomain model and induced by unipolar and bipolar epicardial stimulation in the rabbit heart. (*Top*) Bidomain model predicts VEPs of different pattern for unipolar and bipolar stimuli when electrodes are positioned along or across fiber orientation. (*Bottom*) VEP patterns recorded in the rabbit heart during epicardial stimulation with the same electrode location and polarity as in the top panel. Optically recorded and averaged maps of V_m were obtained from a 5-mm × 5-mm area of anterior epicardium of rabbit heart for unipolar and bipolar anodal and cathodal stimuli. V_m varies from −95 mV (*blue*) to −75 mV (*red*); −85 mV (*white*) represents the resting potential. (*From* Sambelashvili AT, Nikolski VP, Efimov IR. Nonlinear effects in subthreshold virtual electrode polarization. American journal of physiology Heart and circulatory physiology 2003;284:H2368-74; with permission.)

failure via virtual electrode-induced phase singularities (PSs).[43–45]

Fig. 6 shows corresponding VEP patterns recorded during unipolar and bipolar pacing in the rabbit heart for 6 different polarity/electrode location combinations, which mirror computationally predicted VEPs shown in **Fig. 6**. Unipolar pacing thresholds determined in the authors' experiments ranged from 0.15 mA to 0.60 mA for cathodal stimulation and from 0.85 mA to 1.76 mA for anodal unipolar stimulation.[36] This difference is explained by significant difference in depolarized (VC) regions produced by the 2 opposite polarities of stimulation. The most pronounced VEP pattern is observed at 4 ms,[46] which is determined by the time constant for the passive cardiac tissue resistor-capacitor network.

OPTICAL MAPPING OF SINOATRIAL AND ATRIOVENTRICULAR NODES

Normal sinus rhythm originates in the sinoatrial (SA) node and is transmitted from atria to ventricles via the atrioventricular (AV) node. Optical mapping allows detailed reconstruction of excitation of these 2 critical structures in the human and animal hearts. Fedorov and colleagues[47,48] optically mapped human SA and AV nodes with deep-penetration near-infrared fluorescence dyes and demonstrated the presence of specialized conduction pathways connecting these 2 nodes to the nearby atrial myocardium. **Fig. 7** illustrates normal excitation in the human AV node initiated by atrial pacing. **Fig. 7**A shows optical action potentials and their derivatives recorded from sites 1 to 5, during atrial pacing at 60 beats per minute (bpm) (cycle length = 1000 ms). Complex fractionated optical potentials representing asynchronous excitation of different structures within the triangle of Koch can be seen, including AV node, slow pathway (SP), and fast pathway (FP), atrial myocardium, and the bundle of His. Red dots on optical action potential upstrokes correspond to dV/dt peaks. **Fig. 7**B shows activation maps for sequential excitation of the atrial myocardium, the SP and FP, the AV node, and His bundle. Maps are superimposed on the 30 mm^2 × 30 mm^2 optical field of view. The black line demarcates the tricuspid annulus. FP and SP are the substrate for AV nodal reentrant tachycardia.

OPTICAL MAPPING OF ATRIAL FIBRILLATION

Optical mapping data support the hypothesis that acute AF in the structurally normal sheep heart[49–54] and in some patients[55–58] is not a totally random phenomenon. More recent data in animals with persistent and long-term persistent AF have also shown long-lasting (months) signs of organized activity in vivo, which correlated with the presence of rotors in the isolated, Langendorff-perfused, and optically mapped hearts.[59] These data are consistent with new mechanistically based approaches to terminate paroxysmal and persistent AF in patients,[60,61] which have shown high rates of AF termination during the procedure and freedom from AF during follow-up. On the other hand, in long-lasting clinical persistent AF, the theory of multiple random wavelets of activation coexisting to create a chaotic cardiac rhythm is widely accepted,[62] and AF ablative therapy to achieve long-term success rates is more challenging.[61,63] Reentrant activity, which includes anatomic reentries and rotors, vortices, or spiral waves,[64,65] has been shown to underlie various types of ventricular and atrial arrhythmias.[66–68] Although AF may be the result of the breakup of multiple, randomly propagating wavelets that rotate briefly,[69,70] it also may relate to discrete and steady rotor generating waves that break at fixed heterogeneities.[66] These 2 different mechanisms are hypothesized to have different signatures on fibrillation dynamics, the latter showing more organization and stability in its patterns of wave propagation.

The previous sections discuss the utility of the high-spatiotemporal resolution of optical mapping in characterizing features of action potential wave propagation. In recent years, algorithms in the frequency and phase domains were developed to markedly enhance the characterization of complex spatiotemporal patterns of experimental cardiac fibrillation.[49,50,71–75] Transmembrane optical signal at each site exhibited quasiperiodic activity with a strong components at dominant frequencies, typically between 8 Hz and 15 Hz, which were seen as a quasiclosed trajectory in 2-D phase-space that could be represented by phases around the circuit.[71] Spatial phase maps at each instant revealed the sources of fibrillation (rotors) in the form of topological defects, or PSs, at a few sites.[71] Subsequently, the combined use of phase maps with dominant frequency maps constructed using high-resolution optical movies led to the demonstration that fibrillation in isolated animal hearts were characterized by a hierarchy of DF domains where the highest domain (DF$_{max}$) corresponded to the location of the dominant rotor.[49,53,76]

Fig. 8 presents phase maps from experiment verifying the theoretic prediction for the initiation of a wavebreak, secondary to the interaction of a wavefront with a functional obstacle during AF (ie, vortex shedding).[77,78] **Fig. 8** demonstrates

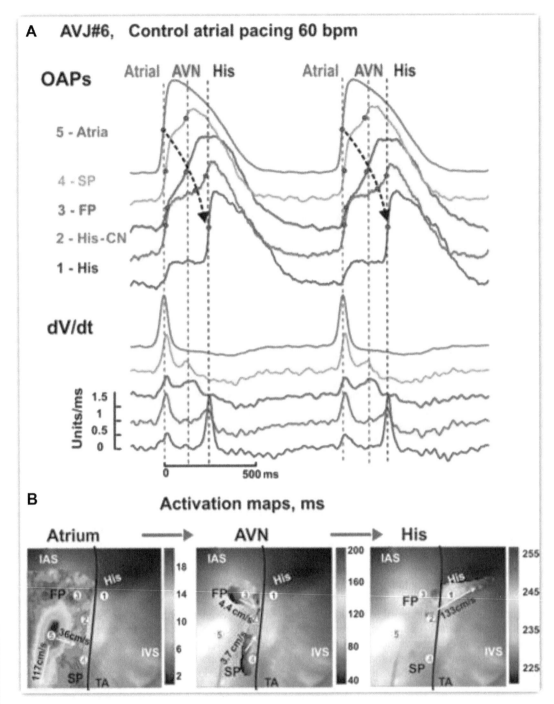

Fig. 7. Visualization of dual pathways in the AV node. Optical mapping of human AV Junction during atrial pacing. (*A*) Optical action potentials and their derivatives recorded from sites 1 to 5 in (*B*), during atrial pacing at 60 bpm (cycle length = 1000 ms). Red dots on OAP upstrokes correspond to dV/dt peaks. (*B*) Separated atrial, AV nodal, and His bundle activation maps superimposed on the OFV (30 mm^2 × 30 mm^2). The black line demarcates the tricuspid annulus. FP and SP are the substrate for AV nodal reentrant tachycardia. (*From* Fedorov VV, Ambrosi CM, Kostecki G, et al. Anatomic localization and autonomic modulation of atrioventricular junctional rhythm in failing human hearts. Circulation Arrhythmia and electrophysiology 2011;4:515-25.)

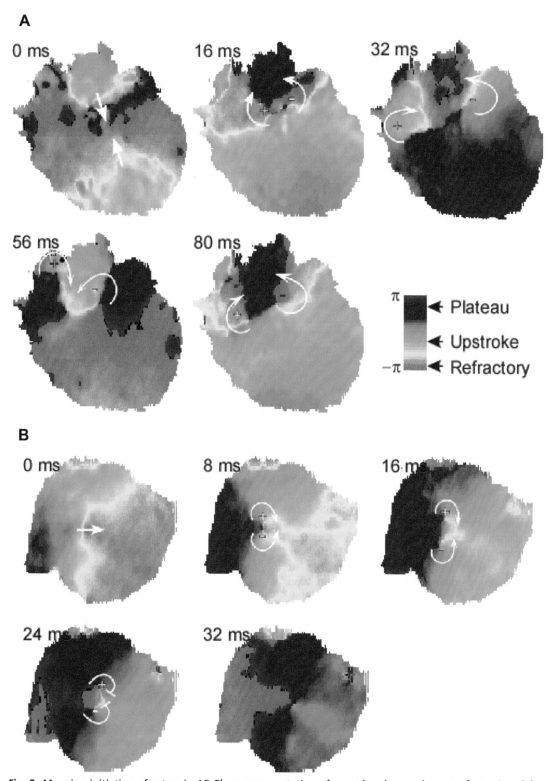

Fig. 8. Mapping initiation of rotors in AF. Phase representation of wave breakup and reentry formation. (*A*) A sequence of phase maps at the indicated times demonstrating generation of figure-8 reentry. (*B*) A sequence of phase maps demonstrating a failure in generating reentry. Color bar scale indicate phase value between -π and π radians with approximated action potential stages (*A*). See text for details. (*From* Chen J, Mandapati R, Berenfeld O, Skanes AC, Gray RA, Jalife J. Dynamics of wavelets and their role in atrial fibrillation in the isolated sheep heart. CardiovascRes 2000;48:220-32; with permission.)

how a pair of PSs is produced at a broken ends of the wavelets[51] on the epicardial surface of the LA and leads to a relative long-lasting episode of a so-called figure-8 reentry (approximately 3 rotations). At 0 ms, there are 2 depolarizing wavefronts present (*green/yellow*). The wave seen at the upper edge of the field of view propagates downward and extinguishes on refractory tissue (*red*) in the center of the field of view. As shown in the frame at 16 ms, the wave on the lower edge of the mapping fields propagates upward and breaks on a functional obstacle (*red*) resulting in 2 PS points (+ and −) of opposite chirality. The maps following 32 ms show the 2 counter-rotating wavelets successfully propagate around and between the 2 PSs (inter-PS distance is 6.8 mm), which serve as a functional isthmus for a figure-8 reentry. The authors' study also found cases of the functional isthmus between the PSs not wide enough to allow propagation establishing a sustained reentry. **Fig. 8** presents phase maps of AF where 2 counter-rotating wavelets, formed after a wavebreak, were unable to complete a full rotation. At 0 ms, the activation wavefront (*green/yellow*) is seen propagating into a heterogeneously recovered region, resulting in 2 wavebreaks, one on each side of the small obstacle of refractoriness in the center of the field (*red*). At 8 ms and 16 ms, the chirality of each of the newly formed PSs is indicated by + and −. At 24 ms, the wavelets have fused and are attempting to propagate between the PS points; the inter-PS distance is 3.3 mm. The 2 counter-rotating wavelets mutually annihilate and the reentry is not completed, as shown in the map at 32 ms. The authors' isolated sheep heart experiments have established that the minimal distance between 2 PSs that allows for the sustenance of a figure-8 reentry in the left atrium is approximately 4 mm.[51] This observation is in good agreement with those of Cabo and colleagues,[78] who in ventricular tissue estimated a critical isthmus of 2.5 mm to 3.5 mm for propagation failure depending on stimulation frequency and fiber orientation. It is, therefore, demonstrated that the mechanism for the generation of reentrant sources during AF could be the collisions of wavefronts with functional obstacles. The fact that the PSs tend to cluster in certain areas[51] indicates that the underlying structure, or other fixed properties of the tissue also are involved in the generation of those obstacles.

The posterior left atrium (PLA) and the left atrial appendage (LAA) are proposed to play a major role in AF maintenance. Endoscopic optical mapping enables quantification of atrial activation patterns in the intact isolated sheep heart during AF with unprecedented details.[59] Phase map movies obtained with the endoscopic approach show that the highest number of rotors is found at the PLA and the junction of PLA with the LAA. Occasionally, when the 3-D equivalent of a rotor (ie, a scroll wave) has a stable center of rotation perpendicular to the surface of the mapping area, it is possible to identify long-lasting rotors whose center of rotation localizes with the highest-frequency domain.[75] **Fig. 9** shows such a rotor located at the PLA with simultaneous fibrillatory conduction at the LAA. The presence of that rotor in the PLA also correlated with a frequency gradient from a high value at PLA to a lower value at the LAA (9 Hz and 6.4 Hz, respectively). The number of rotors was consistently higher in the PLA compared with the LAA,[79] which suggests an essential role for PLA reentry in maintaining the arrhythmia (see **Fig. 9**C). Based on these data, the authors hypothesized that if reentry plays a critical role sustaining stretch-induced AF, then a pharmacologic strategy targeting inward-rectifier K^+ currents that are essential for controlling rotor dynamics, especially I_{K1}, should effectively restore sinus rhythm. Thus, the authors demonstrated that chloroquine, which preferentially blocks I_{K1}, was highly effective on terminating stretch-induced AF. The latter was achieved by significantly increasing the rotor core width before AF termination (see **Fig. 9**D), along with a drastic reduction in the number of rotations observed in the PLA (baseline: 3.2 ± 0.3; before AF termination: 0.7 ± 0.3; $P = .003$).[79]

VENTRICULAR FIBRILLATION IN THE HUMAN HEART

Human left ventricular (LV) wedge preparations were studied by Aras and colleagues.[80] Wedges from the posterolateral LV free wall (**Fig. 10**) perfused via the left marginal artery were dissected, cannulated, and mounted in a tissue chamber with 4 surfaces (epicardium, endocardium, and the 2 transmural sides) facing 4 CMOS cameras of the optical apparatus.[80] Ventricular arrhythmia was induced using the S1S1 pacing protocol after pinacidil administration. **Fig. 10** highlights arrhythmia dynamics from a representative data set, showing wavelets and reentry around a PS. Reentrant arrhythmia was characterized by both rotors and multiple wavelets, and the 4-sided tracking of arrhythmia dynamics suggested a high level of complexity relative to arrhythmic wavefronts creation and propagation, coupled with meandering PS. Only in a few instances were the PSs stable (1%–2%). There was a positive epicardium-endocardium correlation when the reentrant arrhythmia was monomorphic, relative to DF, regularity index, and wavefront count.

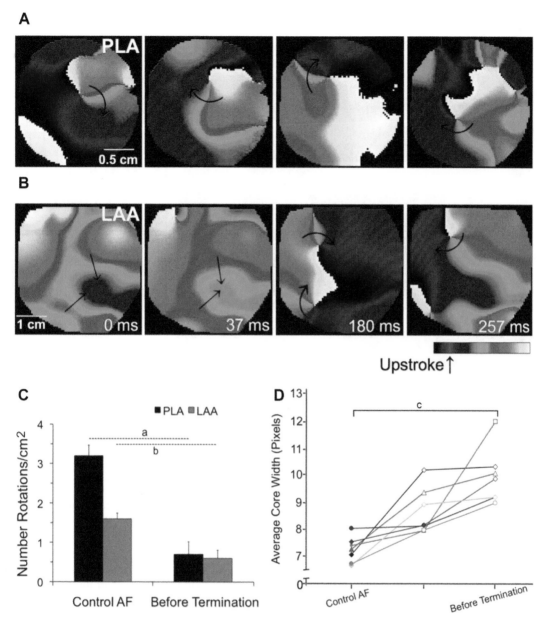

Fig. 9. Rotors and dominant frequency distribution in AF. Simultaneous optical mapping of the (*A*) intact PLA and (*B*) LAA during stretch-induced AF in the isolated sheep heart. (*A*) Sequential endoscopic phase snapshots from the PLA showing a rotor and the drifting of its singularity point. (*B*) Sequential phase snapshots from the LAA. Patterns of activation in the LAA show propagation waves compatible with fibrillatory conduction. Singularity points also are present in correlation with wavebreaks in the fibrillatory conduction region. In this case, the highest DF in the PLA was 9 Hz and in the LAA it was approximately 6 Hz (data not shown), suggesting that the activity in the LAA depends on the rotational activity in the PLA. (*C*) Number of rotations per centimeter squared in the PLA/LAA in control AF and just before chloroquine-induced AF termination. [a] $P = .003$, [b] $P = .0002$. (*D*) Average core width significantly increases in size during chloroquine. [c] $P = .0002$. (*From* Filgueiras-Rama D, Martins RP, Ennis SR, et al. High-resolution endocardial and epicardial optical mapping in a sheep model of stretch-induced atrial fibrillation. Journal of visualized experiments: JoVE 2011; and Filgueiras-Rama D, Price NF, Martins RP, et al. Long-term frequency gradients during persistent atrial fibrillation in sheep are associated with stable sources in the left atrium. Circulation Arrhythmia and electrophysiology 2012;5:1160-7.)

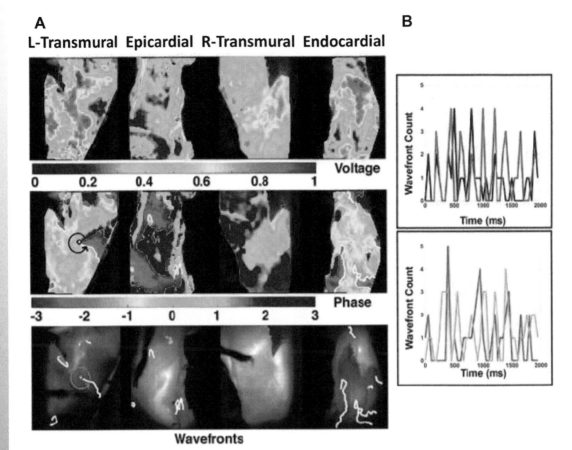

Fig. 10. Panoramic mapping of reentrant VF in ex vivo human heart. (*A*) Representative simultaneous snapshots of voltage, phase, and wavefront maps during reentrant arrhythmia in a human ventricle wedge imaged from 4 different sides. (*B*) Time course of wavefront count at the L-transmural and epicardial maps (*top*) and R-transmural and endocardial maps (*bottom*).[80] (*From* Aras KK, Faye NR, Cathey B, Efimov IR. Critical Volume of Human Myocardium Necessary to Maintain Ventricular Fibrillation. Circulation Arrhythmia and electrophysiology 2018;11; with permission.)

With an increasing complexity of arrhythmia (eg, polymorphic VT or VF) the epicardium-endocardium correlation exhibited an increasing dissociation.

In 1914, Garrey[81] made the observation that "Hearts of large animals fibrillate with great ease and only rarely recover from the fibrillatory state, while small hearts rarely fail to recover." Mines[82] and Garrey[81] postulated that the 1-D wavelength compared with tissue size is a major determinant of reentry maintenance. The usefulness of 2-D wavelength surface area in predicting sustainability of arrhythmia was demonstrated by Lou and colleagues[83] and suggests the important role of wavelength in determining the arrhythmia maintenance. For small animal hearts (eg, rabbit, rat, and mouse), and, for that matter, large animal atrial tissue, wavelength can be approximated as a 2-D metric with longitudinal and transverse components, as long as transmural wavelength is greater than the thickness of the tissue. In the study of Aras and colleagues,[80] wavelength was treated as a 3-D metric with an additional transmural component to account for the sizable (approximately 2 cm) thickness of the LV wall in comparison with transmural wavelength. Thus, a wavelength volume, V_λ, was defined as the product of cardiac wavelengths in longitudinal, transverse, and transmural directions., and the propensity for sustained arrhythmias was correlated with the ratio of the cardiac wedge volume to V_λ. Because wavelength is rate dependent, curvature dependent, and substrate dependent,[34] it is a dynamically varying function of space and time during fibrillation and an arrhythmia vulnerability coefficient κ needs to be calculated ad hoc. The human optical data analyzed by Aras and colleagues[80] showed that there is a critical threshold volume V_T ($V_T = \kappa V_\lambda$) that can predict ventricular arrhythmia vulnerability.

SUMMARY

Optical mapping provides invaluable information on the spatiotemporal patterns of cardiac excitation propagation and is particularly important for better understanding of cardiac stimulation and the complex patterns during fibrillation. The light signals generated by fluorescence of voltage sensitive dyes are a specific and direct probe of the cells' transmembrane potential, which can be mapped over large areas. Optical mapping has become a ubiquitous tool used by numerous experimental cardiology laboratories, due to development of relatively inexpensive off-the-shelf components and open source software solutions.[21] Most recent developments focus on multiparametric optical mapping, which can probe simultaneously the transmembrane potentials and the intracellular calcium[21,84] and promise to expand the mapping into cardiac factors beyond the transmembrane potentials. Continuing challenges in optical mapping include the separation of the cardiac mechanical motion from the propagation of the electrical waves,[85] the 3-D mapping of electrical activity in deep myocardium[86] and the toxicity of the fluorescent dyes preventing clinical and survival in vivo studies.[87,88] Overcoming the limitations and challenges of optical mapping has the potential to transform the way one of the most important health care burdens, cardiac arrhythmias and diseases, is understood and treated.

REFERENCES

1. Camm AJ, Kirchhof P, Lip GY, et al. Guidelines for the management of atrial fibrillation: the task force for the management of atrial fibrillation of the European Society of Cardiology (ESC). Europace 2010; 12:1360–420.
2. Majeed A, Moser K, Carroll K. Trends in the prevalence and management of atrial fibrillation in general practice in England and Wales, 1994-1998: analysis of data from the general practice research database. Heart 2001;86:284–8.
3. Wolf PA, Abbott RD, Kannel WB. Atrial fibrillation as an independent risk factor for stroke: the Framingham Study. Stroke 1991;22:983–8.
4. Stewart S, Hart CL, Hole DJ, et al. A population-based study of the long-term risks associated with atrial fibrillation: 20-year follow-up of the Renfrew/Paisley study. Am J Med 2002;113:359–64.
5. Roth GA, Johnson C, Abajobir A, et al. Global, regional, and National burden of cardiovascular diseases for 10 causes, 1990 to 2015. J Am Coll Cardiol 2017;70:1–25.
6. Heijman J, Guichard JB, Dobrev D, et al. Translational challenges in atrial fibrillation. Circ Res 2018; 122:752–73.
7. Oral H. Mechanisms of atrial fibrillation: lessons from studies in patients. Prog Cardiovasc Dis 2005;48: 29–40.
8. Packer DL, Mark DB, Robb RA, et al. Catheter ablation versus antiarrhythmic drug therapy for atrial fibrillation (CABANA) trial: study rationale and design. Am Heart J 2018;199:192–9.
9. Calkins H, Kuck KH, Cappato R, et al. 2012 HRS/EHRA/ECAS Expert Consensus Statement on Catheter and Surgical Ablation of Atrial Fibrillation: recommendations for patient selection, procedural techniques, patient management and follow-up, definitions, endpoints, and research trial design. Europace 2012;14:528–606.
10. Zheng ZJ, Croft JB, Giles WH, et al. Sudden cardiac death in the United States, 1989 to 1998. Circulation 2001;104:2158–63.
11. Stecker EC, Reinier K, Marijon E, et al. Public health burden of sudden cardiac death in the United States. Circ Arrhythm Electrophysiol 2014; 7:212–7.
12. Buxton AE, Lee KL, Fisher JD, et al. A randomized study of the prevention of sudden death in patients with coronary artery disease. Multicenter Unsustained Tachycardia Trial Investigators. N Engl J Med 1999;341:1882–90.
13. Ideker RE, Smith WM, Blanchard SM, et al. The assumptions of isochronal cardiac mapping. Pacing Clin Electrophysiol 1989;12:456–78.
14. Josephson ME, Horowitz LN, Farshidi A. Continuous local electrical activity. A mechanism of recurrent ventricular tachycardia. Circulation 1978;57:659–65.
15. Haws CW, Lux RL. Correlation between in vivo transmembrane action potential durations and activation-recovery intervals from electrograms. Effects of interventions that alter repolarization time. Circulation 1990;81:281–8.
16. Steinhaus BM. Estimating cardiac transmembrane activation and recovery times from unipolar and bipolar extracellular electrograms: a simulation study. Circ Res 1989;64:449–62.
17. Martinez-Mateu L, Romero L, Ferrer-Albero A, et al. Factors affecting basket catheter detection of real and phantom rotors in the atria: a computational study. PLoS Comput Biol 2018;14:e1006017.
18. Cohen LB, Keynes RD, Hille B. Light scattering and birefringence changes during nerve activity. Nature 1968;218:438–41.
19. Tasaki I, Watanabe A, Sandlin R, et al. Changes in fluorescence, turbidity, and birefringence associated with nerve excitation. Proc Natl Acad Sci U S A 1968;61:883–8.

20. Salama G, Morad M. Merocyanine 540 as an optical probe of transmembrane electrical activity in the heart. Science 1976;191:485–7.

21. Cathey B, Obaid S, Zolotarev AM, et al. Open-source multiparametric optocardiography. Sci Rep 2019;9:721.

22. Morad M, Salama G. Optical probes of membrane potential in heart muscle. J Physiol 1979;292:267–95.

23. Ross WN, Salzberg BM, Cohen LB, et al. Changes in absorption, fluorescence, dichroism, and Birefringence in stained giant axons: : optical measurement of membrane potential. J Membr Biol 1977;33:141–83.

24. Durrer D, Dam Rv, Freud GE, et al. Total excitation of the isolated human heart. Circulation 1970;41:899–912.

25. Cerrone M, Noujaim SF, Tolkacheva EG, et al. Arrhythmogenic mechanisms in a mouse model of catecholaminergic polymorphic ventricular tachycardia. Circ Res 2007;101(10):1039–48.

26. Laughner JI, Ng FS, Sulkin MS, et al. Processing and analysis of cardiac optical mapping data obtained with potentiometric dyes. Am J Physiol Heart Circ Physiol 2012;303:H753–65.

27. Davidenko JM, Pertsov AV, Salomonsz R, et al. Stationary and drifting spiral waves of excitation in isolated cardiac muscle. Nature 1992;355:349–51.

28. Davidenko JM, Kent PF, Chialvo DR, et al. Sustained vortex-like waves in normal isolated ventricular muscle. Proc Natl Acad Sci U S A 1990;87:8785–9.

29. Winfree AT. Electrical instability in cardiac muscle: phase singularities and rotors. J Theor Biol 1989;138:353–405.

30. Frazier DW, Wolf PD, Wharton JM, et al. Stimulus-induced critical point. Mechanism for electrical initiation of reentry in normal canine myocardium. J Clin Invest 1989;83:1039–52.

31. Delgado C, Steinhaus B, Delmar M, et al. Directional differences in excitability and margin of safety for propagation in sheep ventricular epicardial muscle. Circ Res 1990;67:97–110.

32. Zykov VS. In: Winfree AT, editor. Simulation of wave processes in excitable media. 1987. p. 93–112.

33. Cabo C, Pertsov AM, Baxter WT, et al. Wave-front curvature as a cause of slow conduction and block in isolated cardiac muscle. Circ Res 1994;75:1014–28.

34. Kleber AG, Rudy Y. Basic mechanisms of cardiac impulse propagation and associated arrhythmias. Physiol Rev 2004;84:431–88.

35. Sepulveda NG, Roth BJ, Wikswo JP Jr. Current injection into a two-dimensional anisotropic bidomain. Biophys J 1989;55:987–99.

36. Sambelashvili AT, Nikolski VP, Efimov IR. Nonlinear effects in subthreshold virtual electrode polarization. Am J Physiol Heart Circ Physiol 2003;284:H2368–74.

37. Knisley SB, Hill BC, Ideker RE. Virtual electrode effects in myocardial fibers. Biophys J 1994;66:719–28.

38. Neunlist M, Tung L. Spatial distribution of cardiac transmembrane potentials around an extracellular electrode: dependence on fiber orientation. Biophys J 1995;68:2310–22.

39. Wikswo JP Jr, Lin SF, Abbas RA. Virtual electrodes in cardiac tissue: a common mechanism for anodal and cathodal stimulation. Biophys J 1995;69:2195–210.

40. Roth BJ. A mathematical model of make and break electrical stimulation of cardiac tissue by a unipolar anode or cathode. IEEE Trans Biomed Eng 1995;42:1174–84.

41. Sobie EA, Susil RC, Tung L. A generalized activating function for predicting virtual electrodes in cardiac tissue. Biophys J 1997;73:1410–23.

42. Efimov IR, Cheng YN, Biermann M, et al. Transmembrane voltage changes produced by real and virtual electrodes during monophasic defibrillation shock delivered by an implantable electrode. J Cardiovasc Electrophysiol 1997;8:1031–45.

43. Efimov IR, Cheng Y, Van Wagoner DR, et al. Virtual electrode-induced phase singularity: a basic mechanism of defibrillation failure. Circ Res 1998;82:918–25.

44. Lin SF, Roth BJ, Wikswo JP Jr. Quatrefoil reentry in myocardium: an optical imaging study of the induction mechanism. J Cardiovasc Electrophysiol 1999;10:574–86.

45. Lindblom AE, Roth BJ, Trayanova NA. Role of virtual electrodes in arrhythmogenesis: pinwheel experiment revisited. J Cardiovasc Electrophysiol 2000;11:274–85.

46. Latimer DC, Roth BJ. Electrical stimulation of cardiac tissue by a bipolar electrode in a conductive bath. IEEE Trans Biomed Eng 1998;45:1449–58.

47. Fedorov VV, Ambrosi CM, Kostecki G, et al. Anatomic localization and autonomic modulation of atrioventricular junctional rhythm in failing human hearts. Circ Arrhythm Electrophysiol 2011;4:515–25.

48. Fedorov VV, Glukhov AV, Chang R, et al. Optical mapping of the isolated coronary-perfused human sinus node. J Am Coll Cardiol 2010;56:1386–94.

49. Berenfeld O, Mandapati R, Dixit S, et al. Spatially distributed dominant excitation frequencies reveal hidden organization in atrial fibrillation in the Langendorff-perfused sheep heart. J Cardiovasc Electrophysiol 2000;11:869–79.

50. Berenfeld O, Zaitsev AV, Mironov SF, et al. Frequency-dependent breakdown of wave propagation into fibrillatory conduction across the pectinate muscle network in the isolated sheep right atrium. Circ Res 2002;90:1173–80.

51. Chen J, Mandapati R, Berenfeld O, et al. Dynamics of wavelets and their role in atrial fibrillation in the

isolated sheep heart. Cardiovasc Res 2000;48: 220–32.

52. Mandapati R, Skanes A, Chen J, et al. Stable micro-reentrant sources as a mechanism of atrial fibrillation in the isolated sheep heart. Circulation 2000;101: 194–9.

53. Mansour M, Mandapati R, Berenfeld O, et al. Left-to-right gradient of atrial frequencies during acute atrial fibrillation in the isolated sheep heart. Circulation 2001;103:2631–6.

54. Skanes AC, Mandapati R, Berenfeld O, et al. Spatiotemporal periodicity during atrial fibrillation in the isolated sheep heart. Circulation 1998;98: 1236–48.

55. Atienza F, Almendral J, Jalife J, et al. Real-time dominant frequency mapping and ablation of dominant frequency sites in atrial fibrillation with left-to-right frequency gradients predicts long-term maintenance of sinus rhythm. Heart Rhythm 2009;6:33–40.

56. Atienza F, Almendral J, Moreno J, et al. Activation of inward rectifier potassium channels accelerates atrial fibrillation in humans: evidence for a reentrant mechanism. Circulation 2006;114:2434–42.

57. Atienza F, Calvo D, Almendral J, et al. Mechanisms of fractionated electrograms formation in the posterior left atrium during paroxysmal atrial fibrillation in humans. J Am Coll Cardiol 2011;57:1081–92.

58. Sanders P, Berenfeld O, Hocini M, et al. Spectral analysis identifies sites of high-frequency activity maintaining atrial fibrillation in humans. Circulation 2005;112:789–97.

59. Filgueiras-Rama D, Price NF, Martins RP, et al. Long-term frequency gradients during persistent atrial fibrillation in sheep are associated with stable sources in the left atrium. Circ Arrhythm Electrophysiol 2012;5:1160–7.

60. Narayan SM, Baykaner T, Clopton P, et al. Ablation of rotor and focal sources reduces late recurrence of atrial fibrillation compared with trigger ablation alone: Extended follow-up of the CONFIRM trial (conventional ablation for atrial fibrillation with or without focal impulse and rotor modulation). J Am Coll Cardiol 2014;63:1761–8.

61. Haissaguerre M, Hocini M, Denis A, et al. Driver domains in persistent atrial fibrillation. Circulation 2014; 130:530–8.

62. Lee S, Sahadevan J, Khrestian CM, et al. Simultaneous biatrial high-density (510-512 electrodes) epicardial mapping of persistent and long-standing persistent atrial fibrillation in patients: new insights into the mechanism of its maintenance. Circulation 2015;132:2108–17.

63. Weerasooriya R, Khairy P, Litalien J, et al. Catheter ablation for atrial fibrillation: are results maintained at 5 years of follow-up? J Am Coll Cardiol 2011;57: 160–6.

64. Wellner M, Berenfeld O. Theory of reentry. In: Zipes DP, Jalife J, editors. Cardiac electrophysiology - from cell to bedside. 4th edition. Philadelphia: Saunders; 2004. p. 317–26.

65. Wellner M, Berenfeld O, Jalife J, et al. Minimal principle for rotor filaments. Proc Natl Acad Sci U S A 2002;99:8015–8.

66. Jalife J, Berenfeld O, Mansour M. Mother rotors and fibrillatory conduction: a mechanism of atrial fibrillation. Cardiovasc Res 2002;54:204–16.

67. Nattel S, Shiroshita-Takeshita A, Cardin S, et al. Mechanisms of atrial remodeling and clinical relevance. Curr Opin Cardiol 2005;20:21–5.

68. Jalife J, Berenfeld O. Molecular mechanisms and global dynamics of fibrillation: an integrative approach to the underlying basis of vortex-like reentry. J Theor Biol 2004;230:475–87.

69. Moe GK, Rheinboldt WC, Abildskov JA. A computer model of atrial fibrillation. Am Heart J 1964;67: 200–20.

70. Allessie MA, Lammers WJEP, Bonke FIM, et al. Experimental evaluation of Moe's wavelet hypothesis of atrial fibrillation. In: Zipes DP, Jalife J, editors. Cardiac electrophysiology and arrhythmias. Orlando (FL): Grune & Stratton; 1985. p. 265–75.

71. Gray RA, Pertsov AM, Jalife J. Spatial and temporal organization during cardiac fibrillation. Nature 1998; 392:75–8.

72. Jalife J, Berenfeld O, Skanes A, et al. Mechanisms of atrial fibrillation: mother rotors or multiple daughter wavelets, or both? J Cardiovasc Electrophysiol 1998;9:S2–12.

73. Warren M, Berenfeld O, Guha P, et al. IK1 blockade reduces frequency, increases organization and terminates ventricular fibrillation in the Guinea pig heart. PACE 2001;24:647.

74. Berenfeld O, Oral H. The quest for rotors in atrial fibrillation: different nets catch different fishes. Heart Rhythm 2012;9:1440–1.

75. Filgueiras-Rama D, Martins RP, Ennis SR, et al. High-resolution endocardial and epicardial optical mapping in a sheep model of stretch-induced atrial fibrillation. J Vis Exp 2011;(53) [pii:3103].

76. Samie FH, Berenfeld O, Anumonwo J, et al. Rectification of the background potassium current: a determinant of rotor dynamics in ventricular fibrillation. Circ Res 2001;89:1216–23.

77. Starobin JM, Zilberter YI, Rusnak EM, et al. Wavelet formation in excitable cardiac tissue: the role of wavefront-obstacle interactions in initiating high-frequency fibrillatory-like arrhythmias. Biophys J 1996;70:581–94.

78. Cabo C, Pertsov AM, Davidenko JM, et al. Vortex shedding as a precursor of turbulent electrical activity in cardiac muscle. Biophys J 1996;70:1105–11.

79. Filgueiras-Rama D, Martins RP, Mironov S, et al. Chloroquine terminates stretch-induced atrial

fibrillation more effectively than flecainide in the sheep heart. Circ Arrhythm Electrophysiol 2012;5: 561–70.

80. Aras KK, Faye NR, Cathey B, et al. Critical volume of human myocardium necessary to maintain ventricular fibrillation. Circ Arrhythm Electrophysiol 2018;11: e006692.

81. Garrey WE. The nature of fibrillatory contraction of the heart. Its relation to tissue mass and form. Am J Physiol 1914;30:397–414.

82. Mines GR. On dynamic equilibrium in the heart. J Physiol 1913;46:349–82.

83. Lou Q, Li W, Efimov IR. The role of dynamic instability and wavelength in arrhythmia maintenance as revealed by panoramic imaging with blebbistatin vs. 2,3-butanedione monoxime. Am J Physiol Heart Circ Physiol 2012;302:H262–9.

84. Lee P, Bollensdorff C, Quinn TA, et al. Single-sensor system for spatially resolved, continuous, and multiparametric optical mapping of cardiac tissue. Heart Rhythm 2011;8:1482–91.

85. Christoph J, Chebbok M, Richter C, et al. Electromechanical vortex filaments during cardiac fibrillation. Nature 2018;555:667–72.

86. Mitrea BG, Caldwell BJ, Pertsov AM. Imaging electrical excitation inside the myocardial wall. Biomed Opt Express 2011;2:620–33.

87. Dillon SM, Kerner TE, Hoffman J, et al. A system for in-vivo cardiac optical mapping. IEEE Eng Med Biol Mag 1998;17:95–108.

88. Dillon SM, Li KS. In vivo optical mapping of the canine infarct gives first direct evidence of discontinuous activation in ventricular tachycardia. Circulation 1998;98:51.

High-resolution/Density Mapping in Patients with Atrial and Ventricular Arrhythmias

Decebal Gabriel Laţcu, MD*, Nadir Saoudi, MD, FHRS

KEYWORDS

- Ultra–high-resolution density mapping • Atrial tachycardia • Ventricular tachycardia

KEY POINTS

- Multielectrode mapping with smaller and closely spaced electrodes yields a more accurate delineation of pathologic areas in both atria and ventricles.
- Improvedsignal-to-noise ratio and reliable automatic annotation are key points of ultra–high-definition (UHD) mapping.
- UHD mapping helps in diagnosing the precise mechanism of both atrial tachycardia and ventricular tachycardia; the critical areas of arrhythmogenesis are precisely localized.
- This technological advance is widely adopted despite scarce comparative data on long-term efficacy versus point-by-point mapping and is becoming the new standard in electroanatomic mapping.

INTRODUCTION

Contact mapping of cardiac arrhythmias evolved in the past 2 decades from fluoroscopic catheter manipulation and manual detection of the local activation time (LAT) to 3-D point-by-point mapping (PPM) and, recently, to multielectrode mapping (MEM) with reliable automatic annotation of thousands of points in 1 cardiac chamber.[1] These advances were accompanied by progressive decrease of the mapping electrode size, lessening of the electronic noise, and a tremendous progress of the information technology, including software and hardware innovations. Nowadays, the latest mapping tools allow entire chapters of clinical electrophysiology to be rewritten.

WHAT IS HIGH-DEFINITION/ULTRA–HIGH-DEFINITION MAPPING?

For the purpose of this article, when referring to electroanatomic 3-D mapping, the term "point"

refers to both the location of the acquired bipolar electrograms (EGMs) and the EGM itself. The authors acknowledge that contact and noncontact panoramic mapping technologies may yield detailed information about wavefront propagation, but only sequential contact mapping techniques is addressed.

Although there is no consensus definition of the high-definition/ultra–high-definition (HD/UHD) of cardiac mapping, electrophysiology practice changed from low-definition (eg, <100 points for 1 cardiac chamber[2]) to HD (eg, >400 points[2]) or UHD (eg, >15,000 points).[3] Recent reports of UHD mapping of organized arrhythmias yielded figures of 209 points/cm² at the atrial level[3] and 82 points/cm² at the ventricular level.[4] On top of number of points and point density, HD/UHD mapping also allows improved substrate characterization, a better understanding of the arrhythmia mechanism, and a better selection of ablation targets in atrial and ventricular arrhythmias.[3,5]

Conflicts of Interest: Dr D.G. Laţcu received speaking honoraria (modest) from Boston Scientific and travel support from Boston Scientific and Biosense Webster. Dr Bun received speaking honoraria (modest) from Boston Scientific.
Centre Hospitalier Princesse Grace, Avenue Pasteur, 98000 Monaco
* Corresponding author. Cardiologie, Centre Hospitalier Princesse Grace, Avenue Pasteur, 98000 Monaco.
E-mail address: dglatcu@yahoo.com

Card Electrophysiol Clin 11 (2019) 511–524
https://doi.org/10.1016/j.ccep.2019.05.001
1877-9182/19/© 2019 Elsevier Inc. All rights reserved.

HOW TO PERFORM HIGH-DEFINITION/ ULTRA–HIGH-DEFINITION MAPPING
Point-by-Point Versus Multielectrode Mapping

In many cases, reliable activation maps may be performed by PPM. This usually implies the use of a linear mapping catheter with a large-sized electrode (eg, 3.5 mm) designed for radiofrequency delivery. Yet the electrode size is paramount for the resolution/definition of the map. Anter and colleagues[6] studied 30 cases (10 normal and 20 with scar-related atrial tachycardia [AT]) PPM (with a catheter having a 3.5-mm istal electrode and a 2-mm proximal ring electrode, separated by 2 mm [For a more recent version of this catheter-type with slightly different characteristics, please go to https://www.biosensewebster. com/products/carto-3/smarttouch-catheter.aspx]). (Those were compared with MEM using a 20-pole catheter [PentaRay, Biosense Webster, Diamond Bar, CA] Available at: https://www. biosensewebster.com/products/carto-3/pentaray-eco-catheter.aspx]), with 1-mm ring electrodes separated by 2 mm. As expected, MEM had more points (1554 _ 374 vs 366 _ 273; P<.01) and were acquired faster (13 min _ 7 min vs 21 min _ 12 min; P 5 .03). The fifth percentile of the normal bipolar voltage amplitude was similar with the 2 catheters (0.48 mV vs 0.52 mV; P = .65). The advantages of MEM became evident when they found that the surface of the low-voltage areas (defined as bipolar voltage <0.5 mV) was smaller than that of PPM (14.7 cm^2 vs 20.4 cm^2; P = .02) and that the mean bipolar voltage amplitude in these areas was higher using MEM (0.28 mV vs 0.17 mV; P = .01). A better delineation of scars with a more reliable annotation of activation (54% of points for MEM vs 21% for PPM maps; P = .01) in the scar areas was demonstrated. These differences remained significant after normalizing the maps for point density and interelectrode spacing. The investigators concluded that smaller-size electrodes are at least partially responsible for the improved resolution.

The same team[7] demonstrated similar results at the ventricular level in a swine model of normal ventricles and healed myocardial infarction. Although the fifth percentile of the bipolar voltage in normal tissue was similar with the 2 catheters, in swine with healed infarction, the total area of low bipolar voltage amplitude (<1.5 mV) was 22.5% smaller using 1-mm multielectrode catheters (21.7 cm^2 vs 28.0 cm^2; P = .003). In dense scar areas (bipolar amplitude <0.5 mV), this difference was even more important (7.1 cm^2 with the 1-mm electrode catheters vs 15.2 cm^2; P = .003). In this region, MEM had a higher voltage amplitude (0.72 mV

± 0.81 mV vs 0.30 mV ± 0.12 mV; P<.001), with, in 27% of sites, distinct triphasic EGM with the PentaRay compared with fractionated multicomponent EGM recorded with the 3.5-mm electrode catheter. In the same study, cardiac magnetic resonance imaging (MRI) and histology showed improved correlations of the nontransmural scars with MEM maps.

In a recent randomized study[8] of MEM versus PPM for ventricular tachycardia (VT) substrate ablation, the same catheters were used (Navistar, Biosense-Webster, Irvine, CA and PentaRay). Surprisingly, larger bipolar scar areas were obtained with MEM (55.7 cm^2 ± 31.7 cm^2 vs 50.5 cm^2 ± 26.6 cm^2; P = .017); mapping time was similar with MEM (19.7 min ± 7.9 min) and PPM (25 min ± 9.2 min; P = .222). This result might be explained by the use of the 2 techniques in different patients/ ventricles, in a limited number, despite randomization. Although the number of late potential (LP) sites identified within the scar by MEM versus PPM was similar (73 LPs ± 50 LPs vs 76 LPs ± 52 LPs per patient, respectively; P = .965), using the PentaRay, the far-field/LP ratio was significantly lower (0.58 ± 0.4 vs 1.64 ± 1.1; P = .01). Ablation was performed according to the scar-dechanneling technique. For the same acute result in terms of noninducibility, radiofrequency time was shorter with MEM (median interquartile range [IQR] 12 [7–20] min versus 22 [17–33] min; P = .023), attributed to the better discrimination of LP by the PentaRay.

Multielectrode Mapping with Smaller and Closely Spaced Electrodes

In addition to the 5-arm star-shaped PentaRay catheter, discussed previously (coupled with the Carto 3 mapping system [Biosense Webster]), 2 other multielectrode catheters are used for HD/UHD mapping. The Advisor HD grid[9] (Abbott, North Chicago, Illinois), coupled with the EnSite Precision cardiac mapping system (**Fig. 1**B), has equally small ring electrodes (1-mm each) distributed in a 4-by-4 pattern grid on 2.5F splines, with a 4-mm interelectrode distance (center to center). The Rhythmia[1] (Boston Scientific, Marlborough, Massachusetts)) mapping system uses a 64-pole basket mapping catheter (IntellaMap Orion [Boston Scientific] [**Fig. 1**A]), which incorporates small flat, unidirectional, electrodes (0.4 mm^2; 2.5-mm spacing center to center), expected to better suppress noise and far-field signals compared with ring electrodes.

Improving the Signal-to-Noise Ratio by Diminishing the Noise

It is now well established that closely spaced smaller electrodes allow detection of lower-

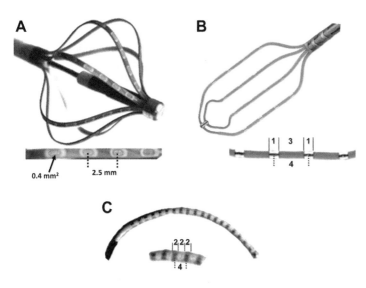

Fig. 1. (*A*) The Intella-Map Orion (Boston Scientific) is a 64-pole basket mapping catheter, which incorporates small flat, unidirectional, electrodes (0.4 mm²; 2.5-mm spacing center to center). Various degrees of deployment allow its use from a linear shape (adapted to small tubular structures as the distal coronary sinus or more distal parts of the pulmonary veins or for epicardial mapping) to a spherical shape). (*B*) The Advisor HD Grid Mapping Catheter, Sensor Enabled (Abbott) is a 16-pole 1-mm ring electrodes catheter with a 4 _ 4 arrangement of the electrodes on a grid preserving the 4-mm interelectrode spacing in 2 directions. The catheter allows for bipolar recordings both along and across the splines to account for directionality and prevent bipolar blindness. Typically, a signal is visualized only when the activation wavefront is propagating parallel to a catheter. The system analyzes the wavefront in 2 perpendicular directions and records the best signal of the 2. (*C*) Steerable duodecapolar catheter (Livewire, 2–2–2 mm spacing, St. Jude Medical). (*Courtesy of* [A] Boston Scientific, Marlborough, MA; with permission; and [B, C] Abbott, Plymouth, MN; with permission.)

amplitude signals (thus improving the density/resolution especially in low-voltage scar areas). The lower threshold of recordable physiologic electric signals is limited by the amplitude of electronic noise, which should be minimized in order to improve the signal-to-noise ratio. Noise and artifacts may have various origins and may bias EGM interpretation. Electromagnetic fields and intermittent connections are the main causes of noise in an electrophysiology laboratory. If cable connections are poor, surface electrocardiogram (ECG) leads and catheter handles can be easily managed; electromagnetic noise sources are more difficult to suppress. A set of measures contributes to noise reduction before the signal amplification process: correct routing of the intracardiac, radiofrequency, and ECG cables without floor contact, isolation of power cables away from signal cables, and careful skin preparation. Intracardiac noise also may be reduced by using an indifferent unipolar electrode inside the inferior vena cava, deep sedation, or general anesthesia.

Despite all these measures, in many laboratories, background noise (BGN) persists at levels that are comparable to the magnitude of the smallest electrical signals from viable tissue within the scar.[10] Noise levels rarely have been the subject of published research.

In a recent study from the authors' group,[3] the electronic noise on the Rhythmia system was measured using the voltage calipers with adequate amplification and speed. From the bipolar EGM acquired during scar-related AT with the Orion catheter, BGN was assessed at 6 prespecified sites for the left atrium (midroof, midposterior wall, posterior mitral annulus, interatrial septum, midanterior wall, and appendage) and 4 prespecified sites for the RA (cavotricuspid isthmus, septum, appendage, and crista terminalis). The BGN also was assessed on the bipolar EGM recorded with a standard decapolar catheter (2-mm ring electrodes and spacing) and on the surface ECG. BGN ranged from 10 μV to 12 μV (0.011 mV ± 0.004 mV) for the basket catheter EGM, without significant differences between sites. This value is much lower than nominal setting of dense scar in the mapping systems (0.03 mV). The small, flat (unidirectional), and closely spaced electrodes of the Orion had less noise than that of the standard decapolar catheter (0.016 mV ± 0.019 mV) and the surface ECG leads (0.02 mV ± 0.01 mV) acquired on the Rhythmia system ($P = .00009$).[3]

This unprecedented low level of BGN opens new possibilities for efficient mapping of viable tissue within scars, by appropriated thresholding of dense scar to lower levels, closer to BGN. UHD mapping becomes now possible in scar areas.

Improved Automatic Annotation and Software Tools for High-density/Ultra–High-density Mapping

The annotation is the detection of the LAT of each point (bipolar EGM), with respect to a preestablished reference. It is obvious that, in the setting of HD/UHD mapping, the very large number of points makes systematic manual check of the annotation (the detection of the LAT) impossible. Reliable automatic annotation thus became mandatory with the advent of HD/UHD mapping.

The first multiple criteria algorithm embedded in a 3-D electroanatomic mapping system to answer this new challenge came with Rhythmia.[1] For annotation of the LAT of each acquired bipolar EGM, the system combines unipolar (maximum negative dV/dt) and bipolar (maximum amplitude) EGM. For fragmented or multiple potential EGM, the system takes into account the timing in the surrounding area to select the potential to use for the timing annotation. In cases of a lack of statistical coherence between neighboring points in an area, no color code is displayed and the area is left gray. Above annotation, cardiac beats are selected automatically for inclusion in the map based on cycle length stability, stable relative timing of 2 reference EGMs, electrode location stability, and respiratory gating. The window of interest (WOI) is automatically set by the system at the cycle length value and centered on the main reference EGM. With these characteristics, in the initial experimental setting,[1] only 0.17% of the acquired EGM were manually reannotated and only for presentation purposes, because blinded examination of all the activation maps (prior to manual annotation of activation time at any site) accurately revealed the site of earliest atrial activation, the location and extent of the lines of conduction block, and the presence or absence of conduction through a gap. This positive initial experience was prospectively confirmed in clinical settings.[3,11,12]

The automated ConfiDENSE HD mapping module (Carto 3 v4) proposes several annotation algorithms with different accuracies in defining the tachycardia mechanism.[13] For the EnSite Precision AutoMap software (Abbott), a multicentric registry[14] revealed arrhythmia-specific adjustments of the nominal mapping thresholds used in clinical practice to collect 8.8-times more electrophysiologically relevant data than manual mapping without increasing mapping time. Ripple mapping (Carto 3), a visualization method that displays each EGM component as a dynamic bar moving out from the surface relative to a fiducial time point on a 3-D map surface, has been used to identify slow conduction channels in AT[15] and VT (within postinfarct scar[16] or in arrhythmogenic right ventricular cardiomyopathy[17]).

In addition to annotation, in case the operators change the reference or the WOI, rapid automatic recalculation of the new LAT for all the acquired points is necessary and provided by some of the systems. Full comprehension of an arrhythmia mechanism (discussed later) also is dependent on the analysis of propagation. Conduction velocity (CV) analysis[3,9,18,19] also brings valuable supplemental information for defining the appropriate target for ablation.

ULTRA–HIGH-DEFINITION MAPPING IN ATRIAL ARRHYTHMIAS
Mechanism of Atrial Tachycardia

Although HD/UHD mapping is used more and more for atrial fibrillation, only organized atrial arrhythmias (stable AT or monomorphic premature atrial complexes) are discussed in this article.

AT, often scar related (either post–AF ablation or incisional), is a challenging arrhythmia. Critical areas of arrhythmogenesis occur often in diseased tissue, where voltage is attenuated often below the BGN. ECG-based diagnosis, entrainment mapping, imaging of the substrate, and detailed knowledge of previously created lesions all are used in the diagnostic of the circuit (or the site of origin in case of a focal source). Except for typical (right isthmus–dependent) flutter, in many cases, these techniques are used as a complement of electroanatomic mapping.

HD/UHD mapping of AT replaced, whenever available, PPM. Very good acute[6] and better long-term results[2] were reported with HD mapping of AT. A shorter mapping time also was demonstrated in these studies with HD mapping.

Precise visualization of the mechanism of AT in the vast majority of cases (ranging from 98%[20] to 100%[3]) became possible with UHD mapping. As a consequence, unusual macroreentrant ATs were found far more frequently than previously reported, accounting for up to one-third of the scar-related ATs. The authors also found a significant number of microreentrant and focal ATs (21%), often not originating from the pulmonary veins. Small (localized) reentries[21] are easily differentiated from pseudoreentries using UHD,[22] with the benefit of avoiding useless ablation.

Critical Isthmus

As a natural consequence of the improvement of mapping, UHD allowed a very precise localization of the critical isthmus.[3] Sites of narrowing of the wavefront and/or slowing of the CV (from 1 m/s to 0.27 m/s; $P<.0001$) were demonstrated to be the appropriate target of ablation with high acute success. In the particular cases of roof or perimitral macroreentries, the critical isthmus proved a practical one for ablation because it is significantly shorter that the anatomic isthmus (roof of left isthmus) in these cases (16.1 ± 8.2 mm vs

33.7 mm± 10.4 mm; $P<.0001$).[23] UHD mapping also brought proof that long-duration (87.8 ms ± 10.7 ms) and low-voltage (0.16 mV ± 0.07 mV) bipolar EGMs are pathognomonic (if both present) for slow conduction,[24] allowing improvement of the interpretation of fragmented potentials.

Supplemental and Future Features of High-definition/Ultra–High-definition Mapping Systems

Special features of the UHD software proved particularly useful. The "show earliest" feature helps identifying precisely the earliest activation site of focal AT (**Fig. 2**). Beyond voltage mapping (discussed previously), UHD activation mapping (in AT or sinus rhythm [SR]) provides considerable help in identifying the substrate of AT (ie, incision lines [**Fig. 3**]) as well as for validating block across previously created ablation lines.[25] Automatic detection of double potential EGM and diatolic potentials are near-future software improvements that will be available (Lumipoint embedded in Rhythmia [**Fig. 4**]).[26,27] The Carto 3 system (v6) with the HD coloring feature provides improved visualization of propagation. An investigational activation mapping software[19] (Coherent Mapping) based on the Carto 3 system, integrating vector and velocity information, further improves the identification of the mechanism of complex

AT (92.5% correct identification vs 70% with standard activation mapping).

Comparison Between High-definition/Ultra–High-definition Mapping Systems for Atrial Tachycardia

To the best of the authors' knowledge there is no randomized comparative trial between the different mapping systems for complex AT mapping and ablation. Such a trial would be difficult to implement due to the different sensor-based location technologies requiring complicated hardware periprocedural switches. Isolated cases have been studied with 2 mapping systems simultaneously (ie, Rhythmia and Ensite Precision) but only comparative images/videos are available online, without any systematic scientific assessment of outcomes.

The first available comparative data came from a multicentric study,[28] which included 20 patients with 24 ATs with a previously failed ablation procedure. In prior procedures, the arrhythmia could not be adequately mapped with Carto 3 or NavX (Abbott) using circular multielectrode or PentaRay catheters. Among these cases, 14 ATs were similar to those previously mapped. The activation map performed with the Rhythmia system was able to define the mechanism and location of the circuit in all 14 cases, yielding a 100% acute ablation success.

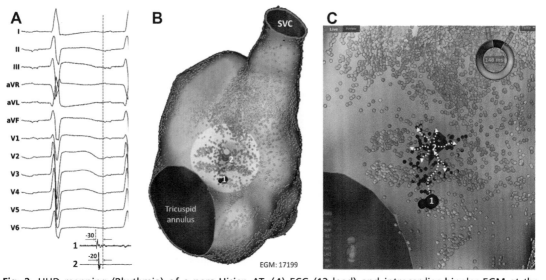

Fig. 2. UHD mapping (Rhythmia) of a para-Hisian AT. (*A*) ECG (12 lead) and intracardiac bipolar EGM at the earliest activation site (EAS) (1) and in the center of the visually earliest (*red*) area (2). (*B*) Septal view of the right atrium and search for the EAS using the show earliest function with the roving (virtual) probe. (*C*) Zoom in the region of the EAS. Activation propagates from the EAS site to site 2 through an insulated fiber, and from site 2 it spreads centrifugally to the entire atrium. Radiofrequency ablation was unsuccessful at site 2 but successful at site 1 (closest to His). SVC, superior vena cava.

A

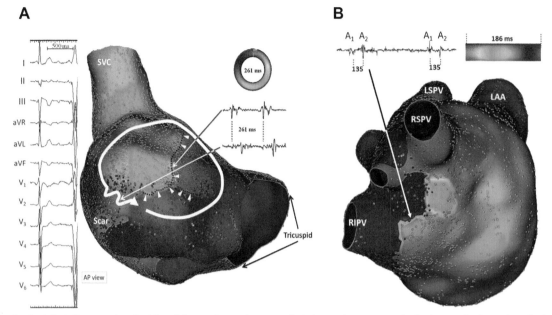

B

Fig. 3. (*A*) UHD map of an incisional flutter (negative wave in V_1), turning counterclockwise on the lateral wall of the RA. The central obstacle of this circuit is represented by the surgical incision line, detected as a double potential line (*black dotted line* and *white arrowheads*). At the lower extremity of this line, there is a site with fragmented and low-voltage potentials, representing the critical isthmus of the tachycardia, and successfully targeted with ablation. (*B*) Right lateral view of the LA, mapped in SR with the Rhythmia system, in a patient with a medical history of mitral valve repair; the surgical report indicated that the incision was performed at the level of the Sondergaard/Waterston interatrial groove, in front of the right pulmonary veins. Locally there is clear-cut separation of the colors coding for the timing of activation, suggesting the presence of a block-line. Double potential EGMs are present along this line, which may represent the substrate of a reentry using one of its extremities as a critical isthmus. AP, Antero-posterior; LAA, left atrial appendage; LSPV, left superior pulmonary vein; RIPV, right inferior pulmonary vein; RSPV, right superior pulmonary vein; SVC, superior vena cava.

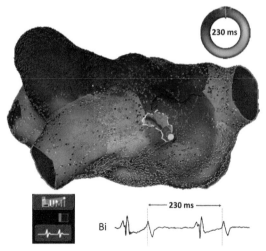

Fig. 4. Superior view of the left atrium in a rrof-dependent atrial flutter (cycle length 230 ms). The "split tool" of Lumipoint automatically highlights the area of double potentials on the roof, thus unmasking the remaining part of the roof as the gap area to be targetted in this case.

Long-term recurrences after AT ablation using UHD mapping (Rhythmia) were compared with HD 3-D mapping (Carto/NavX) in the setting of a retrospective controlled trial.[29] UHD maps had a significantly higher number of points (10,543 ± 5854 per map vs 689 ± 1827 per map; $P<.0001$). Although this did not translate into a significant difference in mechanism identification between the 2 technologies nor a better acute success between groups, there were fewer long-term (1-year) recurrences after AT ablation using UHD mapping (37%) compared with HD mapping (50%, $P = .04$). If electrophysiologists can compensate inadequately mapped AT by entrainment mapping or substrate analysis and ultimately terminate AT with empiric ablation lines (**Fig. 5**), a better long-term result might be the consequence of a better comprehensive approach of AT mechanisms, as diagnosed by UHD mapping. The authors previously reported[3] that in a significant number of AT cases, potential circuits (different from the mapped AT) may be visualized; once the active

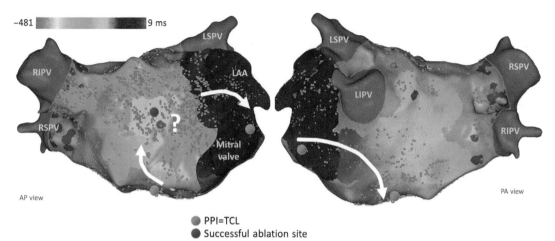

Fig. 5. Activation maps (anteroposterior [AP] and posteroanterior [PA] views) of the LA during a clockwise peri-mitral flutter, using HD mapping (Carto 3 v4, ConfiDENSE module). AP, antero-posterior; LAA, left atrial appendage; LIPV, left inferior pulmonary vein; LSPV, left superior pulmonary vein; PA, postero-anterior; RIPV, right inferior pulmonary vein; RSPV, right superior pulmonary vein. The question mark mark refers to the un-known position of the gap; this is intuitively explained in the legend. Arrows indicate the direction of wavefront propagation. A large scar area is visualized on the anterior wall, with impossible annotation of the EGM in this area, despite a scar setting value of 0.01 mV. The mechanism (perimitral macroreentry) was confirmed by entrain-ment mapping (green tags depict pacing sites with concealed entrainement and a postpacing interval [PPI] equal to the tachycardia cycle length [TCL]). Ablation, therefore, was empirically attempted and finally successful in the scar area (*brown tag*) because this is the expected location of the conduction gap.

AT is interrupted, the potential circuits previously visualized may become active (and subse-quently ablated), but preventive ablation of the critical isthmus of such circuits may avoid future recurrences.

Typical Flutter Rewritten—From Textbooks to Ultra–High-definition Mapping

The advent of UHD mapping of cardiac arrhyth-mias is a historical chance to challenge some cur-rent knowledge. One example in the field of AT is the mapping of typical flutter.[30] By means of UHD mapping, a bicentric series[31] brought new in-sights about the conduction and substrate vari-ability in right atrial macroreentrant tachycardia, mainly in typical flutter. The authors demonstrated, in half of the cases, a significant slowing of the CV within the cavotricuspid isthmus; this has been previously proposed in the literature but was still a subject of debate because only by finely tuned analysis of propagation highly localized regions of conduction slowing in the CTI were visualized.

Pathik and colleagues[31] also contradicted the paradigm of transverse conduction block along crista terminalis. The position of the posterior line of block was, in the majority of patients (72%), post-eromedial to the crista terminalis, at the level of the sinus venosus (as a straight line between the 2 cava veins). This line constitutes, together with the ori-fices of the inferior and superior vena cava and the eustachian ridge, the central posterior boundary of this macroreentry. Other findings of this series are equally interesting, but efforts are still awaited in this field in order to describe the subtle changes of the typical flutter ECG waves with the variations of the breakthrough site in the line of block or the different slow conduction/activation patterns.

Epicardial Bridging of Atrial Tachycardia Diagnosed by Ultra–High-definition Mapping and Use of Entrainement

If the 3-D structure of VT circuits is widely acqui-esced among electrophysiologists and epicardial access for VT ablation commonly used in high-volume centers, epicardial-endocardial dissocia-tion in the atrium has been reported less often. A first experimental study[32] proved that discordant activation between the layers of the atrial wall correlated to transmural differences in fiber orien-tation. This may account for the existence of AT reentrant loops using free-running muscle bundles connecting the epicardial and endocardial sur-faces. In an animal model of atrial fibrillation,[33] pronounced dissociation of electrical activity has been demonstrated between the epicardial layer and the endocardial bundle network. The increase in dissociation is due to the progressive uncou-pling between these structures and correlates with the complexity of the atrial fibrillation substrate.

In stable AT, using UHD mapping, epicardial to endocardial breakthroughs (EEBs) recently were demonstrated.[34] The investigators proposed 3 diagnostic criteria for this phenomenon: (1) the presence of focal endocardial activation with radial spread unaccounted for by an endocardial wavefront, (2) this focal activation is present with the same timing on every tachycardia cycle, and (3) with the EEB site always in proximity to a line of endocardial conduction slowing or block. Moreover, they demonstrated that 80% of unipolar EGM at the EEB site had an rS morphology. If, in this initial series, in 1 only case was the EEB site critical to arrhythmia maintenance, there is now proof that in the case of AT with some part of the circuit located extraendocardially, the EEB site is the most successful ablation site.

This phenomenon often occurs in perimitral flutter, where, despite endocardial mitral block, epicardial bridging connections may persist via the musculature of the coronary sinus[35,36] or the vein of Marshall.[11] These new data demonstrates that endocardial and coronary sinus UHD mapping is now the optimal diagnostic method for complete block at the mitral line, improving the prediction of long-term success in comparison with differential pacing maneuvers.[35]

Because the circuit is not entirely mapped endocardially even by means of UHD mapping, use of entrainment may be useful to demonstrate macro-reentry in these cases. Moreover, entrainment and UHD 3-D mapping provide sometimes critical complementary information because entrainment may unmask visual reentry as passive.[37]

Beyond epicardial to endocardial dissociation in the setting of AT, biatrial UHD mapping also may reveal a dissociation of the 2 sides of the interatrial septum. Thus, true biatrial circuits may occur and 3 different types were reported in a small initial series.[38] The ideal ablation strategy in these situations still needs to be defined.

ULTRA–HIGH-DEFINITION MAPPING IN VENTRICULAR ARRHYTHMIAS
High-definition/Ultra–High-definition Substrate Mapping in Ventricular Tachycardia

HD substrate MEM in scar-related VT was first reported with the use of a steerable linear duodecapolar catheter with 2-mm ring electrodes and a 2-mm interelectrode spacing (**Fig. 1**C).[39–41] In an initial study of 21 patients with postischemic VT, HD mapping with NavX Velocity, several 787 ± 391 and 810 ± 375 points in the left ventricular (LV) endocardium and epicardium were acquired in SR or paced rhythm and maps showed areas of voltage heterogeneity within dense scar

regions, correlated with the presence of LPs. Success of ablation brought proof that these sites were critical for reentrant VT. In a bicentric 17-patient series,[40] the authors used NavX Velocity with manual tagging of the LP sites and entrainment mapping at sites demonstrating diastolic activity on the duodecapolar catheter when the VT was hemodynamically tolerated. The mean number of LV endocardial mapping points was 819 ± 357, with an average mapping time of 31 minutes ± 7 minutes. LPs were seen in all patients during endocardial mapping; the mean number of induced VTs was 2.8 ± 1.6. Ablation was at sites identified by LPs, pacemapping, and/or entrainment with acute success in 94% of patients. The intermediate success rate (free of VT recurrence) was 69%, with an average follow-up of 8 months ± 3 months.

The PentaRay catheter coupled with the Carto system has also been used successfully for HD substrate mapping of VT (**Fig. 6**). In a retrospective study[42] of 26 patients with both ischemic and nonischemic VT, 1085 points ± 726 points were acquired in 55.6 minutes ± 34.4 minutes. The dense scar and patchy areas were well delineated, but the authors questioned the automatic annotation of the fragmented potentials. After a mean ablation time (targeting abnormal potentials within scar areas) of 50.8 minutes ± 30.1 minutes, 65.4% of patients remained arrhythmia-free at 14 months.

A prospective cohort (n = 59) of MEM with the PentaRay in scar-related VT was compared with a control group with PPM (ThermoCool SmartTouch, Biosense-Webster) in a historical cohort (n = 22).[43] Substrate mapping was systematically performed and activation mapping of the induced VT in 39% in the study group. With the PentaRay, the procedure time was significantly shorter (177 min ± 53 min vs 206 min ± 50 min; P = .02) for a similar acute success of VT noninducibility (approximately 70%). This was driven by a significant shortening of the mapping time in the study group (38 min ± 15 min vs 56 min ± 24 min for endocardial LV mapping; P = .003; and 28 min ± 9 min vs 41 min ± 16 min, for epicardial mapping; P = .011). The number of acquired points also was significantly higher in the study group (endocardial MEM, 2150 points ± 1477 points vs PPM 500 points ± 187 points; P<.0001; and epicardial MEM, 3327 points ± 1825 points vs PPM 877 points ± 258 points; P<.0001). This resulted in a higher mapping density (points/cm^2) in the MEM group, especially in the scar area (<0.5 mV): 46.9 points/cm^2 ± 32.3 points/cm^2 versus 8.5 points/cm^2 ± 4.6 points/cm^2 were collected in the endocardial LV scar area

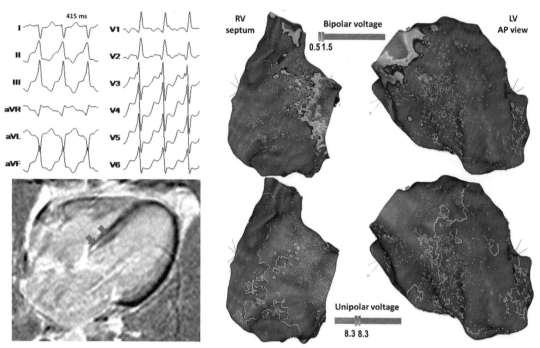

Fig. 6. Right bundle VT in a 58-year old man with a history of syncopal complete AV block. AP, antero-posterior; RV: right ventricle. Cardiac MRI showed late gadolinium enhancement in the midseptum and HD right ventricular (RV) and LV maps acquired with the PentaRay catheter showed normal septal bipolar voltage (*upper panels*) but unipolar maps (*lower panels*) clearly showed substrate abnormalities correlated with the location on the MRI. The exit site of the VT was mapped and successfully ablated on the LV septal side at the upper edge of the unipolar scar area.

(P<.001), and 30.7 points/cm^2 ± 21.9 points/cm^2 versus 8.1 points/cm^2 ± 5.6 points/cm^2 were collected in the epicardial LV scar area (P = .028). In this study, the follow-up duration was not comparable between groups, but it seems that for a similar duration MEM warrants better long-term results.

UHD substrate mapping with Rhythmia was first tested in 2 chronic infarct animal models.[44,45] In the first swine (n = 10) model of myocardial infarction,[44] the authors demonstrated that the fifth percentile of normal bipolar voltage distribution (the lower limit of normality) using the Orion was 1.54 mV. They also showed a better correlation between MRI and catheter scar area measurement for the Orion (r = 0.76 basket vs 0.71 for a linear catheter) as well as the feasibility of the epicardial mapping with the Orion. Most importantly, in 3 animals, poorly tolerated sustained VT was initiated and the circuit was successfully mapped with basket catheter in less than 5 minutes. In the second study,[45] LV endocardial mapping was performed 4.9 months ± 0.9 months after infarction and within 2 weeks of capturing the chronic cardiac MRI. The maps contained 7754 points ± 1960 points with a mean resolution of 2.8 mm ± 0.6 mm. The 3-D MRI signal intensity maps derived from the gadolinium-enhanced images showed a close correlation of scar location and size to the low-voltage areas (defined as bipolar voltage <2 mV). A unipolar voltage of less than 13 mV correlated with transmural extension of scar in MRI, whereas endocardial scar was correlated with cutoffs of unipolar voltage greater than or equal to 15 mV and bipolar voltage less than 1 mV. The recording of LPs also was demonstrated with the Rhythmia system in this experimental study.

In the first clinical series[12] of UHD ventricular substrate mapping with Rhythmia (n = 19), both transseptal and retrograde approaches were used without procedural complications. The authors proposed thresholds of dense scar as less than 0.1 mV and scar border zone as 1.0 mV to 0.1 mV. VT substrate maps (n = 14; median 10,184 points) consistently demonstrated LP with high resolution within the scar areas. The authors also demonstrated feasibility of VT activation maps (n = 25; median 6401 points) with automatic annotation. Ventricular ectopy (VE) timing maps (n = 8) successfully localized the origin of VEs in all, with all accepted beats consistent with clinical VEs. A good long-term result was also reported (median follow-up of 10 months, no arrhythmia recurrence in 75% after VT ablation and 86% after VE ablation).

A second series specifically addressed UHD substrate mapping in human VT (n = 22).[46] If the endocardial and epicardial bipolar voltage scar definition was the same as in the previous study (dense <0.1 mV and border zone 0.1–1.0 mV), the investigators of this series also proposed a unipolar endocardial voltage cutoff for scar less than 4.5 mV. The mean mapping time was 33 minutes ± 4 minutes for substrate maps (10,937 points ± 1923 points) and 9 minutes ± 2 minutes for VT maps (6740 points ± 1140 points). Moving the entire WOI after the end of the QRS complex allowed automatic detection and annotation of LPs in 73% of the substrate maps (but EGM review confirmed them only in 69%).

High-definition/Ultra–High-definition Activation Mapping in Ventricular Tachudardia

The first electrophysiologic characterization of the circuit of post–myocardial infarction reentrant VT (n = 21) by UHD mapping was performed in an animal study (15 swine) by Anter and colleagues.[4] Macroreentrant VTs (n = 18) had often a figure-8 pattern (n = 14). The common channel was characterized by a linear propagation in a 2-D structure bounded by 2 laterally opposing zones of very slow conduction (**Fig. 7**A). Isthmuses were 16.4-mm ± 7.2-mm long and 7.4-mm ± 2.8-mm wide. The axis of the isthmus was uniformly oriented parallel to the long axis of the ventricle (±30°). In contrast with scar-related macroreentrant AT,[3] CV were slow at the inward curvature into the isthmus entrance but was nearly normal at the central isthmus before slowing again at the outward curvature exit (see **Fig. 7**A). Surprisingly, the dimensions of the isthmus defined by entrainment exceeded the dimensions of the isthmus measured by activation mapping by 32% ± 18%. These data suggested that at least parts of the isthmus boundaries are functional and thus corrected an ancient misconception about VT circuits and mapping.[47]

A subsequent animal study from the same team[48] brought proof that the zones of slowest CV during VT (critical zones) exhibited very slow conduction also during SR; these critical areas also may serve as anchor sites for multiple VT. Moreover, the investigators demonstrated that low voltage or LPs are not specific of isthmus sites, probably because dead-end pathways may exist that do not contribute consistently to the main circuits. The positive predictive value of CV slowing greater than or equal to 75% during SR for critical zones was 70%. This predictive value

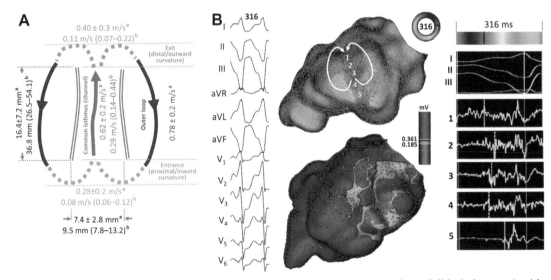

Fig. 7. (A) Sketch of a figure-8 pattern of macroreentrant VT with a common channel (*blue*) characterized by linear propagation in a 2-D structure bounded by 2 laterally opposing zones of very slow conduction (*red double line*). CVs are slow at the inward curvature into the isthmus entrance (*orange*) but are nearly normal at the central isthmus before slowing again at the outward curvature exit (*green*).[4,5] [a] Animal study (mean ± SD),[4] [b] human study (median [IQR]).[5] (B) VT (CL 316 ms) in a patient with a post–myocardial infarction inferior scar. Upper map (inferior view of the LV; activation) shows a figure-8 pattern with multicomponent fragmented potentials at the level of the critical isthmus. Lower map (similar view; bipolar voltage in SR) shows an area of heterogeneity with preserved voltage within the scar, corresponding to the isthmus location. Ablation transecting this area was successful.

was significantly higher than voltage abnormality (21%) or isolated LP (16%) and local abnormal ventricular activities (LAVAs) (14%).

Human data with UHD mapping of VT confirmed many of these new concepts. Thus, in a muticentric series[5] of 31 patients (36 VT), the investigators showed that CV in the VT isthmus slowed at isthmus entrances and exits when compared with the midisthmus (see **Fig. 7**A). The size of the isthmus was bigger than in the animal study, but its orientation was in the majority (78%) approximately longitudinal (±45° to the long axis of the ventricle) and circumferential in 22% of VT. The barriers to conduction in the isthmus seem to be partly functional in 75% of circuits. Median local voltage in the isthmus was low (0.12 mV) during tachycardia and even lower (0.06 mV; $P<.001$) in paced rhythm/SR. The study of the correlation between the EGM timing to surface ECG showed that activation of VT exits occurs approximately 56 ms before QRS onset, or at 77% of the diastolic interval, and the midisthmus is largely activated in diastole, between QRS complexes. Activation of entrance zones is more variable and frequently overlaps with the preceding QRS.

A small human case series[49] (n = 3) of UHD VT activation brought a direct proof for 3-D activation patterns of VT using the complex 3-D distribution of the surviving myocardial bundles in ventricular scars. The investigators elegantly depicted diverging directions of activation in the same area with crossroads or flyover patterns, implying recording of independent multilayer channels.

Ultra–High-definition Mapping of Poorly Tolerated Ventricular Tachycardia

Although hemodynamic support is a valuable option for the mapping of hemodynamically unstable VT, recent reports argue for the utility of rapid UHD mapping in this setting, as discussed in an animal study.[45]

Two human case reports proved the possibility of rapid mapping of hemodynamically unstable VT. In the first,[50] activation mapping had to be discontinued after 3:31 minutes and, even after repeated VT reinduction and subsequent termination, remained incomplete. At that point, 256 beats and 4283 ECGs had been automatically annotated, allowing a reliable visualization of the circuit with successful ablation. In the second,[51] 35 seconds of mapping in the scar zone with the Orion demonstrated the VT circuit with its critical isthmus. A number of 800 points were acquired with Rhythmia during only 28 VT beats. After mapping, the ablation was delivered in SR targeting

the sites with diastolic potentials during VT. Afterward, the clinical VT could not be induced with the same pacing protocol as before the RF applications.

Epicardial Ultra–High-definition Mapping

After a first case-report,[52] demonstrating the feasibility of UHD epicardial mapping using the Orion in the collapsed (linear) state, a multicentric series[53] specifically addressed this issue. In 33 patients, 43 epicardial maps were performed and studied. These included 11 activation maps (17,832 points per map; IQR 7621–32,497; mapping time, 21 min; IQR 9–24 min) and 32 substrate maps (40,149 points per map; IQR 20,926–49,391). The minibasket catheter was advanced to the epicardial space via an 8.5F steerable sheath in all patients. The inner side of the acquired epicardial shell was used for analysis, because it is the one with near-field EGMs measured from the electrodes that were in direct contact with the epicardial surface. The investigators applied the bipolar voltage between 0.1 mV to 1.0 mV as the ventricular low-voltage scar border zone in this study. In 30 of 32 epicardial substrate maps, LAVA was recorded and its location correlated with the scar border zone.

The patients with activation maps underwent epicardial ablation targeting either the isthmus or the earliest activation point, with successful termination of 10 of 11 VTs during radiofrequency delivery. Complete elimination of LAVAs was achieved in 17 of 20 patients; the reason for partial LAVA elimination in the 3 patients was avoidance of coronary vessel or phrenic nerve injury. There were no immediate procedural complications. Two delayed pericardial collections required reinsertion of the pericardial drain 1 day after the procedure, with no long-term sequelae. At 10 months (IQR 4–14), freedom from VT was 64% (7/11) in those patients who had acute termination of VT during radiofrequency delivery plus additional substrate modification and 55% (11/20) in those who had substrate modification only.

SUMMARY

UHD mapping in atrial and ventricular arrhythmias is increasingly adopted by the electrophysiology community. Despite the scarce comparative data on ablation result versus standard mapping, the better understanding of the arrhythmia mechanisms is appealing and this technological advance seems to constitute a no return point in the practice of the clinical and experimental cardiac electrophysiology.

REFERENCES

1. Nakagawa H, Ikeda A, Sharma T, et al. Rapid high resolution electroanatomical mapping: evaluation of a new system in a canine atrial linear lesion model. Circ Arrhythm Electrophysiol 2012;5:417–24.

2. Bun SS, Delassi T, Laţcu DG, et al. A comparison between multipolar mapping and conventional mapping of atrial tachycardias in the context of atrial fibrillation ablation. Arch Cardiovasc Dis 2018;111: 33–40.

3. Laţcu DG, Bun SS, Viera F, et al. Selection of critical isthmus in scar-related atrial tachycardia using a new automated ultrahigh resolution mapping system. Circ Arrhythm Electrophysiol 2017;10:e004510.

4. Anter E, Tschabrunn CM, Buxton AE, et al. High-resolution mapping of postinfarction reentrant ventricular tachycardia: electrophysiological characterization of the circuit. Circulation 2016;134:314–27.

5. Martin R, Maury P, Bisceglia C, et al. Characteristics of scar-related ventricular tachycardia circuits using ultra-high-density mapping. Circ Arrhythm Electrophysiol 2018;11:e006569.

6. Anter E, Tschabrunn CM, Josephson ME. High-resolution mapping of scar-related atrial arrhythmias using smaller electrodes with closer interelectrode spacing. Circ Arrhythm Electrophysiol 2015;8: 537–45.

7. Tschabrunn CM, Roujol S, Dorman NC, et al. High-resolution mapping of ventricular scar: comparison between single and multielectrode catheters. Circ Arrhythm Electrophysiol 2016;9:e003841.

8. Acosta J, Penela D, Andreu D, et al. Multielectrode vs. Point-by-point mapping for ventricular tachycardia substrate ablation: a randomized study. Europace 2018;20:512–9.

9. Masse S, Magtibay K, Jackson N, et al. Resolving myocardial activation with novel omnipolar electrograms. Circ Arrhythm Electrophysiol 2016;9: e004107.

10. Laţcu DG, Bun SS, Casado Arroyo R, et al. Scar identification, quantification and characterisation in complex atrial tachycardia – a path to targeted ablation? Europace 2019;21(Supplement_1):i21–6.

11. Kawamura I, Fukamizu S, Miyazawa S, et al. High-density activation mapping during perimitral atrial tachycardia demonstrates epicardial connection through the vein of marshall. Heart Rhythm 2018; 15:153–4.

12. Viswanathan K, Mantziari L, Butcher C, et al. Evaluation of a novel high-resolution mapping system for catheter ablation of ventricular arrhythmias. Heart Rhythm 2017;14:176–83.

13. De Pooter J, El Haddad M, Wolf M, et al. Clinical assessment and comparison of annotation algorithms in high-density mapping of regular atrial tachycardias. J Cardiovasc Electrophysiol 2018;29:177–85.

14. Sommer P, Albenque JP, van Driel V, et al. Arrhythmia-specific settings for automated high-density mapping: a multicenter experience. J Cardiovasc Electrophysiol 2018;29:1210–20.

15. Luther V, Linton NW, Koa-Wing M, et al. A prospective study of ripple mapping in atrial tachycardias: a novel approach to interpreting activation in low-voltage areas. Circ Arrhythm Electrophysiol 2016;9:e003582.

16. Jamil-Copley S, Vergara P, Carbucicchio C, et al. Application of ripple mapping to visualize slow conduction channels within the infarct-related left ventricular scar. Circ Arrhythm Electrophysiol 2015;8: 76–86.

17. Xie S, Kubala M, Liang JJ, et al. Utility of ripple mapping for identification of slow conduction channels during ventricular tachycardia ablation in the setting of arrhythmogenic right ventricular cardiomyopathy. J Cardiovasc Electrophysiol 2019;30(3):366–73.

18. Laţcu DG, Saoudi N. How fast does the electrical impulse travel within the myocardium? The need for a new clinical electrophysiology tool: the conduction velocity mapping. J Cardiovasc Electrophysiol 2014;25:395–7.

19. Anter E, Duytschaever M, Shen C, et al. Activation mapping with integration of vector and velocity information improves the ability to identify the mechanism and location of complex scar-related atrial tachycardias. Circ Arrhythm Electrophysiol 2018; 11:e006536.

20. Xue Y, Liu Y, Liao H, et al. Evaluation of electrophysiological mechanisms of post-surgical atrial tachycardias using an automated ultra-high-density mapping system. JACC Clin Electrophysiol 2018;4: 1460–70.

21. Frontera A, Mahajan R, Dallet C, et al. Characterizing localized reentry with high-resolution mapping: evidence for multiple slow conducting isthmuses within the circuit. Heart Rhythm 2019;16(5):679–85.

22. Luther V, Sikkel M, Bennett N, et al. Visualizing localized reentry with ultra-high density mapping in iatrogenic atrial tachycardia: beware pseudo-reentry. Circ Arrhythm Electrophysiol 2017;10:e004724.

23. Takigawa M, Derval N, Frontera A, et al. Revisiting anatomic macroreentrant tachycardia after atrial fibrillation ablation using ultrahigh-resolution mapping: implications for ablation. Heart Rhythm 2018; 15:326–33.

24. Frontera A, Takigawa M, Martin R, et al. Electrogram signature of specific activation patterns: analysis of atrial tachycardias at high-density endocardial mapping. Heart Rhythm 2018;15:28–37.

25. Bun SS, Laţcu DG, Delassi T, et al. Ultra-high-definition mapping of atrial arrhythmias. Circulation 2016; 80:579–86.

26. Takigawa M, Martin CA, Derval N, et al. Insights from atrial surface activation throughout atrial tachycardia

cycle length: A new mapping tool. Heart Rhythm 2019. [Epub ahead of print].

27. Martin CA, Takigawa M, Martin R, et al. Use of Novel Electrogram "Lumipoint" Algorithm to Detect Critical Isthmus and Abnormal Potentials for Ablation in Ventricular Tachycardia. JACC Clin Electrophysiol 2019; 5(4):470–9.

28. Anter E, McElderry TH, Contreras-Valdes FM, et al. Evaluation of a novel high-resolution mapping technology for ablation of recurrent scar-related atrial tachycardias. Heart Rhythm 2016;13: 2048–55.

29. Maury P, Champ-Rigot L, Rollin A, et al. Comparison between novel and standard high-density 3d electro-anatomical mapping systems for ablation of atrial tachycardia. Heart Vessels 2019;34(5):801–8.

30. Lațcu DG, Saoudi N. Typical flutter rewritten: from textbooks to ultra-high-definition mapping. JACC Clin Electrophysiol 2017;3:987–90.

31. Pathik B, Lee G, Sacher F, et al. New insights into an old arrhythmia: high-resolution mapping demonstrates conduction and substrate variability in right atrial macro-re-entrant tachycardia. JACC Clin Electrophysiol 2017;3:971–86.

32. Schuessler RB, Kawamoto T, Hand DE, et al. Simultaneous epicardial and endocardial activation sequence mapping in the isolated canine right atrium. Circulation 1993;88:250–63.

33. Eckstein J, Zeemering S, Linz D, et al. Transmural conduction is the predominant mechanism of breakthrough during atrial fibrillation: evidence from simultaneous endo-epicardial high-density activation mapping. Circ Arrhythm Electrophysiol 2013;6: 334–41.

34. Pathik B, Lee G, Sacher F, et al. Epicardial-endocardial breakthrough during stable atrial macroreentry: evidence from ultra-high-resolution 3-dimensional mapping. Heart Rhythm 2017;14:1200–7.

35. Barkagan M, Shapira-Daniels A, Leshem E, et al. Pseudoblock of the posterior mitral line with epicardial bridging connections is a frequent cause of complex perimitral tachycardias. Circ Arrhythm Electrophysiol 2019;12:e006933.

36. Liang JJ, Callans DJ. Continued epicardial conduction after endocardial posterolateral mitral annular linear ablation for perimitral flutter revealed with high-density rhythmia mapping. J Interv Card Electrophysiol 2019. https://doi.org/10.1007/s10840-018-0502-4.

37. Pathik B, Lee G, Nalliah C, et al. Entrainment and high-density three-dimensional mapping in right atrial macroreentry provide critical complementary information: entrainment may unmask "visual reentry" as passive. Heart Rhythm 2017;14: 1541–9.

38. Kitamura T, Martin R, Denis A, et al. Characteristics of single-loop macroreentrant biatrial tachycardia

diagnosed by ultrahigh-resolution mapping system. Circ Arrhythm Electrophysiol 2018;11:e005558.

39. Nakahara S, Tung R, Ramirez RJ, et al. Distribution of late potentials within infarct scars assessed by ultra high-density mapping. Heart Rhythm 2010;7: 1817–24.

40. Tung R, Nakahara S, Maccabelli G, et al. Ultra high-density multipolar mapping with double ventricular access: a novel technique for ablation of ventricular tachycardia. J Cardiovasc Electrophysiol 2011;22: 49–56.

41. Della Bella P, Bisceglia C, Tung R. Multielectrode contact mapping to assess scar modification in post-myocardial infarction ventricular tachycardia patients. Europace 2012;14(Suppl 2):ii7–12.

42. Maagh P, Christoph A, Dopp H, et al. High-density mapping in ventricular tachycardia ablation: a pentaray((r)) study. Cardiol Res 2017;8:293–303.

43. Cano O, Plaza D, Sauri A, et al. Utility of high density multielectrode mapping during ablation of scar-related ventricular tachycardia. J Cardiovasc Electrophysiol 2017;28:1306–15.

44. Tanaka Y, Genet M, Chuan Lee L, et al. Utility of high-resolution electroanatomic mapping of the left ventricle using a multispline basket catheter in a swine model of chronic myocardial infarction. Heart Rhythm 2015;12:144–54.

45. Thajudeen A, Jackman WM, Stewart B, et al. Correlation of scar in cardiac mri and high-resolution contact mapping of left ventricle in a chronic infarct model. Pacing Clin Electrophysiol 2015; 38:663–74.

46. Nuhrich JM, Kaiser L, Akbulak RO, et al. Substrate characterization and catheter ablation in patients with scar-related ventricular tachycardia using ultra high-density 3-d mapping. J Cardiovasc Electrophysiol 2017;28:1058–67.

47. Josephson ME, Anter E. Substrate mapping for ventricular tachycardia: assumptions and misconceptions. JACC Clin Electrophysiol 2015;1: 341–52.

48. Anter E, Kleber AG, Rottmann M, et al. Infarct-related ventricular tachycardia: redefining the electrophysiological substrate of the isthmus during sinus rhythm. JACC Clin Electrophysiol 2018;4: 1033–48.

49. Maury P, Rollin A, Waintraub X, et al. Crossroads or "flyovers" novel insights into ventricular tachycardia mechanisms: the path is twisting. Pacing Clin Electrophysiol 2018;41:1564–7.

50. Kaiser L, Jularic M, Akbulak RO, et al. Catheter ablation of hemodynamically unstable ventricular tachycardia in ischemic cardiomyopathy using high-resolution mapping. Clin Case Rep 2017;5: 389–93.

51. Takigawa M, Frontera A, Thompson N, et al. The electrical circuit of a hemodynamically unstable

and recurrent ventricular tachycardia diagnosed in 35 s with the rhythmia mapping system. J Arrhythm 2017;33:505–7.

52. Hooks DA, Yamashita S, Capellino S, et al. Ultra-rapid epicardial activation mapping during ventricular tachycardia using continuous sampling from a high-density basket (orion(tm)) catheter. J Cardiovasc Electrophysiol 2015;26:1153–4.

53. Shi R, Chen Z, Kontogeorgis A, et al. Epicardial ventricular tachycardia ablation guided by a novel high-resolution contact mapping system: a multicenter study. J Am Heart Assoc 2018;7:e010549.

Reinserting Physiology into Cardiac Mapping Using Omnipolar Electrograms

Karl Magtibay, MASc[a], Andreu Porta-Sánchez, MD, MS[b,c],
Shouvik K. Haldar, MD (Res), MRCP[d], Don Curtis Deno, MD, PhD[e],
Stéphane Massé, MASc[a], Kumaraswamy Nanthakumar, MD, FRCPC[a,*]

KEYWORDS

- Cardiac mapping • Omnipolar • Atrial fibrillation • Ventricular tachycardia • Electrogram direction
- Wavefront orientation • Activation direction • Conduction velocity

KEY POINTS

- Unipolar electrograms are voltage signals that reflect time-varying extracellular currents. Bipolar electrograms provide differential extracellular voltages along an axis and resemble a local directional derivative. Both are based on the fundamental concept of electric fields in tissues. Omnipolar electrograms are derived from a clique, a group of nearby electrodes that generate bipolar signals from multiple directions. They are electrode and catheter-orientation independent.
- Omnipolar electrograms provide wavefront characteristics, such as amplitude, timing, direction, and speed, in physiologically relevant directions located at the center of the electrode clique. This enables determinations of a maximal bipolar voltage amplitude termed OT Vmax, the generalization of peak-to-peak in the presence of directionality, and is not affected by catheter orientation and is less sensitive to electrode distance for small cliques.
- Specialized catheters and three-dimensional mapping system software enable omnipolar electrograms and derived quantities to be generated and displayed in real-time.
- Omnipolar electrograms during atrial fibrillation are significantly less influenced by directional factors, allowing for robust and consistent substrate assessment.
- Mapping the ventricles using an equispaced electrode grid catheter and omnipolar electrograms can provide reliable substrate assessment within infarcted and noninfarcted regions of the ventricles to aid in determining ablation targets, such as a lesion gap or an isthmus.

INTRODUCTION

Cardiac mapping is an essential tool in arrhythmia diagnosis and treatment. Mapping information obtained from signal processing and image display algorithms in present day electroanatomic mapping systems are critically dependent on measured electrograms (EGMs) from catheters. A collection of local activation times (LAT) derived from EGMs within a cardiac chamber

Disclosures: D.C. Deno is an employee of Abbott Laboratories, St. Paul, MN. K. Nanthakumar and S. Massé are consultants for Abbott Laboratories, St. Paul, MN. K. Nanthakumar is a consultant for Biosense Webster, Irving, CA. K. Magtibay, A. Porta-Sanchez, S. K. Haldar have nothing to disclose.

[a] The Hull Family Cardiac Fibrillation Management Laboratory, Toronto General Hospital, University Health Network, 200 Elizabeth Street, Toronto, Ontario M5G 2C4, Canada; [b] Hospital Universitario Quironsalud Madrid, Calle Diego de Velázquez, 1, 28223 Pozuelo de Alarcón, Madrid, Spain; [c] Fundacion Centro Nacional de Investigaciones Cardiovasculares Carlos III (CNIC), Melchor Fernández Almagro, 3, Madrid 28029, Spain; [d] Royal Brompton & Harefield NHS Foundation Trust, Harefield Hospital, Hill End Road, Harefield, Uxbridge UB9 6JH, UK; [e] Abbott Laboratories, One St. Jude Medical Drive, St. Paul, MN 55117, USA
* Corresponding author. 200 Elizabeth Street, GW 3-526, Toronto, Ontario M5G 2C4, Canada.
E-mail address: kumar.nanthakumar@uhn.ca

Card Electrophysiol Clin 11 (2019) 525–536
https://doi.org/10.1016/j.ccep.2019.05.003
1877-9182/19/© 2019 The Authors. Published by Elsevier Inc. This is an open access article under the CC BY-NC-ND license (http://creativecommons.org/licenses/by-nc-nd/4.0/).

characterizes the propagation of electrical waves, whereas its signal amplitude (millivolt) has been used as a surrogate to determine the health of underlying cardiac substrate. These two EGM features are the primary tools for cardiac mapping and, as such, the diagnosis and treatment of arrhythmias.

Traditionally, two types of EGMs are used for cardiac mapping: unipolar and bipolar. Unipolar EGMs are signals from a single electrode with a distant reference electrode providing measurements of change in extracellular voltage over time. Unipolar EGMs are non-directional but are susceptible to low-frequency noise, such as far-field or movement artifacts.[1-3] In contrast, bipolar EGMs are signals from a pair of neighboring electrodes and provide localized measurements of the myocardium. Although bipolar EGMs are less susceptible to low-frequency noise, they are greatly affected by the direction of wavefront propagation relative to the electrode pair[1,2] as shown in **Fig. 1**. Bipolar EGM measurements are also dependent on other parameters, such as electrode distance, electrode size, wavefront speed, and extent of activation.[4-8] Most importantly, neither bipoles nor unipoles can provide wavefront characteristics, such as speed and direction, at a single location or voltages along the wavefront direction.

We recently introduced a novel type of EGM, the omnipolar EGM, for cardiac mapping.[9,10] Omnipolar EGMs combine the strengths of unipolar and bipolar EGMs such that they are direction-insensitive and locally derived. In essence, omnipolar EGMs are orientation-independent, virtual bipolar EGMs that are aligned along the direction of a wavefront that is anatomically and physiologically meaningful. Furthermore, omnipolar EGMs provide localized and time-consistent measures, such as maximal voltage and activation speed and direction, to enable electrophysiologists to create maps that closely represent the underlying physiology of the myocardium.

TROUBLE WITH TRADITION

LATs derived from either unipolar or bipolar EGMs over myocardial surfaces are used to create wave propagation maps to demonstrate activation sequences. There is, however, a continuing debate on the manner of timing annotations (eg, steepest negative or positive slope, minimum, maximum, first and/or last deflection, barycenter) especially in the case of bipolar EGMs because they are affected by numerous factors.[11,12] Unipolar −dV/dt is closely associated with action potential phase 0, rapid depolarization, but in practice, temporal uncertainty results over up to several milliseconds of the downslope of the signal due to local heterogeneities of activation, noise, and low-frequency baseline wander. Bipolar signals are less susceptible to noise (common mode is rejected) and filtering greatly attenuates baseline wander and so are often preferred. However, bipole directional effects may produce several milliseconds of temporal uncertainty of their own, as polarities may reverse and directional influences on amplitude may take effect. This is clearly shown in **Fig. 1** where the -dV/dt of the same wave are temporally different to each other. Also, interoperator differences on timing annotation lead to inconsistencies in LAT values, which therefore affect wave propagation profiles created post hoc. Although the resulting maps are often adequate over large regions and intervals of time, they can create locally unreliable and unreproducible characterizations of activation.

A variety of approaches using combinations of bipoles, unipoles, and time annotation criteria have been implemented for mapping.[13,14] Unfortunately, automatic algorithms incorporating such combined heuristic rules continue to facilitate temporal uncertainty. As such LAT values must be collected over an extended amount of time, over great areas of the myocardium to obtain a broadly accurate depiction of wave propagation. This low-resolution practice is time consuming because it involves spatial mapping first and then post-hoc processing and activation analysis of collected data, without any options for live mapping.

Measurements of peak-to-peak voltages (Vpp) from either unipolar or bipolar EGMs are used to

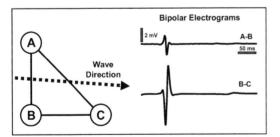

Fig. 1. Problem of directionality. Bipolar electrograms are useful in assessing local characteristics of the myocardium; however, they are catheter-orientation and wave-direction dependent. For a given wave direction within the same area, two orthogonal electrode orientations provide different bipolar electrograms in amplitude and timing. LAT derived at the -dV/dt from these two electrograms have several milliseconds difference from each other. Moreover, the bipolar electrode along the wave direction has a significantly larger bipolar electrogram amplitude compared with a bipolar electrode across a wave.

assess myocardial health and to survey for important substrate features, such as lesion gaps and isthmuses, which were found to be responsible for the maintenance and/or generation of arrhythmia.[15,16] Because unipolar EGMs are greatly affected by far-field effects, this could overestimate true Vpp values. Bipolar EGMs are dependent on orientation such that bipolar electrodes oriented along a wavefront produce an EGM with maximal bipolar Vpp, whereas those oriented across a wavefront measure a minimal bipolar Vpp. Optimizing bipolar Vpp measurements is challenging, especially in vivo, because it requires prior knowledge of the activation direction (AD) and complete control of catheter orientation. In addition to directionality, electrode pairs spaced widely apart, as in ablation catheters, can produce large Vpps and closely spaced electrodes, as seen in modern mapping arrays, produce small Vpps.[6–8] These factors create unreliable and nonreproducible characterization of the cardiac substrate.

Ironically, these EGM features and procedures that are fundamental to current cardiac mapping practices are themselves weaknesses and have not seen major innovation for almost a century. This realization fuels the need for standardized tools and methods that provide measurements with greater physiologic significance. These are the issues that omnipolar EGMs attempt to resolve. In the following section, we provide a description and derivation of omnipolar EGMs targeted to math-friendly clinicians.

OMNIPOLAR ELECTROGRAMS

Omnipolar EGMs take advantage of the directional properties of electric field (E-field) of a traveling wavefront on the surface of the myocardium (Fig. 2A) to produce consistent, physiologically pertinent, beat-by-beat measurements as introduced by Deno and colleagues.[9,10] An intracardiac E-field is analogous to a traditional vectorcardiogram (Fig. 2B) but substitutes voltage signals from catheter electrodes for surface electrocardiogram electrodes. We may understand bipolar catheter signals as manifestations of more fundamental currents and E-fields

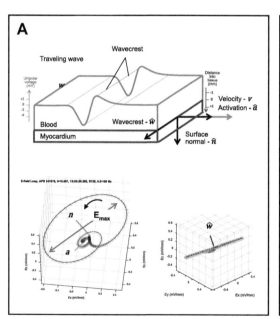
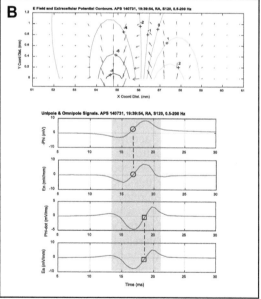

Fig. 2. (A) The traveling wave concept. Omnipolar electrograms are based on the concept of electric fields of a uniform traveling wave. Such a wave represents the activation of propagation of tissues along the surface of the myocardium. Illustrated is a traveling wave with constant velocity v along the a-direction. Representation of extracellular voltages as electric field loops is similar to a traditional vectorcardiogram, which describes the procession of local cardiac activation. (B) Omnipolar electrograms. An electric field drawn as a field of vectors represents the spatial development of extracellular voltages as a wave traverses through an observation window. Such extracellular voltages are represented as an electric field loop that is evolving through time. Characteristics of a traveling wave are maintained in this representation, such as the activation direction and normal-to-surface component. Omnipolar electrograms are derived from these components as presented. (From Deno DC, et al. Orientation-independent catheter-based characterization of myocardial activation. *IEEE Trans Biomed Eng* 2017;64(5):1067–77, with permission).

according to bipole direction and spacing. Omnipolar EGMs are virtual bipolar EGMs computed from nearby but differently directed bipoles. Omnipole signals leverage a local traveling wave model of propagation to avoid directional dependence and instead determine directions and corresponding signals of physiologic significance.

We begin our explanation of omnipolar EGMs and mapping with a simple two-dimensional array of electrodes laid out on a square grid and on a myocardial surface. Adjacent sets of three electrodes are referred to as cliques and produce three bipolar signals, two orthogonal and one diagonal. In keeping with a vector treatment, we note that there are three displacement vectors between electrode pairs and denote them in a 2×3 matrix dX. There is a correspondingly ordered set of unipolar voltage differences (bipoles) among these three electrodes we denote by a 3×1 vector $d\Phi$. Assuming clique electrodes are spaced closely enough that the 2×1 E-field vector E is essentially constant, from physics and matrix algebra we write $d\Phi = -dX^T E$. We then note the least-squares solution for the time-varying E-field using pseudoinverse $(dX^T)^+$ and assuming the electrode locations are effectively unchanged during depolarization is

$$E(t) = -(dX^T)^+ \, d\Phi(t).$$

From the time-varying two-dimensional E-field E(t) we may solve for bipolar voltages in different directions and with different electrode spacings and bring in unipole signals $\Phi(t)$ to determine conduction velocity (CV) and AD in a manner that does not rely on accurate time differences between nearby electrodes. Like the vectorcardiogram, E(t) traces out a loop during depolarization beginning near the origin when isoelectric, changing rapidly during depolarization, and returning to isoelectric when done. We exactly recover constituent bipole voltages when multiplying E(t) by the interelectrode spacing s and projecting the resulting voltage loop V(t) = s E(t) onto the orthogonal bipole directions. So, one interpretation of the E-field loop is that it is a fundamental entity and bipoles in any direction may be obtained from it. We know that when local bipoles are oriented in certain directions, their amplitudes can be much smaller than in other directions. When we gauge the health of myocardium we tend to ask how large can the amplitude be. The proper generalization of peak-to-peak amplitude of an ordinary 1D bipole signal is the span of the voltage loop, a quantity we designate as OT Vmax.

Local propagation speed and direction are determined in a revolutionary way using the relationship between unipole and omnipole signals. If a wavefront near clique electrodes is moving primarily in one direction at a roughly constant speed and producing similar unipolar EGM shapes and amplitudes it satisfies conditions of a traveling wave. The E-field, up to a negative sign, is essentially the spatial derivative of the unipolar potential field. As shown elsewhere,[9,10] traveling waves possess a special relationship between the time and spatial derivatives of their unipolar waveforms. The spatial derivative (in the direction of activation) with units of mV/mm has the identical shape as the temporal derivative $\dot{\varphi}$ (units of mV/ms). They differ by a multiplicative constant, that is, the CV speed. Designating the AD as unit vector $\hat{a}$, we recognize it is possible to determine an AD arrow by finding the angle that maximizes a cross-correlation

$$AD = \hat{a} = \underset{a}{\arg\max}\{xcorr(\dot{\varphi}(t), \boldsymbol{E}(t) \cdot \boldsymbol{a})\}$$

We introduce E_a as shorthand for the E-field signal in the direction of activation $E_a(t) = \boldsymbol{E}(t) \cdot \hat{a}$ and $E_a pp$ for its peak-to-peak amplitude. Bringing back properties of a traveling wave approximation we may now solve for CV speed in units of mm/ms as a ratio of amplitudes.

$$CV = \frac{\dot{\varphi}pp}{E_a pp}$$

This method of determining CV is not dependent on LAT; thus it differentiates itself from the time annotation-based mapping strategies. To conclude, an omnipolar EGM is an E-field based signal obtained from nearby bipolar and unipolar EGMs and electrode locations. Omnipolar EGMs do not depend on catheter-wavefront orientation and are instead linked to relevant anatomic and physiologic directions. Derived characteristics such as signal amplitude and conduction velocity are determined as outlined above and further explained by Deno and colleagues.[9]

VALIDATION OF OMNIPOLAR ELECTROGRAMS

Omnipolar mapping technology (OT) has been validated to rigorous standards using electrical and optical approaches and in various media (ie cardiac myocyte monolayers, cardiac tissue constructs, small and large isolated animal hearts, and diseased isolated human hearts) by Massé and colleagues.[17,18] A physiologic traveling wave was established with a cardiac myocyte monolayer under paced conditions. Each monolayer was electrically mapped on a glass dish with an embedded two-dimensional microelectrode array. Some monolayers were also optically mapped while exhibiting rotational events. Data from these monolayers were processed with the omnipolar algorithm to show a vector field representative of ADs that closely corresponded to optical mapping results. This exercise validated OT AD and the traveling wave concept in real media with electrical and optical waves.

OT was further validated using only optical mapping data gathered from cardiac tissue constructs with perfusion channels. Here we showed that with complex structures coupled with well-behaved waves and reentrant activity, the concept of omnipolar signals from traveling action potential waves holds as well.

For small healthy isolated animal hearts, we presented a novel set up for simultaneous optical and electrical mapping, which has allowed for a direct comparison of electrical measurements with a grid catheter against an optical gold standard (**Fig. 3**A–F). The unique make of the grid catheter allowed us to stitch the catheter on the epicardium while imaging from the gaps separating each spline where myocardial tissues were exposed to a light-sensitive camera. In this study, we found that ADs and CVs calculated from optical mapping data using traditional LAT methods have similar values to the ones calculated from omnipolar EGMs.

We also mapped diseased isolated human hearts during pacing using a high-density electrode plaque with 112 channels arranged in an 8 × 14 grid. Similar to our small isolated animal hearts, even in diseased tissues, we found that ADs and CVs derived from omnipolar EGMs have values similar to those derived with traditional LAT methods using electrical data.

Finally, omnipolar methodology was validated in porcine atria in vivo using the same grid catheter by mapping around the sinoatrial node to represent an activation focus (**Fig. 3**G). The vector fields generated from this study clearly show the utility of E-fields in cardiac mapping.

The previously mentioned studies provide strong proof-of-concept for the use of omnipolar EGMs for determining conduction vectors, which paves the way for its use in preclinical and clinical studies.

OMNIPOLAR MAPPING APPLICATIONS IN THE ATRIA

Voltage assessment is crucial for assessment of health and arrhythmia mechanism in the atria. Evidence from experimental and clinical studies suggest that an underlying atrial fibrotic substrate as delineated by low-voltage areas (LVA) plays a key role in development of atrial fibrillation (AF) drivers and foci that maintain AF.[19–21] Assessing the underlying fibrotic substrate is currently undertaken by creating electroanatomic bipolar voltage maps. However, bipolar voltage amplitude is influenced by several factors, such as electrode characteristics (eg size, spacing, and orientation), wavefront speed and direction, and tissue structure. Omnipolar EGMs offer an alternative to mapping the atria with traditional bipolar EGMs in a manner better suited to complex and time-varying AF mechanisms, such as wave collisions and fractionations.

Haldar and colleagues[22,23] expanded on efforts by Deno and colleagues[10,24] to introduce the concept of maximal bipolar voltage derived from omnipolar EGMs. Intuitively, we expect that bipolar EGMs with maximal Vpp will be measured when the bipole is oriented in the AD, $\hat{a}$. However, the AD must be known first to properly align the bipole and this is not always practical. Instead we rely on EGM signals from a voltage loop V(t), like the E-field loop of **Fig. 2**A, and determine OT Vmax from the maximal span of the loop. This is the proper generalization into two dimensions of the Vpp of a one-dimensional signal. This is challenging to obtain in vivo using traditional methods because it is difficult to align a bipole with the loop's maximal extent. Instead, an omnipolar EGM signal is mathematically determined in any direction in which a virtual bipolar EGM is derived. The derivation of this maximal bipole axis $\hat{m}$ and maximal bipole amplitude Vmax has been previously presented by Haldar and colleagues[23] where it was found to be especially useful when mapping a substrate during AF.

Substrate mapping during AF with traditional bipolar voltages poses significant challenges because of AF's complex mechanism. The presence of wave collisions and fractionation results in low bipolar Vpp, which is exacerbated by orientation-dependence of bipolar EGMs. This results in substrate maps that have unnecessarily large LVA, which could be erroneous targets for radiofrequency ablation. An E-field treatment allows for the calculation of OT EGMs and Vmax to improve the fidelity of atrial substrate maps and better delineate LVA during AF. This may delineate more focused targets for ablation beyond simple pulmonary vein isolation without the need for global mapping to identify electrophysiologic mechanisms that co-locate with LVAs (**Fig. 4**A).

Within the same study, we incorporated information gained from substrate mapping using EGMs with corresponding vector fields to characterize spatial and temporal wavefront organization. As expected, AF omnipole-based vector fields

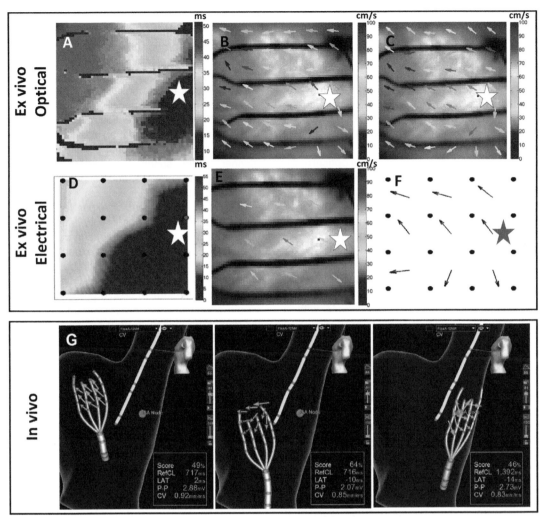

Fig. 3. Validation of omnipolar methodology. (*Top*) The concept of omnipolar electrograms was extensively validated through in vitro, ex vivo, and in vivo experiments. Shown is a simultaneous optical and electrical mapping of the epicardium of an isolated rabbit heart during pacing with the star indicating the pacing location. Traditional LAT-based methods were used to create isochronal maps from optical (*A*) and electrical (*D*) data. LAT-based vector fields were derived from both types of mapping data (*B* for optical and *E* for electrical) showing calculated speed and direction of wave propagation. Finally, omnipole-based vector fields (*C*, *F*) were calculated and were found to be a close match with traditional tools. (*Bottom*) Omnipole-based vector fields were validated in vivo in a porcine atria model using a grid-like catheter (*G*). In this model, it shows that omnipole-based vector fields accurately describe the outward propagation of tissue activation originating from the sinoatrial (SA) node. (*From* Massé S et al. Resolving myocardial activation with novel omnipolar electrograms. *Circ Arrythym Electrophysiol* 2016; 9; with permission).

have great spatial and temporal disorganization. From this we introduced a schema to improve substrate mapping during AF (**Fig. 4**B). This schema uses information of local organization of omnipole-based vector fields to signify coherence. We defined coherence as the organization of a 2 × 2 cluster of omnipolar unit vectors within a mapping area. If the average length of the unit vectors within a cluster is almost 1, it means that all four vectors essentially point in one direction and hence this cluster is included in highly coherent cluster. However, if the average length of the vectors within a cluster is close to 0, it means that vectors point in different, opposing directions, and hence they are included in a noncoherent cluster. Clusters with a high coherence may be included in a resultant voltage map, whereas those less than a certain threshold (<0.5 coherence) were excluded. This schema allows an operator to create a substrate map with better delineation of areas where collision and fractionation occur to better localize radiofrequency ablation treatments.

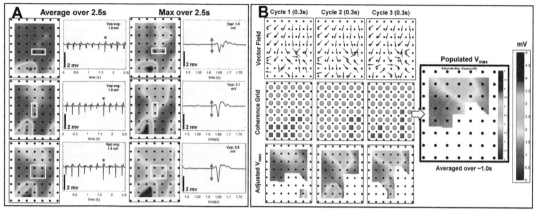

Fig. 4. Mapping atrial fibrillation with omnipolar electrograms. (*A*) Omnipolar electrograms (OT$_{EGM}$s) could aid in defining areas of atrial substrate for ablation during AF. Because of wave fractionation and collisions, in addition to the orientation dependence of traditional bipolar EGMs, mapping substrate during AF yields maps that are generally low voltage. Because OT$_{EGM}$s are catheter- and wave-orientation-independent, it provides a better representation of the substrate throughout the AF cycle since the maximal Vpp is obtained along the activation direction. (*B*) To build more robust substrate maps, we introduced a scheme where the organization of associated omnipolar vector fields are used as a guide to populate a resultant substrate map. Such a map could be used to localize areas of the substrate where wave collisions and fractionation occur as targets for radiofrequency ablation treatments. (*From* Haldar SK, et al. Resolving bipolar electrogram voltages during atrial fibrillation using omnipolar mapping. *Circ Arrhythm Electrophysiol.* 2017; 10(19); with permission).

If implemented in a commercial mapping system, this would provide rapid, high-density, orientation-independent assessment of the underlying atrial substrate.

OMNIPOLAR MAPPING APPLICATIONS IN THE VENTRICLES

The number of ventricular tachycardia (VT) ablation procedures is increasing worldwide. During the last decades, mapping procedures for localizing VT-harboring areas, either by substrate or LAT, have evolved from intraoperative mapping during cardiopulmonary bypass,[25–27] to sequential point-by-point mapping with "large" electrode ablation catheters with 3.5-mm tips,[28–30] and then to high-density, multielectrode mapping.[31–33] Advances in VT substrate mapping commonly rely on the acquisition of large numbers of points to resolve substrate features and is time consuming. However, it is important to recognize that high-density maps do not necessarily better represent underlying myocardial physiology. Traditional unipolar and bipolar EGMs have disadvantages (eg, susceptibility to noise and directionality, respectively) that omnipolar EGMs try to work around, irrespective of map point density. Overcoming these factors is critical when ablating VTs in a hemodynamically unstable patient to minimize procedure time.

Omnipolar EGMs, together with regularly spaced grid catheters, aim to provide physiologically relevant measurements of the substrate and rapidly provide high-density maps. Recent works by Porta-Sanchez and coworkers[34,35] and Magtibay and coworkers[36,37] demonstrated the use of omnipolar EGMs in ex vivo and in vivo mapping of ventricles. Both studies reinforced the concept of catheter-orientation dependence of bipolar measurements especially for voltage/substrate mapping.

Magtibay and coworkers[36,37] ex vivo work focused on building a foundation for omnipolar EGM mapping of ventricular myocardia. This preclinical work reexamined the directional dependence of bipolar EGMs for isolated animal and human hearts using different grid arrays. OT Vmax values provide the maximal bipolar Vpp in any direction along the surface of the myocardium. This was especially useful when delineating diseased tissue to locate lesion gaps or isthmuses that could be responsible for the initiation and/or maintenance of a ventricular arrhythmia (**Fig. 5A**). Because of the nature of omnipolar EGMs, a new voltage threshold for isolating scar area was also developed. Because OT Vmax always yields the maximal bipolar voltage, the established voltage thresholds currently used in clinical practice (0.5 mV for dense scar) may not well-represent the substrate. Magtibay came up with a threshold value of 1.5 mV for dense scar on the epicardium,

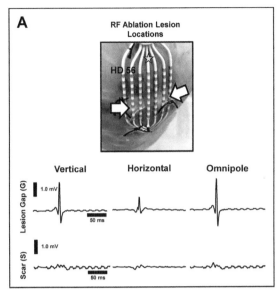

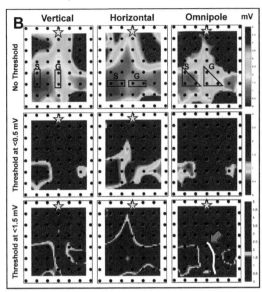

Fig. 5. Ex vivo mapping of the ventricles with omnipolar electrograms. (*A*) Ex vivo work on isolated animal hearts show the advantage of using omnipolar electrograms (OT$_{EGM}$) in mapping the ventricles especially in the presence of an isthmus or lesion gap. Orientation-dependence of bipolar EGMs is re-emphasized such that a lesion gap is misrepresented as a diseased area along one orientation and a normal area along another. OT$_{EGM}$s, however, provide EGMs with maximal voltage values regardless of orientation. (*B*) Translating to substrate maps, bipolar EGMs portray two different profiles of the substrate depending on the orientation examined. OT$_{EGM}$s, however, illustrate a clear delineation between the two lesion islands and the isthmus that exist between them. RF, radiofrequency. (*From* Magtibay K et al. Physiological assessment of ventricular myocardial voltage using omnipolar electrograms. *J Am Heart Assoc.* 2017; 6; with permission).

three times larger than the standard value (1.5 mV). This new threshold achieved fair sensitivity and specificity values of 0.94 and 0.82, respectively (**Fig. 5**B). With this threshold, OT Vmax-based substrate maps closely match diseased areas directly observed on the epicardium compared with bipolar substrate maps.

Magtibay's study also examined the consistency of omnipolar Vmax-based substrate maps for multiple beats and for different rhythms. OT Vmax was more consistent beat-by-beat than traditional bipolar Vpp. OT Vmax-based maps produced more consistent substrate map profiles regardless of rhythm.

Porta-Sanchez and coworkers'[34,35] in vivo work applied grid-like catheters and omnipolar EGMs to a preclinical environment in more realistic scenarios where factors, such as tissue contact and movement, could be detrimental. In this study, pigs with ventricular myocardial infarctions were mapped. Myocardial infarction was achieved by occluding the distal left anterior descending artery with an angioplasty balloon. Images of the whole heart were obtained 4 weeks after myocardial infarction induction using MRI with late-gadolinium enhancement to contrast infarcted against healthy tissues. In vivo mapping was performed using a research version of the Ensite

Precision™ Cardiac Mapping System (Abbott, St. Paul, MN).

In addition to comparing scar areas, this work revisited the orientation dependence of bipolar EGMs. Catheter orientation can make significant differences in substrate maps such that potential isthmuses are only observable along specific bipolar orientations (**Fig. 6**).[38,39] Substrate maps created with bipolar Vpp values have low beat-by-beat consistency on healthy and infarcted areas. However, substrate maps created with OT Vmax values had better beat-by-beat consistency on both areas. OT Vmax-based maps also produced a better representation of the infarcted areas. The surface area of MRI late-gadolinium enhancement scar more closely corresponded to endocardial extent of LVA in OT Vmax electroanatomic maps compared with traditional bipolar maps. This allows for a better, more physiologic in vivo definition of potential VT substrate than traditional bipolar-based substrate maps. Although in this study the omnipolar Vmax threshold developed in Magtibay's work was used, additional in vivo mapping studies should be done to account for variabilities in more clinically realistic cases.

Importantly, Porta-Sanchez's work relied on triangular cliques for calculating E-fields. Previous work with omnipolar EGMs used four closely

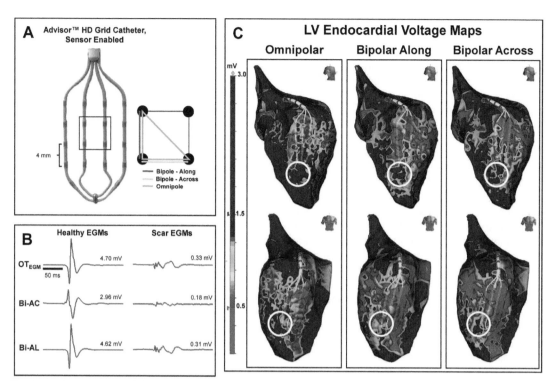

Fig. 6. In vivo mapping of the ventricles with omnipolar electrograms. (*A*) Grid-like catheter was used for mapping the ventricular endocardium of myocardially infracted (MI) porcine model. The bipolar orientations are shown along which their Vpp are calculated (magenta, along; cyan, across). The clique of electrodes used to calculate omnipolar electrograms (*yellow triangle*) are also shown. (*B*) EGMs from both bipolar orientations and electrode cliques are shown. OT$_{EGM}$s is comparable with the bipolar EGM with the largest Vpp but still offers largest Vpp either on scarred or healthy tissues. Again, the orientation dependence of bipolar EGMs is emphasized. (*C*) Voltage maps created from bipolar EGMs from either orientation display stark differences especially within the areas highlighted (*white circle*). OT$_{EGM}$s, however, provide maps that have larger Vpp values, hence better delineation of diseased areas. LV, left ventricular. (*From* Porta-Sanchez A, Magtibay K, Nayyar S, et al. Omnipolarity applied to equi-spaced array for ventricular tachycardia substrate mapping. *Europace* 2019; with permission).

spaced electrodes to comprise a square clique. However, the omnipolar framework allows for a minimum of three electrodes (making a triangular clique) to characterize a traveling wave along a two-dimensional surface. This allows grid-like catheters such as the Advisor™ HD Grid Mapping Catheter, Sensor Enabled™ (Abbott, St. Paul, MN) to quadruple the number and density of map points compared with the original square clique (36 vs 9 points for HD Grid, and decrease map point spacing from 4 to 2 mm). Traditional along spline bipolar measurements only allowed for 12 mapping points for each acquisition. This not only allowed for quicker creation of endocardial maps but also offered a more detailed view on the electrophysiology of myocardium.

FUTURE DIRECTIONS

Deno's seminal work on omnipolar EGMs has paved the way for new and exciting applications

in cardiac mapping. The concepts of traveling waves and E-fields allow us to revisit our understanding of electrophysiology and re-examine our perspective toward reading and interpreting EGMs. Omnipolar EGMs show that one-dimensional signals from electrodes in arbitrary orientations cannot fully evaluate electrophysiologic events. Although appreciated earlier by Kadish and coworkers[39] and Gerstenfeld and coworkers[40,41] it was not yet practical for two- and three-dimensional electrophysiologic signals to be given physiologic and anatomic context in a three-dimensional mapping system. Today, high-density mapping catheters combine with computers with strong graphics and computational abilities and the principles of an omnipolar approach and traveling waves open the door to new understandings of mechanisms and possibly more effective arrhythmia treatments.

Most of the studies reviewed here created substrate maps of voltage to better describe the myocardium using omnipolar EGMs. However, it is important to recognize that omnipolar EGMs also enable local accurate determinations of CV based on the characteristics of a traveling wave, independent of conventional LAT-based methods. Although omnipolar determinations of CV and AD require further and more rigorous in vivo validation, real-time, beat-by-beat, omnipolar AD vectors could be of great use especially in VT cases. The number and density of omnipolar AD vectors feasible with grid-like catheters could enable clinicians to rapidly home in on arrhythmia sources via drag-and-locate strategy[42,43] or rapidly identify reentrant pathways in a drag-and-map approach. In both instances an operator may drag a grid-like catheter within the endocardium, whereas AD vectors and CV speeds are calculated and displayed beat-by-beat. A source may be located by observing that the AD vector field radiates outward in its vicinity and at the source the coherence of direction is least. This method bypasses the need for the creation of global LAT maps and post hoc analysis, which is a time-consuming endeavor. Omnipolar-based AD vectors provide reproducible, real-time, rapid localization of VT sources independent of catheter orientation. This is analogous to a global positioning system style of locating a target on a map.

However, as with any medical diagnostic product, the omnipolar mapping algorithm and related tools must undergo rigorous performance assessments to ensure that the data we obtain from it are robust and trustworthy. We must ask, in what conditions does it fail, how does it fail, and how might we avoid improper characterizations. It is imperative to explore omnipolar algorithm sensitivities (eg, clique type, electrode distance, presence of noise, sampling rate, filter settings) from which to develop confidence metrics to indicate the reliability of data collected and maps created before it is widely adopted into clinical practice.

SUMMARY

Omnipolar EGMs make use of the biophysical E-fields that accompany activation along the surface of the myocardium. A grid-like electrode array provides bipolar signals in orthogonal directions to deliver catheter-orientation-independent assessments of cardiac electrophysiology. Omnipolar EGM features are currently used for two mapping categories: substrate voltage and activation propagation. In addition to comprehensive maps of cardiac chambers, omnipolar algorithms on three-dimensional mapping systems make possible local, beat-by-beat visualizations of maximal bipole voltage and orientation and

CV. OT's E-field loop and traveling wave treatment of omnipolar EGMs enables determination of activation speed and direction, bypassing ambiguous inconsistent LAT annotation. Such abilities have made possible the live mapping of wavefront propagation without time consuming mapping of entire heart chambers.

Studies with myocyte monolayers, isolated animal and human hearts, and anesthetized animals have validated the tenets of omnipolar EGMs. Optical mapping and traditional LAT determinations of conduction speed and direction, under controlled circumstances, were found consistent with those from OT. Omnipolar EGMs from atria and ventricles avoided a tendency for bipole directional mismatch to underestimate voltage, suggesting improvements to delineation of diseased areas of myocardium responsible for the initiation and/or maintenance of arrhythmias. The combination of information from omnipolar-based vectors and voltage values may also aid in localizing areas of wave fractionation and/or collision during fibrillatory episodes. In addition to working to identify clinical benefits of omnipolar EGM, it is also important to compare traditional and omnipolar algorithms looking for situations where one or both seem less trustworthy. Confidence metrics should be developed before OT evaluations of direction and speed are pushed toward real clinical applications. Ultimately, the goal of omnipolar EGMs is to better characterize myocardial substrate through reintroducing the fundamentals of cardiac electrophysiology to avoid catheter-orientation dependence.

REFERENCES

1. Tedrow UB, Stevenson WG. Recording and interpreting unipolar electrograms to guide catheter ablation. Heart Rhythm 2010;8(5):791–6.
2. Stevenson WG, Soejima K. Recording techniques for clinical electrophysiology. J Cardiovasc Electrophysiol 2005;16:1017–22.
3. Blanchard SM, Damiano RJ, Asano T, et al. The effects of distant cardiac electrical events on local activation in unipolar epicardial electrograms. IEEE Trans Biomed Eng 1987;34(7):539–46.
4. Anter E, Josephson ME. Bipolar voltage amplitude: what does it really mean? Heart Rhythm 2016; 13(1):326–7.
5. Josephson ME, Anter E. Substrate mapping for ventricular tachycardia: assumptions and misconceptions. JACC Clin Electrophysiol 2015;1(5):341–52.
6. Behesti M, Magtibay K, Massé S, et al. Determinants of atrial bipolar voltage: inter electrode distance and wavefront angle. Comput Biol Med 2018;102: 449–57.

7. Takigawa M, Relan J, Martin R, et al. Effect of bipolar electrode orientation on local electrogram properties. Heart Rhythm 2018;15:1853–61.

8. Takigawa M, Relan J, Martin R, et al. Detailed analysis of the relation between bipolar electrode spacing and far- and near-field electrograms. JACC Clin Electrophysiol 2019;5(1):66–77.

9. Deno DC, Balachandaran R, Morgan DJ, et al. Orientation-independent catheter-based characterization of myocardial activation. IEEE Trans Biomed Eng 2017;64(5):1067–77.

10. Deno DC, Balachandaran R, Morgan DJ, et al. Omnipolar ablation catheter technology with unique capacity for beat by beat conduction direction and velocity display. Heart Rhythm 2015;12(5):S235.

11. Cantwell CD, Roney CH, Ng FS, et al. Techniques for automated local activation time annotation and conduction velocity estimation in cardiac mapping. Comput Biol Med 2015;65:229–42.

12. Del Carpio Munoz F, Buescher T, Asirvatham SJ. Teaching points with 3-dimensional mapping of cardiac arrhythmias. Circ Arrhythm Electrophysiol 2011;4:e22–5.

13. De Pooter J, Haddad ME, Wolf M, et al. Clinical assessment and comparison of annotation algorithms in high-density mapping of regular atrial tachycardias. J Cardiovasc Electrophysiol 2018;29:177–85.

14. Weiss C, Willems S, Rueppel R, et al. Electroanatomical Mapping (CARTO) of ectopic atrial tachycardia: impact of bipolar and unipolar local electrogram annotation for localization of the focal origin. J Interv Card Electrophysiol 2001;5:101–7.

15. Patel MA, d'Avila A, Neuzil P, et al. Atrial tachycardia after ablation of persistent atrial fibrillation: identification of the critical isthmus with a combination of multielectrode activation mapping and targeted entrainment mapping. Circ Arrhythm Electrophysiol 2008;1:14–22.

16. Anter E, Kleber AG, Rottman M, et al. Infarct-related ventricular tachycardia: redefining the electrophysiological substrate of the isthmus during sinus rhythm. JACC Clin Electrophysiol 2018;4(8):1033–48.

17. Massé S, Magtibay K, Jackson N, et al. Resolving myocardial activation with novel omnipolar electrograms. Circ Arrhythm Electrophysiol 2016;9:e004107.

18. Massé S, Kusha M, Magtibay K, et al. Omnipolar mapping technology: instantaneous wavefront direction and velocity magnitude at catheter tip. Heart Rhythm 2015;12(5):S235.

19. Jadidi AS, Lehrmann H, Keyl C, et al. Ablation of persistent atrial fibrillation targeting low-voltage areas with selective activation characteristics. Circ Arrhythm Electrophysiol 2016;9:e002962.

20. Ghoraani B, Dalvi R, Gizurarson S, et al. Localized rotational activation in the left atrium during human atrial fibrillation: relationship to complex fractionated atrial electrograms and low-voltage zones. Heart Rhythm 2013;10(12):1830–8.

21. Nademanee K, Lockwood E, Oketani N, et al. Catheter ablation of atrial fibrillation guided by complex fractionated atrial electrogram mapping of atrial fibrillation. J Cardiol 2010;55(1):1–12.

22. Haldar SK, Magtibay K, Porta-Sanchez A, et al. Resolving bipolar electrogram voltages during atrial fibrillation using omnipolar mapping. Circ Arrhythm Electrophysiol 2017;10(19):e005018.

23. Haldar SK, Magtibay K, Massé S, et al. Omnipolar mapping to resolve bipolar electrogram voltages during atrial fibrillation. Heart Rhythm 2017;14(5):S259.

24. Deno DC, Bush JC, Morgan DJ, et al. Solving the problem of imprecise atrial voltage mapping with high density fixed spacing grid catheter and omnipolar mapping: in-vivo validation. Heart Rhythm 2017;14(5):S122.

25. Downar E, Parson ID, Mickleborough LL, et al. On-line epicardial mapping of intraoperative ventricular arrhythmias: initial clinical experience. J Am Coll Cardiol 1984;4(4):703–14.

26. Harris L, Downar E, Mickleborough LL, et al. Activation sequence of ventricular tachycardia: endocardial and epicardial mapping studies in the human ventricle. J Am Coll Cardiol 1987;10(5):1040–7.

27. Parson ID, Downar E. Cardiac mapping instrumentation for the instantaneous display of endocardial and epicardial activation. IEEE Trans Biomed Eng 1987;34(6):468–72.

28. Soejima K, Stevenson WG, Sapp JL, et al. Endocardial and epicardial radiofrequency ablation of ventricular tachycardia associated with dilated cardiomyopathy. J Am Coll Cardiol 2014;43(10):1834–42.

29. Delacretaz E, Stevenson WG, Ellison KE, et al. Mapping and radiofrequency catheter ablation of the three types of sustained monomorphic ventricular tachycardia in nonischemic heart disease. J Cardiovasc Electrophysiol 2000;11(1):11–7.

30. Calkins H, Epstein A, Packer D, et al. Catheter ablation of ventricular tachycardia in patients with structural heart disease using cooled radiofrequency energy. J Am Coll Cardiol 2000;35(7):1905–14.

31. Sanders P, Hocini M, Jais P, et al. Characterization of focal atrial tachycardia using high-density mapping. J Am Coll Cardiol 2005;46(11):2088–99.

32. Kumagai K, Ogawa M, Noguchi H, et al. Electrophysiologic properties of pulmonary veins assessed using a multielectrode basket catheter. J Am Coll Cardiol 2004;34(12):2281–9.

33. Anter E, McElderry TH, Contreras-Valdes FM, et al. Evaluation of a novel high-resolution mapping

technology for ablation of recurrent scar-related atrial tachycardias. Heart Rhythm 2016;13(10): 2048–55.

34. Porta-Sanchez A, Magtibay K, Nayyar S, et al. Omnipolarity applied to equi-spaced array for ventricular tachycardia substrate mapping. Europace 2019; 21(5):813–21.

35. Porta-Sanchez A, Magtibay K, Massé S, et al. Equi-spaced electrode array for orientation independent bipolar substrate mapping. Europace 2018; 20(suppl 1):196.

36. Magtibay K, Massé S, Asta J, et al. Physiological assessment of ventricular myocardial voltage using omnipolar electrograms. J Am Heart Assoc 2017;6: e006447.

37. Magtibay K, Massé S, Asta J, et al. Isthmus and lesion gap: the incremental value of omnipoles over high density mapping. Heart Rhythm 2017; 14(5):S528.

38. Magtibay K, Bhaskaran AP, Porta-Sanchez A, et al. Identifying surviving myocardial tracts within infarcted regions in an in-vivo swine model using omnipolar methodology. Can J Cardiol 2018;34: S100.

39. Kadish AH, Spear JF, Levine JH, et al. Vector mapping of myocardial activation. Circulation 1986; 74(3):603–15.

40. Gerstenfeld E, Baerman SA, Ropella K, et al. Detection of changes in atrial endocardial activation with use of an orthogonal catheter. J Am Coll Cardiol 1991;18(4):1034–42.

41. Gerstenfeld E, Sahakian AV, Swiryn S. Evidence for transient linking of atrial excitation during atrial fibrillation in humans. Circulation 1992;86(2):375–82.

42. Magtibay K, Porta-Sanchez A, Nayyar S, et al. Drag and locate strategy for rapid ventricular tachycardia mapping with grid catheter. Heart Rhythm 2018; 15(5):S245.

43. Bhaskaran A, Magtibay K, Massé S, et al. Drag and map strategy for dynamic detection of diseased myocardium: innovative omnipolar application with advisor HD grid. Can J Cardiol 2018;34:S101.

Cardiac MRI and Fibrosis Quantification

Eugene G. Kholmovski, PhD[a,b,c], Alan K. Morris, MSc[a], Mihail G. Chelu, MD, PhD, FHRS[a,d],*

KEYWORDS

• Atrial fibrillation • Ablation • Atrial fibrosis • LGE-MRI

KEY POINTS

• High spatial resolution, timing of data acquisition, contrast dose, and delay between contrast administration and late gadolinium enhancement MRI scan along with appropriate image analysis software are critical to visualize and quantify left atrial fibrosis and scar.
• Left atrial fibrosis is a predictor of outcomes of atrial fibrillation ablation, stroke, and heart failure.
• Imaging of left atrial scar can be used to optimize ablation parameters that lead to durable lesions while avoiding collateral damage to nearby anatomic structures.
• Atrial fibrosis may represent a modifiable risk factor that, when targeted, could improve outcomes of atrial fibrillation ablation, stroke, and heart failure.

INTRODUCTION

Atrial fibrillation (AF) is a major health problem that is closely intertwined in its pathophysiology with stroke and heart failure.[1,2] The mechanisms underlying AF are complex, involving both ectopic activity and reentry through atrial tissue.[3] Atrial remodeling (electric, contractile, and structural remodeling) can either promote triggered activity or create a substrate for reentry. Abnormal local spontaneous discharges from pulmonary veins (PVs) have been identified as a critical trigger for AF.[4] Left atrium (LA) ablation is frequently used to maintain sinus rhythm in patients with symptomatic AF and therefore PV isolation (PVI) has emerged as the cornerstone of any AF ablation.[4,5] In addition, non-PV triggers have been identified with variable frequency from LA and right atrium (RA), superior vena cava, and ligament of Marshall

in paroxysmal, persistent, and long-standing persistent AF.[6,7] Furthermore, atrial fibrosis is an increasingly recognized substrate for AF.[8] Development of imaging techniques using late gadolinium enhancement (LGE) MRI and image analysis software to quantify LA fibrosis[9,10] has allowed significant insights in the role of atrial fibrosis in AF. Atrial fibrosis may provide a pathophysiologic link to stroke and heart failure in patients with and without AF.[11] Furthermore, LA fibrosis seems to be a good predictor of AF ablation outcome.[12] Despite improvement compared with antiarrhythmic drugs, the long-term results of AF ablation remain unsatisfactory with single procedures (16%–29%).[13–16] Multiple studies in patients undergoing a second AF ablation have shown that PV reconnection is the most frequent cause of AF recurrence.[17–20] In addition, progression of atrial fibrosis substrate may explain, at least in

Disclosure: E.G. Kholmovski has equity interest from Marrek Inc. and research funding from Medtronic; A.K. Morris is a shareholder of Marrek Inc.; M.G. Chelu receives research funding from Wavelet Health, Biotronik, Medtronic, and Boston Scientific.
[a] Comprehensive Arrhythmia Research & Management (CARMA) Center, University of Utah, 729 Arapeen Drive, Salt Lake City, Ut 84108, USA; [b] Utah Center for Advanced Imaging Research (UCAIR), University of Utah, Salt Lake City, UT, USA; [c] Department of Radiology and Imaging Sciences, University of Utah, Salt Lake City, UT, USA; [d] Division of Cardiovascular Medicine, Section of Electrophysiology, University of Utah, Salt Lake City, UT, USA
* Corresponding author. Division of Cardiology, University of Utah School of Medicine, 50 North Medical Drive, Salt Lake City, UT 84123.
E-mail address: mgchelu@gmail.com

part, the less-than-ideal results of AF ablation. Furthermore, prior radiofrequency (RF) lesions, including PVI and linear lesions, and/or atrial fibrosis may promote macroreentrant atrial arrhythmias.[21,22] Therefore, both durable PVI and linear ablations are critically dependent on delivering a contiguous, transmural, and durable set of lesions. LGE-MRI has been used to characterize ablation lesions and optimize the efficacy/safety ratio of ablation parameters. Moreover, recent data suggest that targeting areas of fibrosis during AF ablation may improve the outcome of ablation. This hypothesis is currently being explored in a randomized prospective clinical trial, Efficacy of DE-MRI-Guided Fibrosis Ablation vs. Conventional Catheter Ablation of Atrial Fibrillation II (DECAAF II).

This article examines (1) technical aspects of imaging atrial fibrosis/scar by LGE-MRI; (2) use of atrial fibrosis and scar in predicting outcomes, including of AF ablation, stroke, and heart failure; (3) applications of LGE-MRI to assess ablation lesions and optimize ablation parameters while avoiding collateral damage.

TECHNICAL ASPECTS OF FIBROSIS IMAGING AND QUANTIFICATION

Typical cardiac MRI protocols for patients with AF include imaging techniques to assess morphologic (shape and volume), functional (strain, ejection fractions), and structural remodeling (fibrosis/scar) of the LA (**Fig. 1**). Contrast-enhanced magnetic resonance angiography is performed during administration of gadolinium-based contrast agents (GBCAs) and used to define the anatomy of the LA and the PVs. Cardiac cine-MRI is used to evaluate functional characteristic of the LA, such as strain and strain rate of LA wall, and total, passive, and active LA ejection fractions.[23] Three-dimensional (3D) LGE-MRI is usually acquired 20 to 30 minutes after GBCA injection to visualize and quantify atrial fibrosis/scar.

LGE-MRI of LA for fibrosis/scar assessment remains a nontrivial MRI examination. This imaging technique requires well-trained MRI personnel, modern MRI equipment, and specialized pulse sequences and scan protocols.[23] MRI studies for LA fibrosis/scar assessment are usually performed on 1.5-T or 3-T MRI scanners using either conventional torso and spine phased-array coils or specialized cardiac coils.

Assessment of LA fibrosis/scar involves 2 major steps: image acquisition and image processing for fibrosis/scar analysis and quantification.

Late Gadolinium Enhancement MRI Acquisition for Atrial Fibrosis/Scar Quantification

The MRI techniques used by different clinical centers for the assessment of LA fibrosis and postablation scar are similar and are implemented using electrocardiogram-triggered, respiratory-navigated, gradient echo pulse sequence with inversion recovery preparation and fat saturation. By comparison with conventional LGE-MRI of left ventricle (LV), LGE-MRI of LA requires significantly better spatial resolution, patient-specific optimization of scan parameters, strict requirements on contrast dose, and delay between contrast administration and image acquisition[24,25]:

1. LGE-MRI of LA should be performed with high spatial resolution to visualize thin (2–4 mm) LA wall and reduce partial volume effect between the wall and blood pool and the wall and adjacent tissues (**Fig. 2**). Typical voxel size for 3D LGE-MRI of LA is 1.25 × 1.25 × 2.5 mm (reconstructed to 0.625 × 0.625 × 1.25 mm). Larger voxel size reduces contrast between LA wall and blood and makes detection of LA enhancement problematic.

2. Data acquisition for LGE-MRI of LA should be synchronized with cardiac and respiratory motions. To reduce respiration effects on image quality, position of the right diaphragm is measured by MRI navigator, and data acquisition only occurs when the diaphragm is at the position corresponding with the end of the expiration (**Fig. 3**). Typically, data acquisition

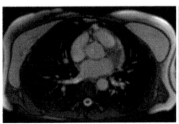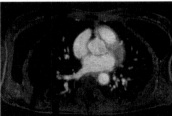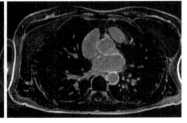

Fig. 1. Cine (*left*), magnetic resonance angiography (*center*), and LGE (*right*) images from MRI study of the LA.

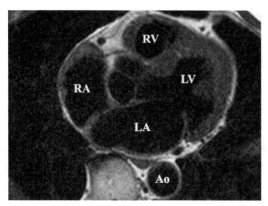

Fig. 2. Thickness of the LA wall (2–4 mm) is much less than thickness of LV wall (8–12 mm). Ao, aorta; RV, right ventricle.

is only performed if displacement of LA is less than 1.5 to 2 mm from baseline.To minimize LA wall blurring caused by cardiac motion (**Fig. 4**), data acquisition is performed during quasistationary phase of LA cardiac cycle and the acquisition is restricted to 10% to 15% of the cardiac cycle (typically, 100–150 milliseconds). There are 2 quasistationary phases of LA cardiac cycle. The earlier one is at the end of LV systole and the late one precedes the atrial kick (atrial systole). The first phase is short (about 10% of cardiac cycle), the other phase is longer (about 20% of cardiac cycle). For patients with regular (sinus) heart rhythm, it is preferable to perform data acquisition during the second (longer) phase and to extend the acquisition to 15% to 20% of cardiac cycle. For patients with arrhythmia, data acquisition should be shortened to 10% to 12% of average cardiac cycle and performed during the first phase because position of the second phase relative to QRS complex is not well determined and is arrhythmia dependent (**Fig. 5**).Image quality of LGE-MRI of the LA depends on the heart rate and rhythm. Arrhythmia may cause

LA wall blurring and ghosting artifacts, which adversely affect visualization/quantification of LA fibrosis/scar. LA scar visibility is significantly lower for patients with a fast (>100 beats per minute) heart rate than for patients with normal heart rate.[26] To achieve good-quality LGE-MRI of the LA for patients with a tachycardic or irregular heart rate, rate control or cardioversion is strongly recommended before MRI examination.

3. The other important requirements for LGE-MRI of LA wall are a dose of extracellular GBCA and delay between contrast administration and LGE-MRI scan. The type of GBCA and the corresponding dose used by various clinical centers for LGE-MRI of LA are provided in **Table 1**. The recommended delay time between contrast administration and LGE-MRI of the LA is between 20 and 40 minutes.[27] Higher contrast doses (>0.2 mmol/kg) and/or shorter delays (<15 mins) result in bright blood signal, making discrimination difficult between LA wall enhancement and blood signal.[24] Longer delays (>40 minutes) result in a poor enhancement of LA fibrosis caused by contrast washout. High-resolution LGE-MR images acquired with correct GBCA dose and delay after GBCA administration should show enhancement not only of LA fibrosis/scar but of the other thin fibrous structures, such aorta wall, valve annulus, and leaflets (**Fig. 6**).

Image Processing for Atrial Fibrosis/Scar Quantification

The main difference between different centers performing assessment of LA fibrosis resides in the processing of the acquired images. There are currently 3 software packages used to process the LGE-MRI images: Corview (Marrek Inc., Salt Lake City, UT), Itk-SNAP Version 2.2.0, and QMass MR Software Version 7.2 (Medis Medical Imaging Systems, Leiden, the Netherlands).

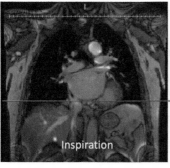
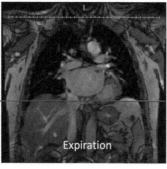

Inspiration   Expiration

Fig. 3. Position of LA considerably changes during patient respiration. Data acquisition for LGE-MRI of the LA should be synchronized with patient respiration to prevent blurring of LA wall. Red line indicates position of LA floor and diaphragm at the end of inspiration.

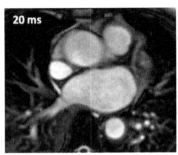 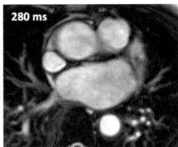 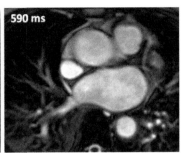

Fig. 4. Frames from cardiac cine-MRI illustrate change in LA wall position during cardiac cycle. Time after R wave shown in top left corner of each frame. Patient had heart rate of 110 beats per minute during cine scan. LA anterior wall moves more than posterior wall. Position of data acquisition relatively to QRS complex of electrocardiogram and duration of data acquisition for LGE-MRI of the LA should be selected so that data acquisition is only performed during stationary phase of LA cardiac cycle.

The main steps of LA fibrosis/scar quantification and visualization are shown in **Fig. 7**:

1. Acquisition of high-resolution LGE-MRI of the LA, as described earlier.
2. Segmentation of the LA wallSegmentation of the LA wall can be performed using manual, semimanual, and automatic methods. Manual segmentation continues to be the most accurate method but it requires well-trained personnel and is time consuming because thin LA wall and antral region of the PVs should be manually traced in each slice of the LGE-MRI volume. Furthermore, mitral annulus, aorta, and left circumflex coronary artery image artifacts should be excluded from the segmentation to minimize detection of false LA enhancement.
3. Quantification of atrial fibrosis/scarTo improve accuracy of LA fibrosis/scar quantification, image intensity inhomogeneity caused by spatially variable sensitivity of receiver coils and nonuniform profile of RF pulses has to be corrected. Inhomogeneity correction map can be estimated from LA blood pool, assuming that intensity of LA blood pool is uniform throughout the LA and any slowly varying deviation from signal uniformity is caused by intensity inhomogeneity. The correction map

estimated from LA blood pool is only applicable for the LA and adjacent regions.Quantification of fibrosis/scar is based on fact that fibrous tissue has higher intensity than normal myocardium and blood in LGE-MRI. Selection of an optimal threshold for accurate detection of LA fibrosis continues to be an active research topic. At present, there are 2 main methods for LA fibrosis quantification. The first method is based on analysis of signal intensity distribution of the segmented LA wall and relies on operator validation of algorithm-selected threshold.[12,25] The operator checks the threshold by visually inspecting the correspondence between enhanced voxels in LGE-MRI images and algorithm-detected fibrosis voxels. Typical threshold values for this method range from 2 to 4 standard deviations greater than the mean intensity of normal myocardium. The second method, known as an image intensity ratio (IIR), normalizes the intensity of the LA wall by the mean value of LA blood pool intensity and uses fixed ranges of IIR values to identify LA fibrosis and scar.[28–31] At present, there is an obvious disagreement between different research centers on what ranges of IIR values should be used for fibrosis and scar identification and quantification. A team from Barcelona University has proposed that LA wall voxels

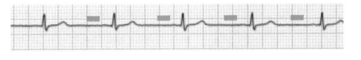

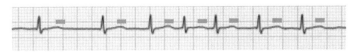

Fig. 5. Recommended position and duration of data acquisition for 3D LGE-MRI of LA for patients with sinus rhythm (*top*) and arrhythmia (*bottom*). Green rectangles indicate data acquisition.

Table 1
Dose of contrast agents used for late gadolinium enhancement MRI of the left atrium

Contrast Agent	Chemical Structure	Dose (mmol/kg)
Dotarem	Macrocyclic, nonionic	0.15–0.2
Gadavist	Macrocyclic, nonionic	0.1–0.2
Magnevist[a]	Linear, ionic	0.2
MultiHance[a]	Linear, ionic	0.1
Omniscan[a]	Linear, nonionic	0.2
ProHance	Macrocyclic, nonionic	0.15–0.2

[a] Indicates contrast agents usage of which was suspended and restricted in the European Union in 2017.

with IIR values between 1.2 and 1.32 be considered as interstitial fibrosis, and LA voxels with IIR greater than 1.32 be considered dense scarring.[31] However, a team from Johns Hopkins University has recommended to use IIR range (0.97, 1.61) to identify LA fibrosis and IIR greater than 1.61 to detect LA postablation scar.[28,29] The discrepancy in IIR ranges between the centers may be attributed to the ratio of image intensities of myocardium and blood pool depending on multiple factors, such as strength of the main field of MRI scanner, type and dosage of GBCA, delay between GBCA administration and LGE scan, patient heart rate and rhythm during LGE scan, patient-specific contrast clearance rate, blood hematocrit, blood oxygenation level, and choice of inversion time (TI) value for LGE scan. Both methods for fibrosis quantification have strong and weak points. The first method uses an operator-adjustable threshold, which accounts for patient-specific and scan-specific variation in contrast between fibrous and normal LA myocardium in a given LGE-MRI scan. The main weakness of this method is the high intra-operator and interoperator variability in quantification of LA fibrosis/scar. The second method has lower operator variability but has a low accuracy of fibrosis quantification for

LGE scans with nonoptimal contrast between LA myocardium and blood. Furthermore, a thorough validation of IIR method for LA fibrosis quantification is required using LGE-MRI data sets from multiple centers.

4. Rendering of the 3D model of LA3D visualization of LA fibrosis/scar is a useful tool that provides clinicians with information about spatial distribution of fibrosis/scar and may serve as a guidance for initial and repeat ablation procedures. Usually, the following color coding is used: healthy tissue is rendered as blue, and tissue with LGE is depicted as green for fibrosis and red for scar (postablation). Representative examples of 3D visualization for LA fibrosis and postablation scar are shown in **Fig. 8**.

ATRIAL FIBROSIS AS A PREDICTOR OF OUTCOMES

A growing body of evidence suggests that atrial fibrosis correlates with outcomes including AF ablation, stroke, and heart failure.

Atrial fibrosis was shown to be detected by LGE-MRI and the degree preablation correlated with the outcome of the ablation.[9] This initial observation was substantiated and further refined in subsequent retrospective and prospective clinical studies. In the only multicenter prospective trial (the DECAAF study) atrial fibrosis quantified in 272 patients was shown to predict arrhythmia recurrence after ablation with operators blinded to the degree of atrial fibrosis.[12] Patients were classified into 4 Utah stages based on the degree of atrial fibrosis: stage I (<10% of the atrial wall), II (≤10% to <20%), III (≤20% to <30%), and IV (>30%) (**Fig. 9**). The arrhythmia recurrence had a graded significant association with the degree of atrial fibrosis (stage I, 15%; stage II, 36%; stage III, 46%; and stage IV, 69%) and was the only variable associated with recurrence in multivariate analyses. Similar recurrence rates were noted at 1-year follow-up in a retrospective study performed in 426 consecutive patients undergoing AF ablation.[32] The degree of atrial fibrosis was shown to be a reliable predictor of long-term AF ablation outcome as well. There was an observed

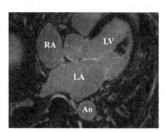
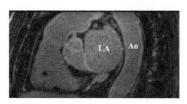

Fig. 6. Representative images from high-resolution 3D LGE-MRI study of the LA. Enhancement of anatomic structures (aorta wall, valve leaflets, and so forth) with high fibrous content is observed. Axial (transverse) and sagittal views are presented.

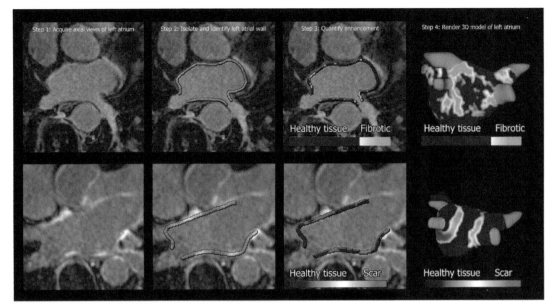

Fig. 7. The main steps of LA fibrosis/scar quantification: acquisition of LGE-MRI of the LA, segmentation of LA wall, quantification of LA fibrosis/scar, and 3D visualization of LA fibrosis/scar. Bottom row, postablation scar; top row, preablation fibrosis.

45% increased risk of recurrence for every 10% increase in atrial fibrosis (hazard ratio [HR], 1.45; 95% confidence interval [CI], 1.20–1.76; $P<.001$) at 5-year follow-up.[33] Virtually all patients with advanced atrial fibrosis had recurrence at 5 years, suggesting the importance of atrial myopathy in the pathogenesis of AF. These findings were supported by findings from another center in a cohort of 165 patients. Patients with LGE less than 35% had favorable ablation outcomes regardless of AF persistence at baseline, whereas those with LGE greater than 35% had a higher rate of AF recurrence in the first year after ablation.[34]

Traditionally, AF is thought to be an independent risk factor for ischemic stroke in nonanticoagulated patients, with cardioembolic stroke occurring 4 to 5 times more frequently in patients with AF relative to those without AF.[35,36] However, several observations have been made challenging the view of a causal relationship between AF and stroke. First, the lack of a consistent temporal relationship between AF episodes and stroke, whereby strokes precede any AF episode, has posed a significant challenge to the concept of AF acting as a trigger.[37,38] Furthermore, the risk of cardiovascular events persists whether sinus rhythm is maintain or there is AF recurrence.[39] Among the multiple factors underpinning the electrical and structural remodeling of the atria in AF, LA fibrosis has been identified as an important factor that may provide a mechanistic link between development of AF and stroke.[40–42] These studies raise the possibility that atrial myopathy could be a precursor and common mechanistic link for both development of AF and thromboembolic events. A study performed in 308 patients identified a significantly higher percentage of LA fibrosis (24.4% ± 12.4% vs 16.2% ± 9.9%; $P<.01$) in patients with a prior history of stroke.[43] When atrial

Fig. 8. 3D visualization of LA fibrosis (*top row*) and postablation scar (*bottom row*). Normal myocardium, blue; fibrosis, green and white; postablation scar, red. Mitral valve and PVs are shown in gray. AP, anteroposterior; PA, posteroanterior.

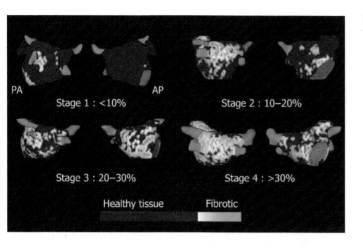

Fig. 9. Representative example of 4 LA fibrosis stages.

fibrosis percentage replaced the stroke in the CHADS2 (congestive heart failure, hypertension, age, diabetes, prior stroke) score, it significantly increased the predictive performance of the score. This finding may be, at least in part, explained by the association between severity of LA LGE and thrombus or spontaneous echocardiographic contrast identified by transesophageal echocardiography.[44] The strongest evidence to date that suggests atrial fibrosis as a precursor for stroke is provided by the study of King and colleagues.[45] Advanced atrial fibrosis was significantly associated with the risk of subsequent stroke or transient ischemic attack (TIA) (HR, 7.08; 95% CI, 2.72–18.45). In addition, a study by Mahnkoph and colleagues[46] found a similar degree of LA fibrosis in patients presenting with a stroke or TIA whether or not they had history of AF, suggesting that the association of LA fibrosis and stroke may extend beyond AF. In addition, atrial fibrosis was higher in patients with AF compared with a group of patients without AF,[47] suggesting that progression of the substrate may precede the development of AF.

There is a significant overlap of pathophysiology and bidirectional interaction between AF and heart failure.[11,48] AF is associated with increased risk of death in patients with heart failure.[49,50] The Catheter Ablation versus Standard Conventional Therapy in Patients with Left Ventricular Dysfunction and Atrial Fibrillation (CASTLE-AF) randomized clinical trial has shown that AF ablation reduced all-cause and cardiovascular mortality and hospitalization from worsening heart failure compared with antiarrhythmic drugs in patients with heart failure and LV ejection fraction less than 35%.[51] The benefit of AF ablation in patients with heart failure compared with amiodarone and rate control, respectively, was observed in 2 other clinical

trials: Ablation vs Amiodarone for Treatment of Atrial Fibrillation in Patients With Congestive Heart Failure and an Implanted ICD/CRTD (AATAC)[52] and Catheter Ablation Versus Medical Rate Control in Atrial Fibrillation and Systolic Dysfunction (CAMERA-MRI).[53] Atrial and ventricular fibrosis may represent one of the important pathophysiologic links between AF and heart failure.[11,54] Patients with heart failure and AF may have a higher degree of atrial fibrosis as detected by LGE-MRI.[55] The risk of developing heart failure, including heart failure with preserved ejection fraction, seems to increase with the degree of atrial fibrosis in patients with AF.[56] In contrast, in a substudy of the CAMERA-MRI trial, diffuse ventricular fibrosis regressed in patients with heart failure in which sinus rhythm was restored with catheter ablation of AF.[57]

ATRIAL SCAR POSTABLATION

LA ablation is frequently used to maintain sinus rhythm in patients with symptomatic AF.[5] However, results of a single AF ablation remain unsatisfactory (16%–29%).[13–16] The unsatisfactory success of AF ablations may be caused by inadequate lesions, progression of atrial fibrosis substrate, or not addressing all potential mechanisms (eg, atrial fibrosis, non-PV triggers). Technological advances in recent years have attempted to overcome prior limitations in lesion delivery by introduction of novel catheters (eg, irrigation, contact force) and mapping technologies that allow a better and more precise customization and annotation of lesion delivery. However, these more powerful technologies have potential risks for collateral damage. In particular, atrioesophageal fistula, albeit a rare complication, is the most dreaded complication because of its high

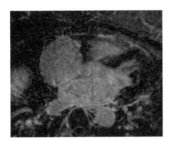
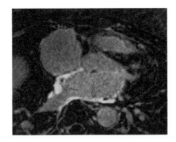

Fig. 10. Preablation and postablation LGE-MRI of the LA. Significant enhancement of the LA wall is easily observed on postablation image (*red arrows* indicate the same area pre- and post- ablation, respectively).

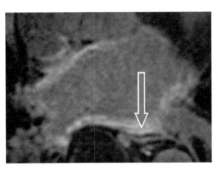
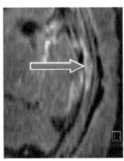

Fig. 11. Detection of ablation injury of esophagus by high-resolution 3D LGE-MRI scan performed acutely (<3 hours) after conclusion of RF ablation procedure for treatment of AF. Red arrows indicate enhancement of anterior wall of esophagus.

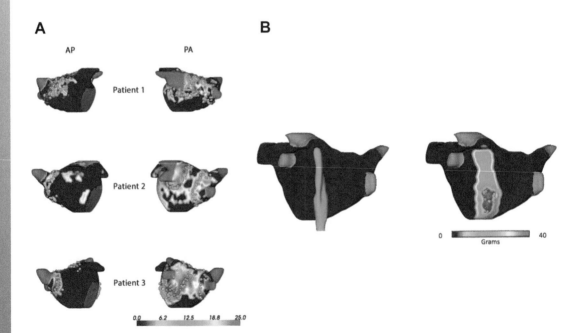

Fig. 12. (*A*) Three patients showing the overlap between lesion tags acquired during ablation and LGE-MRI post-ablation scar at 3 months. Red represents scar. Ablation tags are color coded based on contact force according to the scale. (*B*) Position of esophagus relative to the posterior wall of the LA (*left*) and projection of the esophagus on the posterior wall of the LA (*right*). Red represents the area of esophageal enhancement detected by LGE-MRI within 24 hours of ablation. Ablation tags corresponding with the area of esophageal enhancement are color coded based on contact force according to the scale.

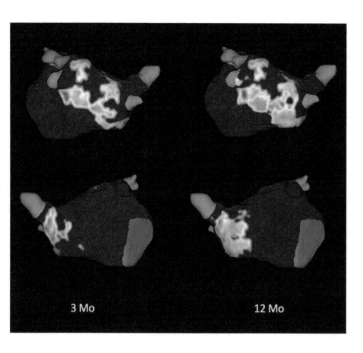

Fig. 13. PA (*top*) and AP (*bottom*) views of LA of the same patient at 3 and 12 months after ablation. Red areas denote scar caused by ablation. Green areas represent new fibrosis identified at 12 months.

3 Mo   12 Mo

fatality rate.[58] LGE-MRI can be effectively used for lesion assessment and quantification of left atrial fibrosis and detection of acute esophageal injury[9,10] (**Figs. 10** and **11**).

Although PVI is used as the cornerstone of any AF ablation,[4,5] durable isolation of the PVs is not frequently achieved. Circumferential scar of all PVs was achieved in only 6.9% in a study of 144 patients.[59] The number of gaps in the PV ablation line did not correlate with the AF recurrence but the total relative gap did correlate with recurrence at 1 year after first PVI.[60] Furthermore, there seems to be a fairly good correlation between gaps in PV lesion sets and sites of electrical reconnection at redo AF procedures.[61] Gaps in PV lines can be identified in real time by MRI, as shown in animal models.[62] In an attempt to obtain durable PVI, other techniques have been proposed to improve the outcomes of PVI: high-power short-duration ablation (HPSD). HPSD may represent a favorable strategy in LA, because there would be a shift toward resistive heating,[63] which would result in shallower lesions in chambers where posterior wall thickness is on average 1.5 to 2.5 mm.[10,64,65] A study comparing a high-power (50 W) short-duration strategy with low-power long-duration strategy found that esophageal thermal injury (ETI) patterns and long-term outcomes are similar but HPSD has shorter procedure time.[66] Furthermore, efforts have been made to delineate the optimal RF ablation parameters to ensure durable lesions while avoiding ETI for the HPSD strategy[67] (**Fig. 12**). Optimal parameters

derived from low-power long-duration strategy have been derived as well using LGE-MRI.[68–70]

Although there is substantial evidence of atrial fibrosis playing a significant role in the pathophysiology of AF and outcomes of AF ablation, it is less clear whether targeting fibrosis may improve outcomes. Residual fibrosis is a strong predictor of arrhythmia recurrence after AF ablation, suggesting that perhaps targeting areas of atrial fibrosis could result in improvement of ablation procedures.[71] This hypothesis is currently being tested in the DECAAF II prospective randomized clinical trial. Note that atrial myopathy is likely a progressive disease and its progression may explain, at least in part, some AF ablation failures. Atrial fibrosis degree was lower in patients without AF compared with those with AF,[47] suggesting a progression of substrate that may precede and eventually lead to the development of AF. Furthermore, new fibrosis formation seems to be a predictor of AF ablation outcome (**Fig. 13**) (Kheirkhahan and colleagues: Left Atrial Fibrosis Progression Detected by LGE-MRI after Ablation of Atrial Fibrillation. Submitted for publication).

SUMMARY

Cardiac MRI is increasingly used to gain insight into the role of atrial fibrosis in outcomes of AF ablation, stroke, and heart failure. In addition, it has been used to better understand the progression of atrial myopathy substrate in patients with AF. Furthermore, atrial fibrosis may provide a mechanistic link between AF and stroke or heart failure. Atrial scar imaging has been helpful in understanding the biophysics of different ablation modalities and defining optimal ablation parameters. Variations in image analysis methods used to define atrial fibrosis have precluded higher uptakes of this specialized imaging technique around the world. Improvements in the spatial resolution, standardization of scan protocols for imaging atrial fibrosis, and development of new and reliable techniques in detecting diffuse fibrosis may further expand the knowledge and understanding of the role of atrial fibrosis in the pathophysiology of different cardiac diseases. Similarly, DECAAF II results may provide a more definitive answer on whether atrial fibrosis modification could improve the outcomes of AF ablation.

REFERENCES

1. Go AS, Hylek EM, Phillips KA, et al. Prevalence of diagnosed atrial fibrillation in adults: national implications for rhythm management and stroke prevention: the AnTicoagulation and Risk Factors in Atrial Fibrillation (ATRIA) Study. JAMA 2001;285(18):2370–5.

2. Miyasaka Y, Barnes ME, Gersh BJ, et al. Secular trends in incidence of atrial fibrillation in Olmsted County, Minnesota, 1980 to 2000, and implications on the projections for future prevalence. Circulation 2006;114(2):119–25.

3. Dobrev D, Nattel S. New antiarrhythmic drugs for treatment of atrial fibrillation. Lancet 2010; 375(9721):1212–23.

4. Haissaguerre M, Jais P, Shah DC, et al. Spontaneous initiation of atrial fibrillation by ectopic beats originating in the pulmonary veins. N Engl J Med 1998;339(10):659–66.

5. Calkins H, Kuck KH, Cappato R, et al. 2012 HRS/EHRA/ECAS expert consensus statement on catheter and surgical ablation of atrial fibrillation: recommendations for patient selection, procedural techniques, patient management and follow-up, definitions, endpoints, and research trial design: a report of the Heart Rhythm Society (HRS) Task Force on Catheter and Surgical Ablation of Atrial Fibrillation. Developed in partnership with the European Heart Rhythm Association (EHRA), a registered branch of the European Society of Cardiology (ESC) and the European Cardiac Arrhythmia Society (ECAS); and in collaboration with the American College of Cardiology (ACC), American Heart Association (AHA), the Asia Pacific Heart Rhythm Society (APHRS), and the Society of Thoracic Surgeons (STS). Endorsed by the governing bodies of the American College of Cardiology Foundation, the American Heart Association, the European Cardiac Arrhythmia Society, the European Heart Rhythm Association, the Society of Thoracic Surgeons, the Asia Pacific Heart Rhythm Society, and the Heart Rhythm Society. Heart Rhythm 2012;9(4):632–96.e21.

6. Santangeli P, Zado ES, Hutchinson MD, et al. Prevalence and distribution of focal triggers in persistent and long-standing persistent atrial fibrillation. Heart Rhythm 2016;13(2):374–82.

7. Zhao Y, Di Biase L, Trivedi C, et al. Importance of non-pulmonary vein triggers ablation to achieve long-term freedom from paroxysmal atrial fibrillation in patients with low ejection fraction. Heart Rhythm 2016;13(1):141–9.

8. Gal P, Marrouche NF. Magnetic resonance imaging of atrial fibrosis: redefining atrial fibrillation to a syndrome. Eur Heart J 2015;38(1):14–9.

9. Oakes RS, Badger TJ, Kholmovski EG, et al. Detection and quantification of left atrial structural remodeling with delayed-enhancement magnetic resonance imaging in patients with atrial fibrillation. Circulation 2009;119(13):1758–67.

10. Badger TJ, Adjei-Poku YA, Burgon NS, et al. Initial experience of assessing esophageal tissue injury and recovery using delayed-enhancement MRI after atrial fibrillation ablation. Circ Arrhythm Electrophysiol 2009;2(6):620–5.

11. Molina CE, Abu-Taha IH, Wang Q, et al. Profibrotic, electrical, and calcium-handling remodeling of the atria in heart failure patients with and without atrial fibrillation. Front Physiol 2018;9:1383.

12. Marrouche NF, Wilber D, Hindricks G, et al. Association of atrial tissue fibrosis identified by delayed enhancement MRI and atrial fibrillation catheter ablation: the DECAAF study. JAMA 2014;311(5):498–506.

13. Weerasooriya R, Khairy P, Litalien J, et al. Catheter ablation for atrial fibrillation: are results maintained at 5 years of follow-up? J Am Coll Cardiol 2011; 57(2):160–6.

14. Rostock T, Salukhe TV, Steven D, et al. Long-term single- and multiple-procedure outcome and predictors of success after catheter ablation for persistent atrial fibrillation. Heart Rhythm 2011;8(9):1391–7.

15. Tilz RR, Rillig A, Thum AM, et al. Catheter ablation of long-standing persistent atrial fibrillation: 5-year outcomes of the Hamburg Sequential Ablation Strategy. J Am Coll Cardiol 2012;60(19):1921–9.

16. Scherr D, Khairy P, Miyazaki S, et al. Five-year outcome of catheter ablation of persistent atrial fibrillation using termination of atrial fibrillation as a procedural endpoint. Circ Arrhythm Electrophysiol 2015;8(1):18–24.

17. Cappato R, Negroni S, Pecora D, et al. Prospective assessment of late conduction recurrence across radiofrequency lesions producing electrical disconnection at the pulmonary vein ostium in patients with atrial fibrillation. Circulation 2003;108(13): 1599–604.

18. Callans DJ, Gerstenfeld EP, Dixit S, et al. Efficacy of repeat pulmonary vein isolation procedures in patients with recurrent atrial fibrillation. J Cardiovasc Electrophysiol 2004;15(9):1050–5.

19. Nanthakumar K, Plumb VJ, Epstein AE, et al. Resumption of electrical conduction in previously isolated pulmonary veins: rationale for a different strategy? Circulation 2004;109(10):1226–9.

20. Ouyang F, Antz M, Ernst S, et al. Recovered pulmonary vein conduction as a dominant factor for recurrent atrial tachyarrhythmias after complete circular isolation of the pulmonary veins: lessons from double Lasso technique. Circulation 2005;111(2):127–35.

21. Parmar BR, Jarrett TR, Kholmovski EG, et al. Poor scar formation after ablation is associated with atrial fibrillation recurrence. J Interv Card Electrophysiol 2015;44(3):247–56.

22. Haissaguerre M, Hocini M, Sanders P, et al. Catheter ablation of long-lasting persistent atrial fibrillation: clinical outcome and mechanisms of subsequent arrhythmias. J Cardiovasc Electrophysiol 2005;16(11): 1138–47.

23. Inoue YY, Alissa A, Khurram IM, et al. Quantitative tissue-tracking cardiac magnetic resonance (CMR) of left atrial deformation and the risk of stroke in patients with atrial fibrillation. J Am Heart Assoc 2015; 4(4) [pii:e001844].

24. Siebermair J, Kholmovski EG, Marrouche N. Assessment of left atrial fibrosis by late gadolinium enhancement magnetic resonance imaging: methodology and clinical implications. JACC Clin Electrophysiol 2017;3(8):791–802.

25. Chubb H, Aziz S, Karim R, et al. Optimization of late gadolinium enhancement cardiovascular magnetic resonance imaging of post-ablation atrial scar: a cross-over study. J Cardiovasc Magn Reson 2018; 20(1):30.

26. Vijayakumar S, Kholmovski EG, McGann C, et al. Dependence of contrast to noise ratio between ablation scar and other tissues on patient heart rate and flip angle for late gadolinium enhancement imaging of the left atrium. J Cardiovasc Magn Reson 2012; 14(Suppl 1):O107.

27. Vijayakumar S, Kholmovski EG, Marrouche NF. Dependence of scar contrast in LGE images of left atrium on the time interval after contrast injection. J Cardiovasc Magn Reson 2011; 13(Suppl 1):P42.

28. Khurram IM, Beinart R, Zipunnikov V, et al. Magnetic resonance image intensity ratio, a normalized measure to enable interpatient comparability of left atrial fibrosis. Heart Rhythm 2014;11(1):85–92.

29. Fukumoto K, Habibi M, Gucuk Ipek E, et al. Comparison of preexisting and ablation-induced late gadolinium enhancement on left atrial magnetic resonance imaging. Heart Rhythm 2015;12(4):668–72.

30. Harrison JL, Sohns C, Linton NW, et al. Repeat left atrial catheter ablation: cardiac magnetic resonance prediction of endocardial voltage and gaps in ablation lesion sets. Circ Arrhythm Electrophysiol 2015; 8(2):270–8.

31. Benito EM, Carlosena-Remirez A, Guasch E, et al. Left atrial fibrosis quantification by late gadolinium-enhanced magnetic resonance: a new method to standardize the thresholds for reproducibility. Europace 2017;19(8):1272–9.

32. McGann C, Akoum N, Patel A, et al. Atrial fibrillation ablation outcome is predicted by left atrial remodeling on MRI. Circ Arrhythm Electrophysiol 2014;7(1): 23–30.

33. Chelu MG, King JB, Kholmovski EG, et al. Atrial fibrosis by late gadolinium enhancement magnetic resonance imaging and catheter ablation of atrial fibrillation: 5-year follow-up data. J Am Heart Assoc 2018;7(23):e006313.

34. Khurram IM, Habibi M, Gucuk Ipek E, et al. Left atrial LGE and arrhythmia recurrence following pulmonary vein isolation for paroxysmal and persistent AF. JACC Cardiovasc Imaging 2016;9(2):142–8.

35. Wolf PA, Abbott RD, Kannel WB. Atrial fibrillation as an independent risk factor for stroke: the Framingham Study. Stroke; a J Cereb Circ 1991;22(8):983–8.

36. Lin HJ, Wolf PA, Kelly-Hayes M, et al. Stroke severity in atrial fibrillation. The Framingham Study. Stroke 1996;27(10):1760–4.

37. Brambatti M, Connolly SJ, Gold MR, et al. Temporal relationship between subclinical atrial fibrillation and embolic events. Circulation 2014;129(21): 2094–9.

38. Martin DT, Bersohn MM, Waldo AL, et al. Randomized trial of atrial arrhythmia monitoring to guide anticoagulation in patients with implanted defibrillator and cardiac resynchronization devices. Eur Heart J 2015;36(26):1660–8.

39. van Gelder IC, Hagens VE, Kingma JH, et al. Rate control versus electrical cardioversion for atrial fibrillation: a randomised comparison of two treatment strategies concerning morbidity, mortality, quality of life and cost-benefit - the RACE study design. Neth Heart J 2002;10(3):118–24.

40. Jalife J, Kaur K. Atrial remodeling, fibrosis, and atrial fibrillation. Trends Cardiovasc Med 2015;25(6): 475–84.

41. Dzeshka MS, Lip GY, Snezhitskiy V, et al. Cardiac fibrosis in patients with atrial fibrillation: mechanisms and clinical implications. J Am Coll Cardiol 2015; 66(8):943–59.

42. Thanigaimani S, Lau DH, Agbaedeng T, et al. Molecular mechanisms of atrial fibrosis: implications for the clinic. Expert Rev Cardiovasc Ther 2017;15(4):247–56.

43. Daccarett M, Badger TJ, Akoum N, et al. Association of left atrial fibrosis detected by delayed-enhancement magnetic resonance imaging and the risk of stroke in patients with atrial fibrillation. J Am Coll Cardiol 2011;57(7):831–8.

44. Akoum N, Daccarett M, McGann C, et al. Atrial fibrosis helps select the appropriate patient and strategy in catheter ablation of atrial fibrillation: a

DE-MRI guided approach. J Cardiovasc Electrophysiol 2011;22(1):16–22.

45. King JB, Azadani PN, Suksaranjit P, et al. Left atrial fibrosis and risk of Cerebrovascular and cardiovascular events in patients with atrial fibrillation. J Am Coll Cardiol 2017;70(11):1311–21.

46. Mahnkopf C, Mitlacher M, Brachmann J. Assessment of left atrial structural remodeling in patients with cryptogenic stroke - lessons learned from LGE-MRI. Journal of Cardiovascular Magnetic Resonance 2016;18(Suppl 1):P202.

47. Siebermair J, Suksaranjit P, McGann CJ, et al. Atrial fibrosis in non-atrial fibrillation individuals and prediction of atrial fibrillation by use of late gadolinium enhancement magnetic resonance imaging. J Cardiovasc Electrophysiol 2019;30(4):550–6.

48. Santhanakrishnan R, Wang N, Larson MG, et al. Atrial fibrillation begets heart failure and vice versa temporal associations and differences in preserved versus reduced ejection fraction. Circulation 2016; 133(5):484–92.

49. Dries DL, Exner DV, Gersh BJ, et al. Atrial fibrillation is associated with an increased risk for mortality and heart failure progression in patients with asymptomatic and symptomatic left ventricular systolic dysfunction: a retrospective analysis of the SOLVD trials. Studies of Left Ventricular Dysfunction. J Am Coll Cardiol 1998;32(3):695–703.

50. Wang TJ, Larson MG, Levy D, et al. Temporal relations of atrial fibrillation and congestive heart failure and their joint influence on mortality: the Framingham Heart Study. Circulation 2003; 107(23):2920–5.

51. Marrouche NF, Brachmann J, Andresen D, et al. Catheter ablation for atrial fibrillation with heart failure. N Engl J Med 2018;378(5):417–27.

52. Di Biase L, Mohanty P, Mohanty S, et al. Ablation versus amiodarone for treatment of persistent atrial fibrillation in patients with congestive heart failure and an implanted device: results from the AATAC multicenter randomized trial. Circulation 2016; 133(17):1637–44.

53. Prabhu S, Taylor AJ, Costello BT, et al. Catheter ablation versus medical rate control in atrial fibrillation and systolic dysfunction: the CAMERA-MRI study. J Am Coll Cardiol 2017; 70(16):1949–61.

54. Nattel S. Molecular and cellular mechanisms of atrial fibrosis in atrial fibrillation. JACC Clin Electrophysiol 2017;3(5):425–35.

55. Akkaya M, Higuchi K, Koopmann M, et al. Higher degree of left atrial structural remodeling in patients with atrial fibrillation and left ventricular systolic dysfunction. J Cardiovasc Electrophysiol 2013; 24(5):485–91.

56. Azadani PN, King JB, Kheirkhahan M, et al. Left atrial fibrosis is associated with new-onset heart failure in patients with atrial fibrillation. Int J Cardiol 2017;248:161–5.

57. Prabhu S, Costello BT, Taylor AJ, et al. Regression of diffuse ventricular fibrosis following restoration of sinus rhythm with catheter ablation in patients with atrial fibrillation and systolic dysfunction: a substudy of the CAMERA MRI trial. JACC Clin Electrophysiol 2018;4(8):999–1007.

58. Ghia KK, Chugh A, Good E, et al. A nationwide survey on the prevalence of atrioesophageal fistula after left atrial radiofrequency catheter ablation. J Interv Card Electrophysiol 2009;24(1):33–6.

59. Badger TJ, Daccarett M, Akoum NW, et al. Evaluation of left atrial lesions after initial and repeat atrial fibrillation ablation: lessons learned from delayed-enhancement MRI in repeat ablation procedures. Circ Arrhythm Electrophysiol 2010;3(3):249–59.

60. Linhart M, Alarcon F, Borras R, et al. Delayed gadolinium enhancement magnetic resonance imaging detected anatomic gap length in wide circumferential pulmonary vein ablation lesions is associated with recurrence of atrial fibrillation. Circ Arrhythm Electrophysiol 2018;11(12):e006659.

61. Bisbal F, Guiu E, Cabanas-Grandio P, et al. CMR-guided approach to localize and ablate gaps in repeat AF ablation procedure. JACC Cardiovasc Imaging 2014;7(7):653–63.

62. Ranjan R, Kholmovski EG, Blauer J, et al. Identification and acute targeting of gaps in atrial ablation lesion sets using a real-time magnetic resonance imaging system. Circ Arrhythm Electrophysiol 2012; 5(6):1130–5.

63. Leshem E, Zilberman I, Tschabrunn CM, et al. High-power and short-duration ablation for pulmonary vein isolation: Biophysical Characterization. JACC Clin Electrophysiol 2018;4(4):467–79.

64. Beinart R, Abbara S, Blum A, et al. Left atrial wall thickness variability measured by CT scans in patients undergoing pulmonary vein isolation. J Cardiovasc Electrophysiol 2011;22(11):1232–6.

65. Hall B, Jeevanantham V, Simon R, et al. Variation in left atrial transmural wall thickness at sites commonly targeted for ablation of atrial fibrillation. J Interv Card Electrophysiol 2006;17(2):127–32.

66. Baher A, Kheirkhahan M, Rechenmacher SJ, et al. High-power radiofrequency catheter ablation of atrial fibrillation: using late gadolinium enhancement magnetic resonance imaging as a novel index of esophageal injury. JACC Clin Electrophysiol 2018; 4(12):1583–94.

67. Chelu MG, Morris AK, Kholmovski EG, et al. Durable lesion formation while avoiding esophageal injury during ablation of atrial fibrillation: lessons learned from late gadolinium MR imaging. J Cardiovasc Electrophysiol 2018;29(3):385–92.

68. Andreu D, Gomez-Pulido F, Calvo M, et al. Contact force threshold for permanent lesion formation in

atrial fibrillation ablation: a cardiac magnetic resonance-based study to detect ablation gaps. Heart Rhythm 2016;13(1):37–45.

69. Park CI, Lehrmann H, Keyl C, et al. Mechanisms of pulmonary vein reconnection after radiofrequency ablation of atrial fibrillation: the deterministic role of contact force and interlesion distance. J Cardiovasc Electrophysiol 2014; 25(7):701–8.

70. Sohns C, Karim R, Harrison J, et al. Quantitative magnetic resonance imaging analysis of the relationship between contact force and left atrial scar formation after catheter ablation of atrial fibrillation. J Cardiovasc Electrophysiol 2014;25(2):138–45.

71. Akoum N, Wilber D, Hindricks G, et al. MRI assessment of ablation-induced scarring in atrial fibrillation: analysis from the DECAAF study. J Cardiovasc Electrophysiol 2015;26(5):473–80.

Fibrosis and Ventricular Arrhythmogenesis
Role of Cardiac MRI

Mohammad Shenasa, MD

KEYWORDS

- Arrhythmias • Conduction • Fibrosis • Imaging • Magnetic resonance • Myocardial fibroblasts
- Sudden cardiac death • Ventricular arrhythmias

KEY POINTS

- Cardiac fibrosis is defined as a significant increase in the collagen volume fraction of myocardial tissue and is due to increased numbers of cardiac fibroblasts.
- Cardiac fibrosis plays an important central role in the pathophysiology of many cardiovascular abnormalities, such as coronary artery disease (CAD), ischemia, cardiomyopathies, heart failure (HF), hypertension, congenital heart disease, and many others.
- Electrophysiologically, myocardial fibrosis produces anisotropic conduction, inhomogeneity, and conduction delay, which predisposes to conduction block and reentrant arrhythmias.
- Several markers are currently available to detect myocardial fibrosis, including image-based methods, such as cardiac MRI (CMRI), cardiac computed tomography, echocardiography, and biomarkers.
- CMRI is the most commonly used imaging technique and its surrogate, late gadolinium enhancement cardiac magnetic resonance (LGE-CMR), provides markers for tissue characterization, disease progression, and arrhythmic events.
- Furthermore, LGE-CMR can be used as a risk marker of occurrence of ventricular tachycardia (VT), ventricular fibrillation (VF), sudden cardiac death (SCD), and implantable cardioverter defibrillator (ICD) implantation for primary prevention in high-risk patients.

PATHOPHYSIOLOGY OF MYOCARDIAL FIBROSIS
What Is Cardiac Fibrosis?

Definition: fibrosis is defined as excess deposit of collagen in extracellular matrix within the myocardial tissue.[1,2] Many pathologic conditions that are involved in the atrial or ventricular myocardium will cause myocardial fibrosis. The most common among them are shown in **Box 1**.

Myocardial fibrosis is due to the increase in number of cardiac fibroblasts (CFs), within the myocardial tissue that generate collagen biomarkers such as C-terminal propeptide of type I procollagen. CFs account for approximately 20% of cardiac cells. At the cellular level, CFs initiate signals that are involved in the production of mRNAs, which participate in the pathogenesis of many diseases,[2] as shown in **Box 1**. Idiopathic fibrosis without any recognized cause is now known as an independent

Disclosure: There are no conflict of interests relevant to this article.
Heart and Rhythm Medical Group, Department of Cardiovascular Services, O'Connor Hospital, San Jose, CA 95030, USA
E-mail address: mohammad.shenasa@gmail.com

Card Electrophysiol Clin 11 (2019) 551–562
https://doi.org/10.1016/j.ccep.2019.06.002
1877-9182/19/© 2019 Elsevier Inc. All rights reserved.

Box 1
Cardiac pathologic conditions that induce myocardial fibrosis

1. Idiopathic fibrosis
2. Coronary artery disease, acute myocardial infarction, myocardial ischemia, postmyocardial infarction
3. Hypertension, LVH, HHD
4. Diastolic dysfunction
5. Inherited cardiomyopathies, such as HCM, DCM, ARVD/C, and so forth
6. Inherited cardiac channelopathies such as Brugada syndrome
7. Ischemic and nonischemic cardiomyopathies
8. Heart failure: HFrEF and HFpEF
9. Valvular heart disease, such as aortic stenosis
10. Congenital heart disease and adult congenital heart disease
11. Sarcoidosis, Chagas disease, amyloidosis
12. Myocarditis
13. Diabetic cardiomyopathy
14. Inflammatory diseases
15. Athletic heart
16. Obesity and metabolic syndrome
17. Sleep apnea
18. Chemotherapy and radiation induced
19. Others

Abbreviations: ARVD/C, arrhythmogenic right ventricular dysplasia/cardiomyopathy; DCM, dilated cardiomyopathy; HCM, hypertrophic cardiomyopathy; HFpEF, heart failure with preserved ejection fraction; HFrEF, heart failure with reduced ejection fraction; HHD, hypertensive heart disease; LVH, left ventricular hypertrophy.

entity that has been observed in patients with sudden cardiac death (SCD).[3,4]

González and colleagues[2] described the developmental pathways and phases in myocardial interstitial fibrosis seen in different cardiovascular pathologic conditions. Fibroblasts, through cell signaling and genetic pathways, cause diffuse deposits of collagen within the myocardial matrix. Felisbino and McKinsey[5] also reported the genetic regulation of CF and pathways that lead to cardiac fibrosis. Histologic studies obtained from biopsies demonstrated the presence of collagen fibers and micro scars that precipitate the genesis of reentrant arrhythmias.[1,6]

ELECTROPHYSIOLOGICAL EFFECTS OF MYOCARDIAL FIBROSIS

Myocardial fibrosis and disease progression increases with age.

Electrical propagation in the myocardium is generally anisotropic; that is, conduction is faster parallel to the myocardial fibers compared with perpendicular direction.[7]

Similarly, under normal conductions, impulse propagation is continuous and uniform, whereas myocardial fibrosis causes discontinuous propagation and nonuniform conduction, which results in slow conduction, electrogram fractionation, and unidirectional block, which in turn precipitates reentry to occur.[7–10]

The detailed biophysical and cellular effects of fibrosis are beyond the purpose of this review. The readers are referred to articles by Kleber and Janse[8] and Spach and colleagues.[10]

Fig. 1 demonstrates the effect of fibrosis on myocardial conduction and local electrograms; note zigzag and slow conduction on the left panel and electrogram fractionation on the right panel.

FIBROSIS AND VENTRICULAR ARRHYTHMIAS AND SUDDEN CARDIAC DEATH

Late gadolinium enlacement cardiac magnetic resonance (LGE-CMR) imaging plays an important role in detection, mechanisms, tissue characterization, and response to therapy in patients at risk of ventricular arrhythmias (VAs) and SCD.

Neilan and colleagues[11] have recently reported LGE-CMR in patients who survived an episode of sudden cardiac arrest. A total of 147 patients with aborted sudden cardiac arrest were identified and underwent LGE-CMR before implantable cardioverter defibrillator (ICD) implantation. Ten patients had known diagnosis (acute myocardial infarction, 6; hypertrophic cardiomyopathy (HCM), 1; sarcoidosis, 1; and myocarditis, 2). Importantly, 137 patients had no clear diagnosis before LGE-CMR scanning. The underlying causes were identified based on LGE-CMR in most patients. Patient diagnoses based on LGE-CMR are shown in **Fig. 2**. Furthermore, patients who had positive LGE-CMR scan had significantly higher arrhythmic events and lower survival compared with those with negative LGE-CMR results as shown in **Fig. 3**.[11]

Similarly, Aljaroudi and colleagues[12] have reported on the role of LGE-CMR in risk stratification of SCD in a variety of cardiac pathologic conditions such as HCM, dilated cardiomyopathy (DCM), arrhythmogenic right ventricular dysplasia/cardiomyopathy (AVRD/C), viral

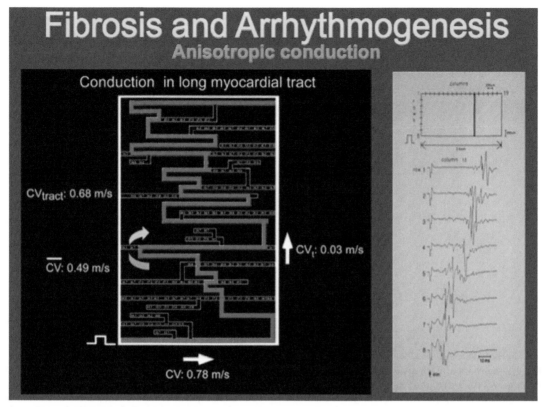

Fig. 1. Demonstration of conduction slowing and zigzag propagation (left panel) and fractionated electrograms (right panel). (*From* Kleber A, Janse M. In Shenasa et al, eds. Cardiac Mapping 5th Edition, chapter 29. 2019. Wiley; with permission.)

myocarditis, sarcoidosis, amyloidosis, hemochromatosis, postpartum cardiomyopathy, and Duchenne muscular dystrophy. The investigators further reported that LGE-CMR provided valuable information in identification of high-risk individuals for SCD in a variety of specific pathologic conditions. They concluded that myocardial fibrosis was an independent marker for VA and SCD.

TECHNIQUES FOR DETECTION OF MYOCARDIAL FIBROSIS AND DISEASE PROGRESSION

There are several markers that can detect myocardial fibrosis.

1. Image based
   a. Cardiac MRI (CMRI) and its surrogate, late gadolinium enlacement (LGE)
   b. Cardiac computed tomography
   c. Echocardiography
2. Biomarker based

In this article, only the role of LGE-CMR in detection and assessment of myocardial fibrosis and its relation to VA and SCD in certain specific pathologic conditions is discussed.

ROLE OF LATE GADOLINIUM ENLACEMENT CARDIAC MAGNETIC RESONANCE IN EVALUATION OF MYOCARDIAL FIBROSIS

Gadolinium (Gd) is an element in the periodic table with an atomic number of 64. Gd is toxic to mammals, except in its chelated form, with a half-life of 90 minutes. Gd is used as an intravenous MRI contrast agent. Gd does not enter the intact cell membrane; however, it accumulates in extracellular cell space. Therefore, when extracellular space expands, the number of Gd atoms is increased.

The roles of CMRI and LGE-CMR in specific pathologic conditions and related arrhythmias is discussed below.

MYOCARDIAL FIBROSIS IN PATIENTS WITH INHERITED CARDIOMYOPATHIES

Several clinical syndromes are related to inherited cardiomyopathies, such as HCM, DCM, and ARVD/C.[13]

Hypertrophic Cardiomyopathy

HCM is the most common genetic cardiac disease with an autosomal dominant pattern. The most

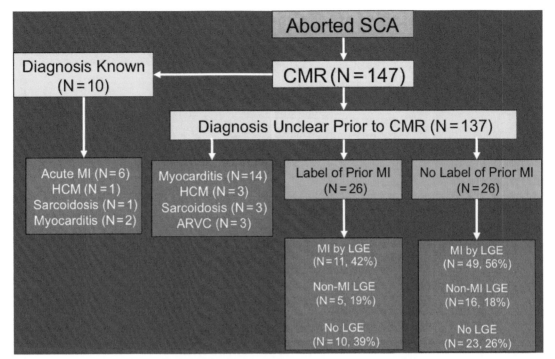

Fig. 2. Flowchart of patients with aborted sudden cardiac arrest, who were diagnosed according to LGE-CMR findings. ARVC, arrhythmogenic right ventricular cardiomyopathy; CMR, cardiac magnetic resonance; HCM, hypertrophic cardiomyopathy; LGE, late gadolinium enhancement; MI, myocardial infarction; SCA, sudden cardiac arrest. (*Reprinted from JACC:* Cardiovascular Imaging, Volume 8, Issue 4, Thomas G. Neilan, Hoshang Farhad, Thomas Mayrhofer et al, Late gadolinium enhancement among survivors of sudden cardiac arrest, Pages 414–423, Copyright 2015, *with permission from* Elsevier.)

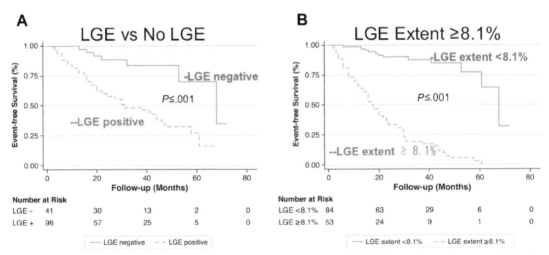

Fig. 3. Event-free survival separated according to the presence and extent of LGE. Kaplan-Meier curves displaying event-free survival in cohorts according to (*A*) the dichotomous presence of absence of LGE and (*B*) an extent of LGE of ≥8.1% or <8.1% of the volume of the left ventricle. ARVC, arrhythmogenic right ventricular cardiomyopathy; CMR, cardiac magnetic resonance; HCM, hypertrophic cardiomyopathy; LGE, late gadolinium enhancement; MI, myocardial infarction; SCA, sudden cardiac arrest. (*Reprinted from* JACC: Cardiovascular Imaging, Volume 8, Issue 4, Thomas G. Neilan, Hoshang Farhad, Thomas Mayrhofer et al, Late gadolinium enhancement among survivors of sudden cardiac arrest, Pages 414–423, Copyright 2015, *with permission from* Elsevier.)

common genetic mutations are found in beta-myosin heavy chain and myosin-binding protein C gene.[14,15] The presentation of patients with HCM is related to arrhythmic events, atrial fibrillation (AF), ventricular tachycardia (VT), and SCD, and/or progression to heart failure (HF). Syncope and presyncope are also common and maybe related to the hemodynamic effects of septal hypertrophy or arrhythmias. Myocardial fibrosis plays a central role in HCM from a preclinical stage to its end stage with HF and cardiac transplantation.

LGE-CMR imaging has significantly improved our understanding of the diverse natural history, presentation, and management strategies in patients with HCM.[15,16] LGE-CMR imaging demonstrates a variety of morphologic patterns and phenotypes in patients with HCM, such as (1) asymmetric septal hypertrophy, (2) focal hypertrophy, (3) apical aneurysm, (4) localized transmural fibrosis, (5) left ventricular (LV) lateral wall

hypertrophy, and (6) preclinical forms of HCM, in which in some cases appear as genotype positive and phenotype negative. These patterns of HCM morphologies were recognized using LGE-CMR imaging. Maron and colleagues[15] demonstrated these image characteristics using LGE-CMR techniques. Furthermore, LGE-CMR imaging as well as genetic testing provided better selection of patients at high risk of arrhythmias and sudden death, and identification of patients who may benefit from primary prevention of ICD implantation as well as screening of family members who may be carriers of the disease.[17–20]

Ho and colleagues[19] demonstrated the role of myocardial fibrosis in HCM. HCM is caused by a genetic abnormality in the cardiac sarcomere, which causes myocardial disarray and results in reentry.[21–23] The degree of myocardial fibrosis detected by LGE-CMR imaging is related to the development of VA. **Fig. 4** A and B demonstrate LGE-CMR images in 2 different patients with

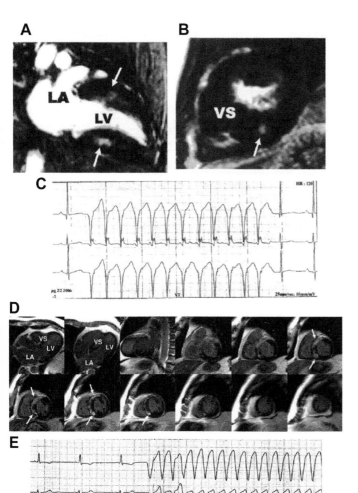

Fig. 4. (*A* and *B*) Demonstrate presence of focal fibrosis in a patient with hypertrophic cardiomyopathy and nonsustained ventricular tachycardia. Arrows denote the presence of fibrosis detected on LGE-CMR. (*C*) Holter recording from a patient with image of *A* and *B* showing nonsustained VT. (*D*) CMR imaging showing areas of late gadolinium enhancement (*arrows*). (*E*) Holter electrocardiography recorded and episode of monomorphic sustained VT during syncope that let to hospital admission. LA, left atrium; LV, left ventricle; VS, ventricular septum. (*Reprinted from* The American Journal of Cardiology, Volume 110, Issue 8, Simon Greulich, Julia Schumm, Stefan Grün, et al, Incremental Value of Late Gadolinium Enhancement for Management of Patients With Hypertrophic Cardiomyopathy, Pages 1207–1212, Copyright 2012, *with permission from* Elsevier.)

HCM and nonsustained and sustained VT, respectively, recorded during Holter monitoring.

The electrophysiological pathways leading to VA and SCD with HCM is illustrated in **Fig. 5.**[24]

LGE-CMR imaging is useful to identify patients at risk of VT and SCD, and in selecting high-risk patients for primary prevention of ICD implantation. Therefore, LGE-CMR imaging has been used as a marker to identify the patient's risks of VT/ventricular fibrillation (VF) and ICD shocks (**Fig. 6**).[25]

The American College of Cardiology/American Heart Association guidelines on prevention of SCD in high-risk patients with HCM was recently published.[26] These guidelines suggest considering prophylactic implanted ICDs in high-risk patients or at the risk of VT/VF and SCD.

Fibrosis and Arrhythmogenesis in Patients with Dilated Cardiomyopathy

DMC encompasses different pathologic conditions, including (1) ischemic dilated cardiomyopathy, (2) nonischemic cardiomyopathy, and (3) a juvenile genetic form of DCM. The 3 syndromes commonly share progressive symptoms of congestive HF, LV dilatation, and reduced LV systolic function with reduced left ventricular ejection fraction (LVEF). However, because of significant pathologic differences, LGE-CMR imaging provides distinct pathologic patterns of myocardial fibrosis. Wu and colleagues[27] reported on the use of LGE-CMR in patients with nonischemic cardiomyopathy. In their study, 60 patients with nonischemic cardiomyopathy and LVEF of less than 35% were investigated before ICD implantation for primary prevention of SCD. The results of that study showed that patients with positive LGE-CMR imaging findings had an 8-fold higher risk of arrhythmic events. Their conclusion was that LGE-CMR was useful in detection of myocardial fibrosis, which appears as a surrogate for increased risk of cardiac outcome. Regardless of the above causes, the pathways and mechanisms of disease progression leading to end-stage HF and the need for cardiac transplant is similar, which is due to decreased myocardial energetics, mitochondrial dysfunction, oxidative stress, increased apoptosis leading to increased interstitial collagen deposits, increased matrix,

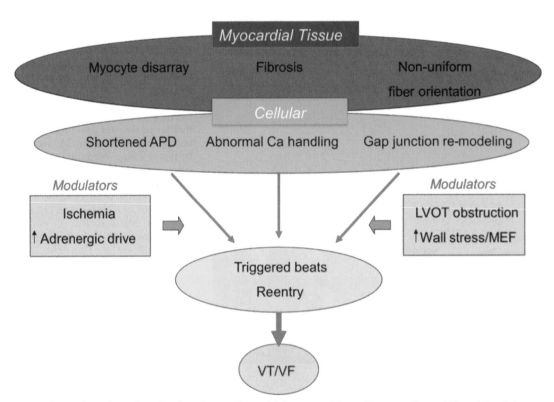

Fig. 5. Electrophysiological mechanisms in a patient with hypertrophic cardiomyopathy and fibrosis leads to ventricular tachycardia and fibrillation. (*From* Lambiase PD, McKenna WJ. Hypertrophic cardiomyopathy: Risk stratification and management of arrhythmia. In Shenasa et al, eds. Cardiac Mapping, 4th Edition, 2012. Wiley; with permission.)

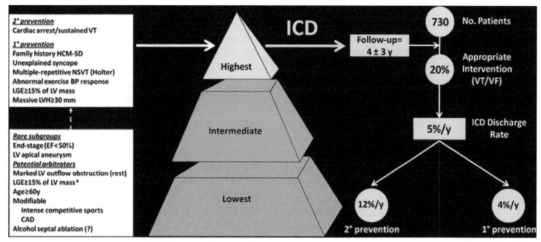

Fig. 6. Use of LGE-CMR imaging as a tool for identifying risk of VT and SCD and in selecting high-risk patients for primary prevention of implantable cardioverter defibrillators (ICD) implantation. [a] Extensive LGE can be a primary risk marker, but also an ICD decision arbitrator when assignment of high-risk status is ambiguous based on conventional risk markers. BP, blood pressure; CAD, coronary artery disease; EF, ejection fraction; HCM, hypertrophic cardiomyopathy; LV, left ventricle; NSVT, nonsustained ventricular tachycardia; SD, sudden death; VF, ventricular fibrillation; VT, ventricular tachycardia; y, years. (*Adapted from* Maron BJ, Ommen SR, Semsarian C, et al. Hypertrophic cardiomyopathy: present and future, with translation into contemporary cardiovascular medicine. J Am Coll Cardiol 2014;64:83–99.)

metalloproteinase, leading to myocardial fibrosis and remodeling and arrhythmia.

In patients with DCM, the presence of focal myocardial fibrosis, particularly in the septal and mid wall region, provides prognostic information regarding the risk of VT, and also helps to identify patients who might benefit from ICD implantation.[28]

Fibrosis and Arrhythmogenesis in Patients with Arrhythmogenic Right Ventricular Dysplasia/Cardiomyopathy

ARVD/C is an inherited cardiomyopathy that involves most of the right ventricular (RV) free wall with fibrofatty deposits in the RV. These patients usually present with arrhythmias, such as AF, VT/VF, and SCD, as well as syncope and symptoms of right HF. The role of LGE-CMR in the diagnosis, prognosis, and risk stratification of arrhythmias and selection of high-risk patients for ICD therapy is well investigated. VAs in these patients are due to the presence of patchy scars, and the VT circuits may be localized both endocardially and/or epicardially. Therefore, catheter ablation may be necessary in both regions.[29]

Fibrosis and Arrhythmogenesis in Patients with Heart Failure

Several experimental and clinical investigations have demonstrated that interstitial fibrosis plays an important role in myocardial remodeling and structural changes leading to myocardial

remodeling and HF, and subsequently development of arrhythmias. This phenomenon is related to both the syndrome of HF, ie, HF with preserved and also with reduced LV ejection fraction (HF with preserved ejection fraction [HFpEF] and HF with reduced ejection fraction [HRrEF])[2]

Complex cellular and genetic mechanisms, including biomarker interplay in the development of fibrosis leading to HF. Discussion of the detailed mechanism(s) is beyond the scope of this review and the readers are referred to other articles for further reading.[2,5]

FIBROSIS AND ARRHYTHMOGENESIS IN CORONARY ARTERY DISEASE

LGE-CMR imaging is useful in the evaluation and characterization of myocardial structure and the risk of VA (scar-related VT) and SCD. Similarly, LGE-CMR is useful for image-based visualization of scar morphologies and localization of reentry circuits, as well as assessment of catheter ablation for VT.[30]

VALVULAR HEART DISEASE
Late Gadolinium Enlacement Cardiac Magnetic Resonance in Valvular Heart Disease, Especially Aortic Stenosis

Several reports suggest that this imaging technique provides useful information in assessment of patients with aortic stenosis and risk of adverse events. The LGE-CMR in these patients usually shows focal fibrosis and a linear LV mid wall fibrosis. **Fig. 7** demonstrates the pathophysiology of myocardial fibrosis in aortic stenosis.[31]

LGE-CMR imaging is also useful for risk stratification of surgical and transcatheter aortic valve replacement.[31] Barone-Rochette and colleagues evaluated 154 consecutive patients for surgical or transcatheter aortic valve replacement. The study demonstrated that fibrosis was present in 29% of patients undergoing surgical aortic valve replacement and 51% of patients undergoing transcatheter aortic valve replacement. The results further showed that the presence and magnitude of fibrosis detected by LGE-CMR served as an independent predictor of cardiac and all-cause mortality.[31] It is assumed that development of fibrosis in patients with aortic stenosis is due to the development of LVH.

ROLE OF LATE GADOLINIUM ENLACEMENT CARDIAC MAGNETIC RESONANCE IN DETECTION OF FIBROSIS IN PATIENTS WITH CONGENITAL HEART DISEASE AND ADULT CONGENITAL HEART DISEASE

LGE-CMR provides specific patterns of fibrosis and scar tissue in patients with congenital heart disease that also have prognostic implications, as well as guiding management. For example, the test has been used mostly in patients with tetralogy of Fallot, in which fibrosis was detected in the RV lateral wall at the ventriculotomy region and on Fontan procedure.[32–36]

CARDIAC RESYNCHRONIZATION THERAPY

Cardiac resynchronization therapy (CRT) is well established in patients with HFrEF and left bundle branch block who have LV electrical and mechanical dyssynchrony. These patients benefit from CRT implantation. LGE-CMR imaging is useful to identify areas of myocardial fibrosis and scar tissue to avoid implantation of an LV lead in scar and fibrotic regions. Furthermore, LGE-CMR is a useful imaging technique to identify appropriate candidates for CRT.[37,38]

CARDIAC SARCOIDOSIS

Cardiac sarcoidosis is part of systemic sarcoidosis and is due to a process of granulomatosis. Patients with cardiac sarcoidosis often present with a variety of arrhythmias, most commonly, complete heart block, AF, LV tachyarrhythmias, and SCD. Although, the FDG-PET is widely used,

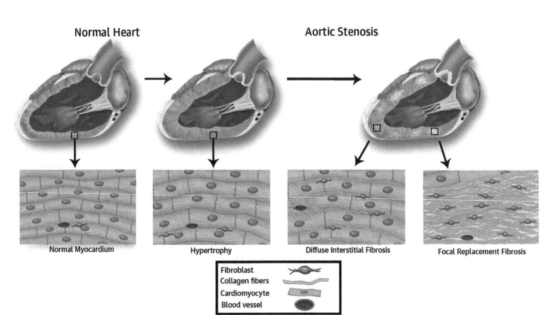

Fig. 7. Pathophysiology of myocardial fibrosis in aortic stenosis. In response to the chronic pressure overload of severe aortic stenosis, the left ventricle reacts by compensatory concentric hypertrophic remodeling. This phenomenon involves not only increased myocyte volume (*second panel from the left*) but also coordinated remodeling and increased extracellular matrix, with development of both diffuse interstitial and focal replacement fibrosis. Diffuse interstitial fibrosis consists of increased deposition of collagen in interstitial spaces (*third panel from the left*). Focal replacement fibrosis consists of replacement of myocytes by fibrotic tissue (*right panel*). This latter form of fibrosis can be detected by late gadolinium enhancement on cardiac magnetic resonance. (*Reprinted from* Journal of the American College of Cardiology, Volume 64, Issue 2, Giles Barone-Rochette, Sophie Piérard, Christophe De Meester de Ravenstein, et al, Prognostic significance of LGE by CMR in aortic stenosis patients undergoing valve replacement, Pages 144–154, Copyright 2014, *with permission from* Elsevier.)

LGE-CMR imaging has increasingly been used, especially in patients with ventricular tachyarrhythmias who are being considered for catheter ablation and ICD implantation. The LGE-CMR demonstrates the presence of myocardial fibrosis where sarcoid granulomas are located in the heart. At time of writing, LGE-CMR imaging is considered to be a noninvasive biopsy for cardiac sarcoidosis. Furthermore, LGE-CMR imaging is used for determining patient response to immunotherapies.[39–41]

CARDIAC AMYLOIDOSIS

Cardiac amyloidosis is caused by increased deposits of immunoglobulin light chain amyloses, also known as primary amyloidosis and transthyretic amyloidosis.[42,43]

The pathophysiology and biochemistry of amyloidosis is well described elsewhere. The amyloid deposits within atria or ventricle cause myocardial fibrosis and enhanced development of atrial arrhythmias and VAs and SCD.[43]

LGE-CMR has been of interest in the understanding of the pathophysiology as well as management of patients with amyloidosis. Similar to other causes of fibrosis, CMRI using LGE-CMR provides specific patterns, such as diffuse subendocardial fibrosis that involves both the RV and LV endocardium as well as atrial tissue. This LGE-CMR pattern on CMRI demonstrates a sensitivity of 93% and specificity of 70% in patients with cardiac amyloidosis.[44]

FIBROSIS AND ARRHYTHMOGENESIS IN ATHLETES (ATHLETES HEART)

Athletic activities produce LV geometry changes, as well as fibrosis, which increases the risk of atrial arrhythmias and VAs. The cardiac changes are due to LVH and cardiac dilatation depending on the type of sport. CMR is an excellent technique that can measure the RV and LV volumes and mass, as well as global and regional architectural changes and contractile function. LGE-CMR is capable of identifying fibrosis and can differentiate patients with LV hypertrophy, HCM, early ARVD/C, and infiltrative myocardial diseases, such and Anderson-Fabry syndrome. Interestingly, stopping athletic activity will reverse LV remodeling and other structural changes, whereas LVH due to other pathologic conditions will not change with sport secession.[45]

OTHER CARDIOVASCULAR PATHOLOGIC CONDITIONS

Myocardial fibrosis plays an important role in the following pathologic conditions: myocarditis,[46] chemotherapy and radiation-induced, obesity, sleep apnea, and others These condition produce inflammation, which leads to remodeling and fibrosis that result in AF and VA. Some of them are also shown in **Box 1**.

CLINICAL APPLICATIONS OF LATE GADOLINIUM ENLACEMENT CARDIAC MAGNETIC RESONANCE IN PATIENTS WITH VENTRICULAR ARRHYTHMIAS AND SPECIFIC CARDIAC PATHOLOGIC SUBSTRATES

1. Risk stratification and prognosis of sudden death selection of patients suitable for primary prevention of device implant, such as ICD or CRT
2. Coronary artery disease, ischemic heart disease, acute myocardial infarction, and scar characterization
3. Cardiomyopathies
   a. Ischemic cardiomyopathy
   b. Non-ischemic cardiomyopathy
   c. Dilated cardiomyopathy (DCM)
   d. Hypertrophic cardiomyopathy (HCM)
   e. Arrhythmogenic right ventricular dysplasia/cardiomyopathy (ARVD/C)
   f. Non-compaction cardiomyopathy
   g. Other cardiomyopathies: Fabry disease, hemochromatosis, amyloidosis
4. Hypertension, hypertensive HD, LVH, diastolic dysfunction
5. Heart failure with reduced ejection fraction (HRrEF)
6. Heart failure with preserved ejection fraction (HFpEF)
7. Congenital heart disease and adult congenital heart disease
8. Sleep apnea
9. Obesity and metabolic syndrome
10. Athletes, athletic heart
11. Myocarditis, sarcoidosis, Chagas disease
12. Inherited channelopathies such as Brugada syndrome[47]
13. Alcohol consumption
14. Chemotherapy and radiation-induced cardiomyopathy[48]
15. Postcardiac transplant follow-up
16. Regenerative cell therapy[49]

Myocardial fibrosis, detected on LGE-CMR is the final common pathway in the genesis of AF, VT/VF, and SCD, as discussed earlier. Inflammation, fibrosis and remodeling lead to arrhythmias (**Fig. 8**).

FUTURE DIRECTIONS

In future, advanced methods of fibrosis detection and quantification, such as diffuse tensor imaging,

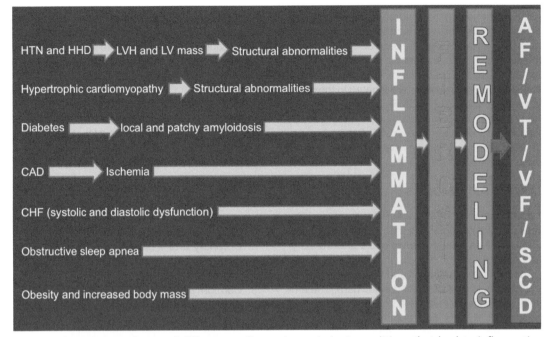

Fig. 8. Final common pathways of different cardiovascular pathologic conditions that lead to inflammation, fibrosis, remodeling, and arrhythmias. AF, atrial fibrillation; CAD, coronary artery disease; CHF, congestive heart failure; HHD, hypertensive heart disease; HTN, hypertension; LV, left ventricle; SCD, sudden cardiac death; VF, ventricular fibrillation; VT, ventricular arrhythmia.

may improve specificity and sensitivity of LGE-CMR in specific substrates.[50–54]

SUMMARY

Fibrosis plays an important role in the pathogenesis of atrial arrhythmias and VAs. Fibrosis causes anisotropic impulse propagation, conduction delay, and predisposition to reentrant arrhythmias and SCD. There are several specific imaging markers for fibrosis, such as LGE detected by CMRI, which provides a specific pattern in a variety of cardiac pathologic conditions and arrhythmias. LGE-CMR is a well-established technique for tissue characterization in a variety of cardiovascular pathologic conditions. The magnitude of LGE detected on CMR correlates with the amount of fibrosis and propensity to arrhythmogenesis. LGE-CMR may also be used as an imaging marker for risk stratification of SCD, VA, AF, and ICD/CRT indication, as well as assessment of catheter ablation of arrhythmias and the possibility of arrhythmia recurrence in many diseases, such as CAD, ischemic and nonischemic HCM, DCM, ARVD/C, and others.

ACKNOWLEDGMENTS

The author wish to thank Dr Seyed-Mostafa Razavi for his assistance in the preparation of this article.

REFERENCES

1. Judd RM, Kim RJ. Extracellular space measurements with CMR imaging. J Am Coll Cardiol 2012; 5:908–10.
2. González A, Schelbert EB, Díez J, et al. Myocardial interstitial fibrosis in heart failure: biological and translational perspectives. J Am Coll Cardiol 2018; 71:1696–706.
3. John BT, Tamarappoo BK, Titus JL, et al. Global remodeling of the ventricular interstitium in idiopathic myocardial fibrosis and sudden cardiac death. Heart Rhythm 2004;1(2):141–9.
4. Hookana E, Junttila MJ, Kaikkonen KS, et al. Increased type I collagen synthesis in victims of sudden cardiac death due to idiopathic myocardial fibrosis. Ann Med 2014;46:318–23.
5. Felisbino MB, McKinsey TA. Epigenetics in cardiac fibrosis: emphasis on inflammation and fibroblast activation. JACC Basic Transl Sci 2018;3:704–15.
6. Echegaray K, Andreu I, Lazkano A, et al. Role of myocardial collagen in severe aortic stenosis with preserved ejection fraction and symptoms of heart failure. Rev Esp Cardiol (Engl Ed) 2017;70:832–40.
7. Cardinal R, Vermeulen M, Shenasa M, et al. Anisotropic conduction and functional dissociation of ischemic tissue during reentrant ventricular tachycardia in canine myocardial infarction. Circulation 1988;77(5):1162–76.
8. Kleber AG, Janse MJ. Fibrosis and arrhythmogenesis. In: Shenasa M, Hindricks G, Callans DJ, et al,

editors. Cardiac Mapping. 5th edition. Hoboken, NJ: Wiley Blackwell; 2019. p. 375–82.

9. Valderrábano M. Influence of anisotropic conduction properties in the propagation of the cardiac action potential. Prog Biophys Mol Biol 2007;94:144–68.

10. Spach MS, Dolber PC, Heidlage JF. Properties of discontinuous anisotropic propagation at a microscopic level. Ann N Y Acad Sci 1990;591:62–74.

11. Neilan TG, Farhad H, Mayrhofer T, et al. Late gadolinium enhancement among survivors of sudden cardiac arrest. JACC Cardiovasc Imaging 2015;8(4): 414–23.

12. Aljaroudi WA, Flamm SD, Saliba W, et al. Role of CMR imaging in risk stratification for sudden cardiac death. JACC Cardiovasc Imaging 2013;6(3):392–406.

13. Watkins H, Ashrafian H, Redwood C. Inherited cardiomyopathies. N Engl J Med 2011;364:1643–56.

14. Spirito P, Seidman CE, McKenna WJ, et al. The management of hypertrophic cardiomyopathy. N Engl J Med 1997;336(11):775–85.

15. Maron BJ, Ommen SR, Semsarian C, et al. Hypertrophic cardiomyopathy: present and future, with translation into contemporary cardiovascular medicine. J Am Coll Cardiol 2014;64(1):83–99.

16. Greulich S, Schumm J, Grün S, et al. Incremental value of late gadolinium enhancement for management of patients with hypertrophic cardiomyopathy. Am J Cardiol 2012;110:1207–12.

17. Ho CY. Genetics and clinical destiny: improving care in hypertrophic cardiomyopathy. Circulation 2010; 122:2430–40.

18. Landstrom AP, Ackerman MJ. Mutation type is not clinically useful in predicting prognosis in hypertrophic cardiomyopathy. Circulation 2010;122:2441–9.

19. Ho CM, Lopez B, Coelho-Filho O, et al. Myocardial fibrosis as an early manifestation of hypertrophic cardiomyopathy. N Engl J Med 2010;363:552–63.

20. Sanaani A, Fuisz A. Cardiac magnetic resonance for diagnosis and risk stratification. Cardiol Clin 2019; 37:27–33.

21. Maron BJ, Maron MS. Hypertrophic cardiomyopathy. Lancet 2013;381(9862):242–55.

22. Ariga R, Tunnicliffe EM, Manohar SG, et al. Identification of myocardial disarray in patients with hypertrophic cardiomyopathy and ventricular arrhythmias. J Am Coll Cardiol 2019;73:2493–502.

23. McKenna WJ, Moon JC, Sulaiman A. Understanding the myocardial architecture of hypertrophic cardiomyopathy for clinical care. J Am Coll Cardiol 2019; 73:2503–5.

24. Lambiase PD, McKenna WJ. Hypertrophic cardiomyopathy: risk stratification and management of arrhythmia. In: BM Shenasa M, Breithardt G, editors. Cardiac mapping. 4th edition. Oxford (England): Wiley; 2013.

25. Maron BJ. Historical perspectives on the implantable cardioverter-defibrillator and prevention of sudden death in hypertrophic cardiomyopathy. Card Electrophysiol Clin 2015;7:165–75.

26. Maron MS, Rowin EJ, Wessler BS, et al. Enhanced American College of Cardiology/American Heart Association strategy for prevention of sudden cardiac death in high-risk patients with hypertrophic cardiomyopathy. JAMA Cardiol 2019. https://doi.org/10.1001/jamacardio.2019.1391.

27. Wu KC, Weiss RG, Thiemann DR, et al. Late gadolinium enhancement by cardiovascular magnetic resonance heralds an adverse prognosis in nonischemic cardiomyopathy. J Am Coll Cardiol 2008; 51:2414–21.

28. Nazarian S, Bluemke DA, Lardo AC, et al. Magnetic resonance assessment of the substrate for inducible ventricular tachycardia in nonischemic cardiomyopathy. Circulation 2005;112:2821–5.

29. Zghaib T, Ghasabeh MA, Assis FR, et al. Regional strain by cardiac magnetic resonance imaging improves detection of right ventricular scar compared with late gadolinium enhancement on a multimodality scar evaluation in patients with arrhythmogenic right ventricular cardiomyopathy. Circ Cardiovasc Imaging 2018;11:e007546.

30. Ashikaga H, Sasano T, Dong J, et al. Magnetic resonance-based anatomical analysis of scar-related ventricular tachycardia: implications for catheter ablation. Circ Res 2007;101(9):939–47.

31. Barone-Rochette G, Pierard S, De Meester de Ravenstein C, et al. Prognostic significance of LGE by CMR in aortic stenosis patients undergoing valve replacement. J Am Coll Cardiol 2014;64(2):144–54.

32. Babu-Narayan SV. The role of late gadolinium enhancement cardiovascular magnetic resonance in the assessment of congenital and acquired heart disease. Prog Pediatr Cardiol 2010;28:11–9.

33. Vasanawala SS, Hanneman K, Alley MT, et al. Congenital heart disease assessment with 4D flow MRI. J Magn Reson Imaging 2015;42:870–86.

34. Yim D, Riesenkampff E, Caro-Dominguez P, et al. Assessment of diffuse ventricular myocardial fibrosis using native T1 in children with repaired tetralogy of Fallot. Circ Cardiovasc Imaging 2017;10 [pii:e005695].

35. Sathananthan G, Harris L, Nair K. Ventricular arrhythmias in adult congenital heart disease: mechanisms, diagnosis, and clinical aspects. Card Electrophysiol Clin 2017;9:213–23.

36. Hernández-Madrid A, Paul T, Abrams D, et al, ESC Scientific Document Group. Arrhythmias in congenital heart disease: a position paper of the European Heart Rhythm Association (EHRA), Association for European Paediatric and Congenital Cardiology (AEPC), and the European Society of Cardiology (ESC) Working Group on Grown-up congenital heart disease, endorsed by HRS, PACES, APHRS, and SOLAECE. Europace 2018;20:1719–53.

37. Prinzen FW, Vernooy K, Auricchio A. Cardiac re-synchronization therapy: state-of-the-art of current applications, guidelines, ongoing trials, and areas of controversy. Circulation 2013;128:2407–18.

38. Obeng-Gyimah E, Nazarian S. Cardiac magnetic resonance as a tool to assess dyssynchrony. Card Electrophysiol Clin 2019;11:49–53.

39. Lau J, Syed HJ, Ellenbogen KA, et al. Atrial fibrillation and ventricular tachycardia in a patient with cardiac sarcoidosis. J Innov Card Rhythm Manag 2018; 9:3016–21.

40. Birnie DH, Sauer WH, Bogun F, et al. HRS expert consensus statement on the diagnosis and management of arrhythmias associated with cardiac sarcoidosis. Heart Rhythm 2014;11:1305–23.

41. Kandolin R, Lehtonen J, Airaksinen J, et al. Cardiac sarcoidosis: epidemiology, characteristics, and outcome over 25 years in a nationwide study. Circulation 2015;131(7):624–32.

42. Lane T, Fontana M, Martinez-Naharro A, et al. Natural history, quality of life, and outcome in cardiac transthyretin amyloidosis. Circulation 2019. https://doi.org/10.1161/CIRCULATIONAHA.118.038169.

43. Donnelly JP, Hanna M. Cardiac amyloidosis: an update on diagnosis and treatment. Cleve Clin J Med 2017;84:12–26.

44. White JA, Kim HW, Shah D, et al. CMR imaging with rapid visual T1 assessment predicts mortality in patients suspected of cardiac amyloidosis. JACC Cardiovasc Imaging 2014;7:143–56.

45. Galderisi M, Cardim N, D'Andrea A, et al. The multi-modality cardiac imaging approach to the Athlete's heart: an expert consensus of the European Association of Cardiovascular Imaging. Eur Heart J Cardiovasc Imaging 2015;16:353.

46. Lurz P, Luecke C, Eitel I, et al. Comprehensive cardiac magnetic resonance imaging in patients with suspected myocarditis: the MyoRacer-trial. J Am Coll Cardiol 2016;67:1800–11.

47. Rudic B, Schimpf R, Veltmann C, et al. Brugada syndrome: clinical presentation and genotype—correlation with magnetic resonance imaging parameters. Europace 2016;18(9):1411–9.

48. Galán-Arriola C, Lobo M, Vílchez-Tschischke JP, et al. Serial magnetic resonance imaging to identify early stages of anthracycline-induced cardiotoxicity. J Am Coll Cardiol 2019;73:779–91.

49. Malliaras K, Smith RR, Kanazawa H, et al. Validation of contrast-enhanced magnetic resonance imaging to monitor regenerative efficacy after cell therapy in a porcine model of convalescent myocardial infarction. Circulation 2013;128:2764–75.

50. Sosnovik DE, Nahrendorf M, Weissleder R. Molecular magnetic resonance imaging in cardiovascular medicine. Circulation 2007;115(15):2076–86.

51. Mekkaoui C, Sosnovik DE. Diffusion Magnetic Resonance Imaging Tractography of the Heart. In: Shenasa M, Hindricks G, Callans DJ, et al, editors. Cardiac Mapping. 5th edition. Hoboken, NJ: Wiley Blackwell; 2019. p. 1113–23.

52. Sosnovik DE. Molecular Magnetic Resonance Imaging in Cardiac Electrophysiology. In: Shenasa M, Hindricks G, Callans DJ, et al, editors. Cardiac Mapping. 5th edition. Hoboken, NJ: Wiley Blackwell; 2019. p. 1124–31.

53. Shenasa M, Shenasa H, Rahimian J. Principles of Diffusion Tensor Imaging of the Myocardium: Clinical Applications. In: Shenasa M, Hindricks G, Callans DJ, et al, editors. Cardiac Mapping. 5th edition. Hoboken, NJ: Wiley Blackwell; 2019. p. 1096–112.

54. Basser P, Mattiello J, LeBihan D. MR diffusion tensor spectroscopy and imaging. Biophys J 1994;66: 259–67.

Printed and bound by CPI Group (UK) Ltd, Croydon, CR0 4YY

03/10/2024

01040306-0017